The Merger

The Merger:

M.D.s AND D.O.s IN CALIFORNIA

Sibylle Reinsch, Ph.D., Michael Seffinger, D.O.,
and Jerome Tobis, M.D.

LIBRARY OF CONGRESS CONTROL NUMBER:		2008905855
ISBN:	HARDCOVER	978-1-4363-5439-4
	SOFTCOVER	978-1-4363-5438-7

This book was printed in the United States of America.

To order additional copies of this book, contact:
Xlibris Corporation
1-888-795-4274
www.Xlibris.com
Orders@Xlibris.com
50851

CONTENTS

Preface

M.D.s and D.O.s in California

If you are interested in the recent history of the medical professions, this book is for you. If personal narratives of historical events speak to you as a second layer of documentation, this book is for you. If you are aware that in America there exist two separate yet equal, fully licensed physicians, M.D.s and D.O.s, you might be interested in learning about their unique relationship in California. If you know little about D.O.s, this book will give you a picture of their approach to patient care and to their M.D. colleagues.

The osteopathic profession in California has a unique history, as it differs dramatically from the profession's history in the rest of the nation. More than 100 years ago, a small pioneering group of osteopathic physicians established in Southern California the Pacific School of Osteopathy to graduate physicians and surgeons with the ability to acquire an unlimited license. Since then, the educational, research, and regulatory arenas of osteopathy have seen in California low points of near elimination and high points of recognition.

Cultures are based on firm beliefs in the truth of their understanding of the world. Often they collide with those who respect different truths. Similarly, the medical culture in California went through collisions between osteopathic and allopathic medicine, often in response to competition and antagonism. Which values and beliefs about each other's profession were held so fervently in California that prompted the unique event of absorbing the osteopathic profession into allopathic mainstream medicine?

This project explores the events, unique to California but with repercussions nationwide, of a merger between osteopathic and allopathic medicine. In 1962, the relatively small medical organization of fully licensed osteopathic physicians (the California Osteopathic Association) merged with the much larger mainstream medical profession (the California Medical Association). What were the incentives for a fully licensed parallel healthcare profession to forfeit its identity and philosophy? What key players and leaders emerged? How did the individual practicing physician think and feel about the merger?

While about two thousand osteopathic physicians changed to the M.D. degree, about two hundred D.O.s residing in California did not merge but persevered in their battle to restore the licensing power of their profession in California. What social and personal motivational sources sustained this group for over a decade? How has osteopathy's unique history affected medical education and professional relations, nationwide and internationally?

Answers to these questions have emerged in historical narratives by key persons figuring in the events. Most of them have not written about their lives and their social and political surroundings at the time of the merger and its repercussions. Many never learned the long-term outcomes of their endeavors. Our multidisciplinary research team transcribed in-depth interviews to capture the thoughts and feelings among individuals who played significant roles from the 1940s to the '70s. With the approval of the Institutional Review Board of the University of California, Irvine for the protection of the participants' rights, we asked 35 physicians, administrators, lawyers and lobbyists to provide their historical narratives and their suggestions for future directions.

Our objective has been to give an unbiased account, listening equally to representatives of allopathy, osteopathy, and politics. Inspired by Dr. Gevitz' cogent academic analysis of osteopathic medicine in America (Gevitz, 2004), this book presents personal perceptions of events, integrated with documented descriptions, stored in archives, to facilitate the reader's understanding and analysis. The work has been based on the assumption that it is necessary to get inside historical events by capturing the thoughts and feelings of key persons in the context of their time and situation.

Many allopathic and osteopathic physicians contributed to California's pursuit of a constructive relationship between M.D.s and D.O.s. Yet, their contributions have hardly been acknowledged, nor can this book do justice to their work. We tried to convey what we have learned.

Most participants were involved in creating the history that now provides the foundation for our current and future practice of medicine in California. Our narrators belonged to the responsible parties of California's recent medical history; without them, the world would be different, and medical relationships in California would be different. They were the movers and shakers of their time. They seized opportunities in a particular place at a particular time, and the world moved through them and because of them, like a vortex of time. They made their imprint on the nature of the two professions in this state. They are not the only ones, but they are those that have been pointed out by others as having made a difference.

Every discussion about politics and medicine at nationwide professional meetings on manual medicine seems to turn to the "merger" in California. People use it for every argument, be it as a warning sign for losing one's professional allegiance and identity, or be it as a sign of respect and acceptance of each other's medical tradition.

Often, inaccurate accounts are given, though, that might hinder constructive relations between the professions. A detailed personal description is missing of the social and political climate in California in the 1900s that can facilitate a broader understanding of the complexity of the M.D.—D.O. relationship. How could the merger be shrouded in mystery only 40 years later?

Motives to merge differed among the various forces. Maybe there were disappointments about unexpected outcomes or unfulfilled promises. Maybe time moved on with little opportunity to learn from the professions' cultural heritage. But people still live who witnessed the merger era and often played key roles in the events. Their medical practice has been shaped by the events, whether they integrated themselves with mainstream medicine or whether they persevered as osteopathic physicians and surgeons. They have insights to share that contribute to a fuller understanding of these historical events and their consequences.

We embedded the historical narratives in the documentation of archival texts, including the unpublished "*History of Osteopathy in California*" by Dain Tasker, D.O. and files maintained by Forest J. Grunigen, M.D. and Louis Chandler, D.O., as well as documents collected by many other key players. The richness of the interviews allows us to liven up these archival historical documents and point toward promising venues for mutual understanding and respect among D.O.s and M.D.s. The narratives provide suggestions for collaboration in education and research.

For nearly forty years, the 41st Medical Trust at the University of California, Irvine has aimed to support research on osteopathic manipulation, which had been one of the incentives for merging the medical professions. Members of the 41st Medical Trust committee presently include Victor Passy, M.D. as Chair, Jen Yu, M.D., Ph.D., Stanley van den Noort, M.D., Dolores Grunigen, Richard Kammerman, M.D., Robert Steedman, M.D., and Leonard Kitzes, Ph.D. A grant by the 41st Medical Trust has made possible this documentation of osteopathic and allopathic medicine in California.

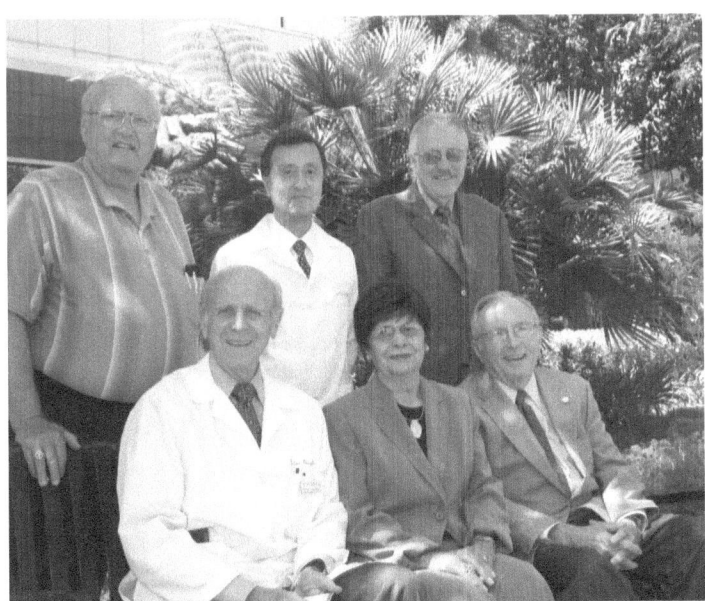

Figure 1. "The 41st Medical Trust Committee, 2007:
Standing from left to right: Richard Kammerman, M.D., Jen Yu, M.D.,Ph.D.,
Robert Steedman, M.D. Seated from left to right:
Victor Passy, M.D., Dolores Grunigen, B.A., Stanley van den Noort, M.D."

Chronology of the M.D.—D.O. Relationship in California

Pioneering Osteopathy (1890s to 1920s)

- **1892: American School of Osteopathy** founded by **Andrew Taylor Still, M.D.** in Kirksville, Missouri.
- **1895: Aubrey C. Moore, D.O.** (Diplomat of Osteopathy) graduated from the ASO and moved to California.
- **1896: Dr. Moore** and **B.W. Scheurer**, M.D. started the first osteopathic college outside of Missouri, the **Pacific Sanitarium and School of Osteopathy** in Anaheim.
- **1898: San Francisco College of Osteopathy** opened. The Pacific Sanitarium and School of Osteopathy, now called the **Pacific School of Osteopathy (PSO)**, was the first school to grant the **D.O.** (*Doctor* **of Osteopathy**) degree to two M.D. students.
- **1899:** The first graduates of PSO without advanced standing were granted a **Doctor of Osteopathy** degree.
- **1900:** The Pacific School of Osteopathy moved to Los Angeles and established the first osteopathic clinic in California for teaching and training. The **Osteopathic Association of the State of California (OASC)** was formed (became the California Osteopathic Association (COA) 1917-1962).
- **1901: Dain Tasker** was elected president of OASC. **AB 230 became law** by the statutes of limitations, establishing the **Board of Osteopathic Examiners**. It allowed for D.O.s, who graduated from a state osteopathic licensing board accredited college, to practice osteopathy, which at that time was limited to a drugless and non-surgical scope of practice. There were separate licensing boards for M.D.s, homeopaths, and eclectic practitioners as well.
- **1903**: **South Pasadena Osteopathic Sanitarium** opened, with Dain Tasker, D.O., as Director. The Pacific School moved to South Pasadena too but kept the free clinic in LA.

- **1904:** The PSO declared bankruptcy and a new non-profit school was established, the **Pacific College of Osteopathy (PCO)**, which returned to Los Angeles. It was chartered to offer both the D.O. and the M.D. degrees.
- **1905: The Los Angeles College of Osteopathy (LACO)** was established by faculty from the Des Moines S. S. Still College of Osteopathy as a for-profit institution.
- **1906:** The Los Angeles County Osteopathic Medical Society, sponsored by Dr. Dain Tasker, was formed to "consolidate those who were opposed to the Los Angeles College of Osteopathy group". The San Francisco earthquake badly damaged the San Francisco College of Osteopathy.
- **1907:** Dr. Tasker was elected President of OASC. The osteopathic state licensing board did not accredit the LACO and refused to let its graduates sit for its examination. The LACO faculty filed a lawsuit and won. The osteopathic practice act was declared unconstitutional and repealed. The legislature enacted a new Medical Practice Act to regulate all of the health professionals in the state under one composite licensing board consisting of 5 allopaths (regular M.D.), 2 osteopaths, 2 homeopaths and 2 eclectic practitioners. The Medical Practice Act of 1907 repealed the previous Medical Practice Acts of 1876 and 1901. This act provided for the issuance of three different forms of certificates by the Board of Medical Examiners of the state of California: First, a certificate authorizing the holder to practice medicine and surgery; second, a certificate authorizing the holder to practice osteopathy; and third, a certificate authorizing the holder to practice any other system or mode of treating the sick and afflicted, not otherwise referred to. The 1907 Medical Practice Act allowed D.O.s to have an unlimited physician and surgeon license if he or she took the required curriculum and passed the requisite examinations. Only M.D.s or D.O.s were allowed to sit for that examination, however, since the other professions were not complete schools of medicine and surgery.
- **1910:** Dain Tasker, D.O. became the only D.O. to be president of the composite state licensing board. The American Osteopathic Association (AOA) threatened the PCO it would remove accreditation unless the school dropped granting the M.D. degree; PCO acquiesced and only provided the D.O. degree thereafter. Clement Whiting, D.O., dean of PCO, enabled the first D.O.s to care for patients at the L.A. County outpatient maternity clinics.
- **1912:** The D.O. school in San Francisco closed.
- **1913:** The **Medical Practice act of 1913** was enacted under which medicine and surgery is still practiced in California today. The Medical Practice Act of 1907 was repealed. A ten-person board was appointed by the governor and three types of licenses were issued: Physician and Surgeon, Drugless Practitioner, and License by Reciprocity. **Clement Whiting, D.O.,** dean of PCO and intermediary between the two osteopathic colleges in Los Angeles, was killed upon being struck by a car on his way to a meeting between each of the two osteopathic college's Board of Trustees to discuss merging.

- **1914:** The two osteopathic schools in Los Angeles, the PCO and the LACO, merged to form a non-profit institution, **The College of Osteopathic Physicians & Surgeons (COP&S).**
- **1916:** Four COP&S graduates were appointed as **interns to the Los Angeles County Hospital.**
- **1917:** An amendment to the 1913 Medical Practice Act enabled D.O.s licensed under the previous acts to take an oral examination to raise the license from that of drugless to that of physician and surgeon. The OASC was renamed as **COA.**
- **1918: University of Southern California (USC) closed** (until 1928) leaving COP&S and the **College of Medical Evangelists** as the only medical schools remaining open in Southern California. The **American College of Surgeons (ACS)** began on-site inspections and accreditation of hospitals.
- **1919:** One third of the 31 interns at L.A. County Hospital were D.O.s. The **Council on Medical Education of the American Medical Association (AMA)** threatened the L.A. County Hospital with removal of accreditation unless any association with osteopaths was discontinued, i.e., not allowing D.O.s to be interns. The **state composite licensing board** also declared that COP&S was no longer accredited and graduates could not sit for licensure exams. COP&S filed suit against the state licensing board and prevailed, forcing the licensing board to allow D.O.s to sit for the exam.
- **1922:** Proposition 20 was passed as an initiative by the people of the state of CA, creating a separate osteopathic licensing board. (A separate chiropractic licensing board was also created on the same ballot by the same process). D.O.s applied for the right to admit and attend patients at the L.A. County Hospital, and have post graduate training, i.e., internships and residencies. In order for the M.D.s to maintain accreditation from the AMA, however, the D.O.s had to be in a segregated building and attend patients separately from the M.D.s.
- **1923:** Agreement signed between the osteopathic profession and the L.A. Board of Supervisors granted D.O.s the right to care for patients at a segregated Unit II and instituted post-graduate training at the L.A. County Hospital. This was the only County Hospital in the world that allowed D.O.s on staff until the 1950s.

Osteopathic Medicine as segregated medical profession (1928 to 1960)

- **1928:** The communicable diseases building at the L.A. County Hospital was renovated to accommodate the D.O. physicians in a segregated unit, called Unit II, and the M.D. unit was called Unit I. There was a tunnel adjoining the two units for housekeeping and food services. USC re-opened its medical school.
- **1929:** The ACS removed its accreditation of Unit I until a newer Unit I was built and the M.D.s were physically and administratively separated from the D.O.s. The AOA mandated that all osteopathic colleges implemented into their

curricula education about materia medica and pharmacology. The name of the profession changed from "Osteopathy" to "Osteopathic Medicine."

- **1930:** The L.A. Board of Supervisors allocated funds for a new and much larger, more modern Unit I facility, physically separated from Unit II.
- **1931: Forest Grunigen** graduated from COP&S.
- **1932: Louis Chandler, D.O.** noticed that between 1928 and 1932, the morbidity and mortality statistics for Unit II were less than Unit I, implying superior care, not inferior care, as M.D.s usually assumed.
- **1933:** Construction of the new Unit I was completed. Dr. Chandler had his data analysis of the M.D. vs D.O. care of L.A. County patients published in an article in the **Journal of the American Osteopathic Association.** Nevertheless, the segregation policy persisted.
- **1934:** Unit II was renamed to **Los Angeles County Osteopathic Hospital (LACOH),** though the nickname of "Unit II" remained. L.A. County Hospital 20 story acute facility was built with 2,500 beds.
- **1935:** The **ACS re-approved accreditation** for **Unit I** of the L. A. County Hospital.
- **1938:** President **Carle Phinney, D.O**. of COP&S died in office, throwing the institution into turmoil as to its direction.
- **1939:** A merger between USC and COP&S was proposed by COP&S alumni. A member of the USC Presidential cabinet, **Ballentine Henley, JD**, was selected as the new President of COP&S, the first non-D.O. to fill this position.
- **1940: A merger between the California Osteopathic Association (COA) and California Medical Association (CMA)** was promoted by COP&S alumni, including **Forest Grunigen, D.O.**
- **1943: Forest Grunigen, D.O.** elected president of COA on the platform of unifying the osteopathic and allopathic professions in California. **Grunigen** appointed a **Fact Finding Committee** to lead merger talks with **CMA's Committee on Other Professions. Merger agreement was made between CMA and COA,** but not accepted as valid by the AMA, medical specialty societies or the AOA. **Grunigen** and his colleagues **(Vincent Carroll, D.O., Glen Cayler, D.O., and Dorothy Marsh, D.O.)** moved into national professional politics to promote a merger of the AOA and AMA, or at least to obtain permission from the national organizations to enable the state associations to handle the negotiations between the two professions according to their own discretion.
- **1944:** Alumni of COP&S engaged in obtaining an M.D. degree from **Metropolitan University** in Los Angeles, a diploma mill (not accredited by licensing boards) set up in Los Angeles to provide M.D. degrees to D.O.s upon taking some courses and an examination.
- **1947: John Cline, M.D.** was elected as CMA President.
- **1948: COA delegates** went to the AOA to request that graduates of Metropolitan University have their AOA membership revoked; the AOA created a policy

to revoke membership if D.O.s took an M.D. degree from an institution not accredited by a state licensing board. **Forest Grunigen, D.O.** served on the AOA Board of Trustees along with **Vincent Carroll, D.O.**

- **1950: Mark Twain Hospital** was built in San Andreas, California. **Senator Stephen Teale, D.O.** wrote into the bond measure for that hospital in 1948 that there will be no discrimination of D.O.s who wanted to admit and care for patients there. **It was the first such hospital built anywhere by a state bond measure mandating non-discrimination against D.O.s.**

- **1951: Vincent Carroll, D.O.,** from Laguna Hills, CA, elected **President of the AOA** at the 54th AOA Annual Convention in Chicago. **John Cline, MD**, from San Francisco, CA, became **AMA President**. The two Californians, along with Forest Grunigen, formally began a national campaign to **merge the AMA and AOA. Formal talks began between AMA and AOA representatives.** The American College of Physicians, the American Hospital Association, the American Medical Association, and the Canadian Medical Association joined with the American College of Surgeons (ACS) to create the Joint Commission on Accreditation of Hospitals (JCAH), an independent, not-for-profit organization whose primary purpose was to provide voluntary accreditation of hospitals. The AOA or osteopathic hospitals were not included.

- **1952: Past AMA President Cline** created an **AMA Committee for the Study of Relations between Osteopathy and Medicine** to seek information about osteopathy. The AOA appointed a **Conference Committee** to correspond with like committee at AMA. **L.A. County Board of Supervisors** voted to build a **new L.A. County Osteopathic Hospital.**

- **1953: College of Osteopathic Physicians and Surgeons** received a contract of $120,000 per year for 14, 358 hours of service in the **Los Angeles County Osteopathic Hospital.**

- **1952-1955:** Meetings of **AOA-AMA** conference committees and **visitations** to five osteopathic colleges, including **COP&S**, by the **Cline Committee** were held.

- **1954:** $9,000,000 bond measure passed by the Los Angeles voters for the building of a new **Los Angeles County Osteopathic Hospital**.

- **1955: Report of Cline Committee** was given to AMA House of Delegates at Atlantic City meeting. Majority report reflected visits of educators and requested acceptance of osteopathic physicians and their institutions, and removal of the "cult" label; this was **rejected by the AMA House** in favor of the minority report by **Milford Rouse, M.D**. Unless the AOA and its institutions remove statements in their brochures and catalogs related to the "osteopathic concept" and "A.T. Still", the AMA voted to **maintain the "cult" label and considered it unethical for M.D.s to interact professionally with D.O.s.** Informal, unofficial, but regular meetings between the **COA Fact Finding Committee (Seth Hufstedler as Counsel)** and the **CMA Committee on Other Professions (Howard Hassard as attorney)** began.

- **1956:** The cornerstone, with a time capsule embedded, of the new **L.A. County Osteopathic Hospital** was laid. **Grace Bell, D.O.** was appointed as the first Dean of COP&S, the first woman as dean of an American osteopathic medical school and of a U.S. co-ed medical institution.
- **1958:** The **AOA** and its institutions removed reference to the "osteopathic concept" and "A.T. Still" from their brochures and catalogs in order to comply with the AMA demands. The **L.A. County Osteopathic Hospital** was dedicated.
- **1959:** The new **L.A. County Osteopathic Hospital** was opened; a ten-story structure with 500 beds. The AMA received a report from its judicial council. Council recommendations were amended in Reference Committee and on the floor of the House of Delegates. Action called for appointment of liaison committee to talk with AOA committee. Judicial council recommended to accept D.O.s and allow M.D.s to associate with them in their schools and institutions, and remove the "cult" label. California's M.D.s told AMA House and committee that overall action was unnecessary because California D.O.s wanted to become M.D.s and that discussions were underway between the professions. **Warren Bostick, M.D.,** delegate from the CMA, proposed an amendment to **only accept interaction with D.O.s who were in the process of changing their school to an accredited M.D. institution and who practiced only scientific medicine. This was approved. AOA** House of Delegates at their annual meeting reaffirmed the **"separate and distinct"** status of osteopathic profession. **California delegates opposed. AMA** appointed committee to meet with AOA committee.
- **1960:** AOA House of Delegates resolved that any state society entering negotiations with another profession concerning unification or merger is subject to possible revocation of charter by AOA. COA House of Delegates voted to **continue negotiations with the CMA.** Official, formal negotiations between the **Fact Finding Committee of the COA** and the **CMA Committee on Other Professions** began. **Osteopathic Physicians and Surgeons of California (OPSC)** formed in opposition to the merger and COA. **Richard Eby, D.O.** was elected founding president. **AMA-AOA committees** met twice with no resolution.

The COA/CMA merger and its aftermath (1961-1974)

- **1961:** COA charter was revoked** by the AOA. **OPSC was accepted** as the new state association representing the AOA in California. **COA/CMA merger was completed.** The Board of Trustees of COP&S changed the name of its school to the **California College of Medicine (CCM).**
- **1962:** CCM was **accredited by the AMA** on Feb. 15. The faculty of CCM, led by **Grace Bell**, the Founding Dean of the College, were the **first to receive the M.D. degree** on March 7. (**Grace Bell, M.D.** became the first female Dean of an American M.D. granting Medical School). CCM took over the Los Angeles

County Osteopathic Hospital, whose name reverted to "**Unit II**" once again. CCM graduated its first class of M.D.s in June, and granted M.D. degrees to approximately 2,000 D.O.s in July. **The COA became the 41ˢᵗ Medical Society** which became part of the **CMA** in August. **Proposition 22** was passed by the voters in November, which **limited the power of the osteopathic licensing board** so that it could no longer grant new licenses to D.O.s, and would transfer its duties to the medical licensing board when the number of D.O.s re-certifying annually decreased to less than 40.

- **1964:** The **41ˢᵗ Medical Society** established the **41ˢᵗ Medical Trust** to direct funds from the sale of osteopathic property and COA membership dues and donations to **integration of D.O.s with M.D.s** and **to research osteopathic (musculoskeletal) manipulation**. Thanks to political efforts of **Senator Stephen Teale**, now M.D., the State legislators voted to accept **CCM** as part of the **University of California**, effective January 1, 1964.

- **1964: Warren Bostick, M.D.,** dean of CCM, became the **Founding Dean of the University of California at Irvine College of Medicine.** Dr. Grunigen and Dr. Bostick unsuccessfully campaigned through the AMA nationwide to effect mergers of state medical and osteopathic associations and eliminate U.S. osteopathic medicine completely.

- **1966: First D.O. promoted to Medical Officer in U.S. Armed Forces.** Former D.O. specialists still had difficulty in getting accepted into M.D. specialty societies unless they were trained in M.D. residency programs.

- **1967: First D.O. civilian commissioned as Medical Officer in U.S. Armed Forces. Forest Grunigen, M.D.** became the first, and only, former D.O. president of the M.D. licensing board of California.

- **1968: CCM relocated to UC Irvine campus;** USC leased the 2 buildings adjacent to the L.A. County Hospital from UC Regents. USC took over the patient load and faculty of the old osteopathic hospital and renamed it **Women's Hospital of the Los Angeles County Hospital.**

  D'Amico et al (osteopathic physicians from out of state and commissioned Medical Officers in the military), with the support of OPSC, filed a law suit against the **Attorney General of the State of California, and the Medical and Osteopathic Licensing Boards**, for civil rights infraction, restricting trade of osteopathic practice. **AMA** allowed D.O.s to become members of state and county M.D. societies.

- **1969: AMA** allowed D.O.s to become members of the AMA. D.O.s were accepted as residents in allopathic post graduate training programs. The AOA began to rebuild and grow: the first of many new osteopathic colleges in about 50 years was established at Michigan State University and became the first state supported osteopathic college.

- **1970: American Hospital Association** accepted hospitals with D.O.s on staff and **Joint Commission on Accreditation of Hospitals** recognized D.O.s as qualified members of hospital medical staffs. The **American Academy of Family Physicians (AAFP)** accepted its first former D.O., **Richard Ryder, M.D.,** as member.

- **1974: California Supreme Court** ruled in favor of **D'Amico et al** and restored licensing power of the osteopathic licensing board. The first new osteopathic physician and surgeon licenses were granted to over 340 qualified out of state D.O.s since 1962. Efforts to build a hospital on the campus of CCM at UC Irvine, subsidized in part by the sale of the buildings across from L.A. County Hospital to USC and assets of the 41st Medical Society Trust, were unsuccessful. CCM continued to use Orange County General Hospital in Orange, CA as its main training hospital.
- **1975: CMA** opened its membership to qualified D.O.s.

D.O.s return to California (1978-1982)

- **1978: College of Osteopathic Medicine of the Pacific (COMP) opened in Pomona, CA,** with **Philip Pumerantz, Ph.D.** as president.
- **1979: AOA** allowed its members to join the AMA and specialty societies outside the osteopathic profession. **CMA** proposed legislation enabling D.O.s to be licensed by either the **Board of Medical Quality Assurance (BMQA)** or the **Board of Osteopathic Examiners** failed to pass.
- **1980: BMQA** attempted to change its regulations enabling it to license D.O.s, but **Attorney General** stated it would be illegal to do so as BMQA could not accredit osteopathic schools.
- **1981: The Journal of the American Medical Association** published the first American randomized clinical trial on an osteopathic manipulation procedure for patients with low back pain, carried out at **UC Irvine CCM,** with funding from the **41st Medical Trust**, under the direction of **Jerome Tobis, M.D.**
- **1982: COMP** graduated its first class. The first osteopathic internships and residencies opened since 1962.

M.D.s and D.O.s work side by side in California (1982- present):

- **1983:** 41st Medical Trust Funds were transferred to the California College of Medicine Support Foundation. **OPSC** began a string of anti-discrimination legislation to protect the rights of osteopathic students and physicians in obtaining clerkships, training and employment throughout the state. It was settled in court that an osteopathic physician must use the D.O. designation unless he or she applied to the Board of Medical Examiners in 1962 for permission to use the M.D. degree.
- **1986: UC Irvine Family Medicine Residency** began to accept D.O.s into its post-graduate training program. **UC Irvine Physical Medicine & Rehabilitation Residency** had accepted D.O.s into its Residency program already earlier.

- **1989: Anti-D.O. discrimination** laws in California were finally in place.
- **1991: M.D.s and D.O.s** began to associate in combined business ventures and medical groups as Health Maintenance Organizations put economic pressures on both groups.
- **1992: The American Academy of Family Physicians** began to accept D.O.s who trained in AOA approved family practice residency programs as members.
- **1995-6: Josiah Macy Foundation** sponsored a two year symposium looking at the current and future status of the relations between M.D.s and D.O.s in America.
- **1996: The College of Osteopathic Medicine of the Pacific (COMP)** became part of **Western University of Health Sciences** in Pomona, CA.
- **1997: Touro University College of Osteopathic Medicine**, in the San Francisco Bay Area, became the second osteopathic college in the state of CA. **The 41st Medical Society was dissolved on 7-31-1997.**
- **1999: CMA** resolved to work with **OPSC** on issues of common concern of physicians in California.
- **2004: Cynthia Stotts, D.O.,** a COMP graduate (1988), became the first female and the first D.O. President (Chief) of Medical Staff (which includes approximately 2,000 M.D.s, 40 D.O.s, about 900 interns and residents, and 200-400 medical students, as well as allied health professionals) at the Los Angeles County/USC Hospital in its 158 year history.
- **2005: CMA** resolved to oppose consolidation [efforts led by the Governor] of the Medical Board of California with the Osteopathic Medical Board of California. **41st Medical Trust** funded narrative history project on D.O.-M.D. relations in California.
- **2006: Cynthia Stotts, D.O.** became the first physician to be elected for a second two-year term as **Chief of Staff** at **LA County/USC Hospital.**
- **2007-present:** All hospitals in the state allow mixed M.D.-D.O. staff and allopathic post-graduate training programs accept both D.O.s and M.D.s. However, osteopathic post-graduate training programs only accept D.O.s. **University of California Irvine School of Medicine, Western University of Health Sciences College of Osteopathic Medicine** and **Touro University College of Osteopathic Medicine** continue to thrive in California, and **CMA** and **OPSC** interact on a regular basis on common issues. D.O.s can become voting members of CMA, but M.D.s cannot become voting members of OPSC. There are still two separate licensing boards, one for D.O.s and one for M.D.s.

Participants in the collection of historical narratives

(Abbreviations are explained below)

Allen, Ethan, D.O.
Founding Chair of the Board of COMP, Former President of OPSC

Alloy, Paul, M.D.
Facilitated awarding a UCI College of Medicine graduate certificate to former D.O.s and participated in the approval process for COMP

Chesky, Stuart, D.O., J.D.
First osteopathic Director of Medical Education in California after the merger (1982)

Dilworth, Donald, D.O.
Co-founder of COMP, former President of OPSC

Dowell, Emery, M.S.
California Hospital Association, worked with Senator Stephen Teale

Eby, Richard, D.O.
Founding President of OPSC, co-founder of COMP

Frymann, Viola, D.O., F.A.A.O.
Co-founder of COMP, former President of OPSC, President of the Board and Medical Director of the Osteopathic Center for Children and Families, San Diego

Grunigen, Dolores, B.S., B.A.
Worked on California Medical Licensing Board in getting former D.O.s licensed as M.D.s

Golanty, Stanley, M.D.

Former Academic Dean of Education at Pacific Hospital, Long Beach

Haldeman, Scott, M.D., Ph.D., D.C.

Trained in Neurology at UC Irvine, participated in research funded by the 41st Medical Trust, raised attention nationally and internationally to the science of musculoskeletal manipulation and helped the U.S. Government establish healthcare policies on its clinical application

Hufstedler, Seth, LL.B.

Legal counsel for COA, 41st Medical Society, and 41st Medical Trust

Kamajian, Steven, D.O.

Graduate of the Philadelphia College of Osteopathic Medicine in 1978, first clinical instructor for third year medical students at COMP and osteopathic physician for many faculty members, staff and students since 1981; Chief of Staff at Glendale Adventist Hospital

Kammerman, Richard, M.D.

Graduate of COP&S in 1956, presently Clinical Professor in the Department of Family Medicine at UCI CCM, Past President of the Orange County Osteopathic Society and the Orange County Medical Association, Past President of the Voluntary Faculty Association at the Orange County Medical Center, Past President of COP&S/CCM Alumni Association, member of 41st Medical Trust Committee

Kasovac, Mitchell, D.O.

Former Dean of COMP, former President of AOA

Korneff, Allen, M.S.

Former CEO and President of Downey Regional Medical Center, amalgamated Rio Hondo Hospital (osteopathic) with Downey Hospital (allopathic) which maintains osteopathic family medicine and osteopathic manipulative medicine residency programs (only one in the state)

Krpan, Donald, D.O.

Former dean of COMP, former Provost of Western University of Health Sciences, former president

24

	of OPSC and AOA, President of Osteopathic Medical Board of California
MacCracken, Betsy, M.D., M.P.H.	Graduate and faculty of COP&S, served at the Los Angeles County Department of Public Health, in charge of pediatric health care
Menkes, Alan, D.O.	Graduate of the Philadelphia College of Osteopathic Medicine in 1967, joined initial efforts to start COMP in 1976, and became the first professor and chair of the Department of Medicine
Michael, Jay, M.S.	Lobbyist for CMA, worked with Senator Teale in Sacramento, CA
Nelson, Thomas, M.D.	Founding Chair of Pediatrics at the University of California Irvine College of Medicine
Norcross, Robert, M.D.	Graduate of COP&S in 1951, surgeon at Bay Harbor Hospital in Lomita, his two sons graduated from COMP
Passy, Victor, M.D.	Graduate of COP&S in 1959, Active Professor Emeritus of Otolaryngology at UC Irvine School of Medicine, Chair of 41st Medical Trust Committee, Past President of CCM Alumni Association
Pumerantz, Philip, Ph.D.	Founding President of Western University of the Health Sciences in Pomona, CA
Ryan, William, D.O.	One of the first osteopathic physicians commissioned in the U.S. Navy (1967), stationed in San Diego, CA; first D.O. hired by Kaiser Permanente of Southern California, and first D.O. to be accepted as a partner in Kaiser Permanente Medical Group.
Ryder, Richard, M.D.	Graduate of COP&S in 1960, first former D.O. to be a member of AAFP

Seffinger, Michael, D.O.

Graduate of MSU-COM, faculty of COMP, chair of the AAFP CME spinal manual medicine programs, participated in research funded by the 41st Medical Trust, initiated this history project by collecting documents and narrative histories, and stimulated cataloguing the documents archived at UC Irvine and WUHS

Steedman, Robert, M.D.

Graduate of COP&S in 1959, member of 41st Medical Trust Committee, past president of COP&S/CCM Alumni Association, Clinical Voluntary Associate Professor at UC Irvine, trained under both D.O. and M.D. attendings, and trained both D.O. and M.D. students

Stotts, Cynthia, D.O.

Graduate of COMP in 1988, interned at Pacific Hospital of Long Beach, trained at L.A. County-USC Medical Center in Pediatrics/Internal Medicine/Allergy/Immunology, pediatric intensivist, first female and first D.O. Chief of Staff at L.A. County-USC Medical Center

Taylor, James, M.D.

Graduate of COP&S in 1958, trained at USC, Assistant Professor of Anesthesiology at UCI CCM, practiced at Bay Harbor Hospital in Lomita, CA

Tobis, Jerome, M.D.

Graduate of Chicago Medical School, former Chair of Dept. Physical Medicine & Rehabilitation at UCI CM, conducted first randomized clinical trial on osteopathic manipulation therapy in the United States

Ulansey, Seymour, M.D.

Graduate of COP&S and Metropolitan University (1940s), Co-owner of mixed staff Hollywood Hospital, financially supported both CCM and COMP

Van den Noort, Stanley, M.D.

Graduate of Harvard Medical School, former Dean of UCI CM, former Chair of the Dept. of Neurology, oversaw research funded by the 41st

	Medical Trust, member of the 41st Medical Trust Committee
Vinn, Norman, D.O.	Past President of OPSC, first Vice-President of the AOA, helped the osteopathic medical profession to adapt to managed care
Weyuker, Matt	Executive Director Emeritus of OPSC, lobbyist for COMP
Wykle, John, M.D.	Graduate of COP&S in 1941, shared a medical practice with Senator Teale for several years

Abbreviations stand for:

AAFP	American Academy of Family Physicians
AOA	American Osteopathic Association
CCM	California College of Medicine
CMA	California Medical Association
COMP	College of Osteopathic Medicine of the Pacific
MSU-COM	Michigan State University, College of Osteopathic Medicine
OPSC	Osteopathic Physicians and Surgeons of California
UCI CM	University of California, Irvine, College of Medicine
WUHS	Western University of Health Sciences

Chapter 1

If medicine is allopathy, what is osteopathy?

For over a century now, organized medicine in America has had two separate and distinct divisions: regular medicine and osteopathic medicine. Regular medicine is characterized by medical doctors who have an M.D. degree and is often referred to as "allopathy". Osteopathic medicine is characterized by osteopathic doctors who have a D.O. degree and is often referred to as "osteopathy". Members of both professions are legally recognized by federal and state governments and by the military as physicians and surgeons with full practice privileges.

There are over 650,000 M.D. and 55,000 D.O. physicians in America. In many communities in America patients have the option of being treated by a D.O. or an M.D. Yet many Americans do not know about this enriched spectrum of care. The objective of this chapter is to provide brief definitions of the two professions and overviews on their respective historical development in California.

Allopathy: Definition and use of the term

Webster's dictionary defines allopathy as a method of treating disease with remedies that produce effects different from those caused by the disease itself. At least historically, allopathy provided healing by using these methods. For example, if the disease caused the body to become hot with a fever, allopathic treatments would have included remedies that lowered the body's temperature. The German physician Dr. Hahnemann (1755-1843) had coined the term allopathy, in comparison to his healing art which he called homeopathy because he used natural substances that were known to cause similar symptoms as the afflicted and, upon ingestion of diluted solutions of these substances, the body would be able to heal itself. Osteopathic physicians have continued to use the term allopathy for regular medicine. M.D.s who were former D.O.s might use the term, but M.D.s generally do not refer to themselves as allopathic physicians.

Organized regular medicine, however, uses the term "allopathy" on some of its professional organization websites, like the American Medical Association (AMA) referring to M.D. students as allopathic medical students, usually in the context of medical education to describe equal opportunities and fees for students of allopathic and osteopathic medicine. The AMA glossary provides no definition per se for allopathy but uses the term frequently together with osteopathy and medical education.

Presently, the Association of American Medical Colleges describes the type of medicine they teach as allopathic. In the late 1980s and 1990s, however, the term allopathy was used in juxtaposition to alternative and complementary medicine (Gundling, 1998). In a *Commentary*, Dr. Grundling expressed her concern that to patients the term might indicate an "inflexible philosophy of care" (page 2168) and one of many systems of care from which to choose. The choice of an unlimited licensed physician in the U.S. presently is, however, only to be made among two, namely doctors with an M.D. degree and those with a D.O. degree.

The meaning of words changes over time. Concerns about alternative medicine in the 1990s brought about a revival of Dr. Hahnemann's term but some M.D. physicians seemed to feel offended by the term. With the resurgence of popularity of alternative or complementary medicine adjunctive to mainstream medicine, potential negative connotations of allopathy seem to have dissolved.

The increasing representation of osteopathic medicine in the formerly strictly allopathic organizations might also be a reason for using the term allopathy on the respective websites. For example, for the past 40 years, D.O.s have been allowed to become members of the AMA, and many D.O.s are members of the M.D. medical and surgical specialty colleges.

One more reason for the continued popularity of the term allopathy might be its uniqueness. Other terms like traditional medicine, conventional medicine, Western medicine, scientific medicine, or orthodox medicine have been used or proposed. The older term "regular medicine" for allopathy might be the most exact one to use, but currently the term has lost distinction since many D.O.s practice allopathically as well as osteopathically, and many M.D.s are interested in osteopathic manipulative medicine. In this book we will use the terms "mainstream" and "allopathic" medicine interchangeably because of the greater number of M.D.s than D.O.s practicing in the United States at present.

Allopathy: Mainstream medicine today

The vision and ethics of the medical profession are reflected in adaptations of the Hippocratic Oath, usually taken as part of the medical school graduation ceremonies. With changing cultural and social awareness in the 1970s, many allopathic medical schools around the country developed modern versions of the traditional oath or arrived at alternative pledges about the duties of a doctor. In California in 1976, the oath of allopathic medicine was adapted by the "Class of 1976" of the College of Medicine at the University of California, Irvine where it is still in use.

> *I solemnly promise, as a physician, to practice my profession to the best of my ability.*
> *I will use my knowledge and skills to aid in the prevention, diagnosis, and treatment of medical diseases.*

I will try to help my patients to understand disease, treatment and prognosis.

I will encourage my patients to participate in decisions relating to their lives.

I will endeavor to alleviate their fears, and recognize that occasionally the most meaningful treatment may be to listen with kindness and understanding.

I will treat my patients with dignity and I will give them the respect and privacy which I would hope to receive if I were ill.

I will keep their trust and preserve confidentiality.

I will understand that a patient's sense of self-esteem is essential to good health.

I will value life as I strive to understand the process of dying.

I will respect the wisdom of my teachers and will share my knowledge with others.

I will strive to further my education and develop habits that promote further intellectual growth.

I will be proud to practice medicine to the best of my ability and humble enough to call for assistance when necessary.

I will encourage and cooperate with all others involved in the care of my patients so that others may perform their duties effectively and with consideration.

I will live and practice medicine for people rather than for things.

I desire that my empathy will never be subservient to skill and knowledge.

I see my ability to be a good physician as a gift to be shared with humanity.

Professional standards in allopathic medicine are guarded by the American Medical Association with its respective State Associations. In California, this Association was formed 150 years ago. In an attempt to set standards for medical practice, 76 physicians founded the Medical Society of California in 1856. The society grew and was reorganized in 1932 as the California Medical Association (CMA). Shortly after the reorganization—and the likely increase in sociopolitical status of the Association—the CMA became a key player with the California Osteopathic Association (COA) in negotiating their professional relations. As described in the following chapters of this book, the CMA—COA relationship took unique turns, compared to the relations between M.D. and D.O. medical associations in the rest of the country.

The mission statement of the CMA includes efforts to promote the science and art of medicine, the health and well-being of patients, the protection of public health, and the betterment of the profession. According to the CMA website, it is presently the largest state medical association in the U.S. and a leader in the socioeconomics of medicine nationwide. Leadership and professional competence were of equal importance in the last century when the CMA sought to merge with the California Osteopathic Association, as explained in chapters 4 and 5.

Allopathy in California: A brief historical review

California in the 1800's had sparse medical care available since it was a western frontier of the United States. At military outposts, medical care might be available through a medical officer. In Christian missions that were built along the Spanish highway, the local inhabitants could turn to the mission padres for medical support to the extent that it was available.

By the mid 19th century, there was a westward move associated with the gold rush and individual physicians who had arrived with their families probably provided care as best they could. The knowledge gained from medical discoveries in Europe at that time had not yet reached America and certainly not remote California. Many of these physicians were poorly trained, either acquiring their knowledge in a commercial—for—profit school or working in a doctor's office under a type of apprenticeship. As many as 250,000 people are estimated to have migrated to California at that time, by far exceeding the capacity of the limited medical care available.

M.D.s often used harsh treatments in the 1850s, for symptoms whose causes were not understood. Blood letting seemed a panacea for every illness, and a mercury compound was often given in combination with blood letting. Medical texts existed as well as a pharmacology, called *materia medica*, but they rarely were based on investigation. The inadequate quality of care even under medical supervision reflected the level of medical art and science of that day.

These conditions of desperate need for medical care, combined with a fear of harsh treatments, favored the creation of self-styled healers. Quacks, i.e. untrained and uneducated salesmen, often recognized the plight of sick and injured people and took advantage of that market. But there were also serious alternative methods proposed for diagnosis and healing, including homeopathy, eclectic medicine, and naturopathy. While physicians distrusted alternative methods, the general public often distrusted the allopathic drugs in use at that time, and showed instead an interest in osteopathy with its rare use of drugs (Dain Tasker, D.O., unpublished manuscript).

Even at the beginning of the 20th century, American medicine had still not yet acquired the scientific standards of inquiry nor applied many of the principles of physiology and pathology that had evolved in Western Europe. With the exception of a few university medical schools such as Johns Hopkins, the training of medical students was generally of low quality.

In California, though, several allopathic medical colleges opened in the late 19th and early 20th century and soon achieved academic quality: *Toland Medical College* opened in San Francisco in 1864 and joined a decade later with the University of California; the *University of Southern California* (USC) established a College of Medicine in Los Angeles in 1884, the first in southern California; and *Cooper Medical College* opened in 1891 in northern California and transferred to Stanford University in 1908. Soon after the turn of the century, two more allopathic medical colleges opened in southern California: the *College of Physicians and Surgeons* was chartered in 1903 and became affiliated with

USC in 1909; the *College of Medical Evangelists*, later named *Loma Linda University* School of Medicine, opened in 1909 and was the first to offer four academic years of study and experience in a hospital setting.

In 1910, **Abraham Flexner,** a public school principal and brother of a highly respected pathologist, was chosen by the Carnegie Foundation to survey the American medical schools and recommend change to improve medical education. This project was undertaken at the behest of the Council on Medical Education, an instrument created by the American Medical Association (AMA). The AMA was committed to allopathic medicine and an AMA official accompanied Flexner throughout most of his 90-day trip to visit 69 medical schools (http://www.unmc.edu/Community/ruralmeded/flexner.htm, accessed 07/13/08).

Flexner was probably strongly influenced by his experience with European standards of medical education. He doubted the validity of any approach to medical care other than allopathy. Any other approach, he deemed quackery. Medical schools that taught these courses were threatened with loss of accreditation if they did not drop them. Eventually, all complied or closed their schools.

Flexner favored the AMA platform that there were far too many physicians being trained. His report resulted in discrimination against women, African Americans and other minorities. Three out of the five Negro medical schools in the U.S. were closed, including Leonard Medical School in North Carolina, the first medical school for African-Americans in the United States to offer a four-year curriculum. Rising costs associated with implementing the changes recommended in the Flexner Report forced Leonard Medical School to close in 1918 (www.mclibrary.duke.edu). Rural areas were often left without medical care. Only upper middle class candidates could afford to enter the profession because of the sharp rise in tuition.

Within a decade after the Flexner Report on Medical Education was published in 1910, the majority of medical schools had closed, and by 1935 only 66 medical schools existed. However, the American Osteopathic Association was able to bring several of the osteopathic schools into compliance, and neither of the two osteopathic medical schools that existed in Los Angeles in 1910 had to close their program. They had to merge, though, in 1914 to stay in business. The San Francisco College closed in 1912, as described in Chapter 2.

Osteopathy: Origins and definition

> In 1900, Dain Tasker, D.O. advised "*to let osteopathy be free to grow. Let every osteopath be an investigator and let him discover as much new truth as he can, and let osteopathy be broad enough to receive this new truth.* He defined osteopathy as "*the science of treating the body, viewed from an anatomical and physiological standpoint, without the use of drugs . . . . The story of the development of osteopathy in California should stress the conservative, ethical and dignified administration of the first law. This approach created in the public an attitude of respect and confidence*" (Dain Tasker, D.O., unpublished manuscript).

Osteopathy is a healing profession that is unique to America. The founder of osteopathy, an allopathic physician by training, aimed to improve upon medicine, as practiced in his day and his part of the country. While Dr. Andrew Taylor Still, the founder, did not intend to advocate a separate and alternative science of healing, social and political forces created such separation.

D.O.s are fully trained and unlimited licensed physicians who can specialize in family practice or in any other specific field of medicine. Osteopathic medicine has the objective to treat people, rather than only their symptoms. Together with M.D.s, D.O.s are the only physicians in the United States licensed to perform surgery and prescribe medication. Like M.D.s, D.O.s are complete physicians. That means the medical care provided by D.O.s includes diagnosing the cause of illness, preventing diseases, and when necessary performing surgery and prescribing medication. Delivery of babies and comprehensive management of patients in hospitals and nursing homes are also in the purview of these physicians.

Many D.O.s seek additional training, including osteopathic manipulation treatment, that enables them to focus on their patients' physical structure and function, and the body's ability for self-repair. They believe all parts of the body are interrelated and a problem in one area or system is likely to impact the function elsewhere in the body.

Osteopathic Manipulative Treatment, or OMT, is a technique in which D.O.s use their hands to help diagnose and treat an injury or illness. It is a non-invasive therapy that can be used with, or sometimes in place of, medication or surgery. OMT helps treat structural abnormalities allowing the physician to relieve joint restrictions and malalignments. Unlike massage therapy, osteopathic manipulative treatment is a deeper technique that addresses musculoskeletal problems. It is an added expertise that D.O.s can offer patients.

While osteopathic medicine is a fully licensed medical profession, separate from and equal to traditional medicine (allopathy), it is still a minority profession, providing about 16% of physicians nationwide. **The osteopathic medicine oath** seems to emphasize the profession's integrity.

> *I do hereby affirm my loyalty to the profession I am about to enter.*
>
> *I will be mindful always of the great responsibility to preserve the health and life of my patients, to retain their confidence and respect, both as a physician and as a friend who will guard their secrets with scrupulous honor and fidelity, to perform faithfully my professional duties, to employ only those recognized methods of treatment consistent with good judgment and with my skill and ability, keeping in mind always nature's law and the body's inherent capacity for recovery.*
>
> *I will ever be vigilant in aiding in the general welfare of the community, sustaining its laws and institutions, not engaging in those practices which will in any way bring shame or discredit upon myself or my profession. I will give no drugs for deadly purposes to any person, though it may be asked of me.*
>
> *I will endeavor to work in accord with my colleagues in a spirit of progressive cooperation and never by word or by act cast imputations upon them or their rightful practices.*

> *I will look with respect and esteem upon all those who have taught me my art. To my colleague I will be loyal and strive always for its best interests and for the interests of the students who will come after me. I will be ever alert to further the application of basic biologic truths to the healing arts and to develop the principles of osteopathy which were first enunciated by Andrew Taylor Still.*

The osteopathic oath was modified from the Oath of Hippocrates in 1938 by a committee of prominent and respected members of the osteopathic profession. Dr. Frank E. MacCracken, an osteopathic physician from California, had suggested adapting the oath specifically for the osteopathic profession. Parenthetically, Dr. Frank MacCracken is the father of Dr. Betsy MacCracken who contributed her personal narratives to several chapters in this volume. In the 1930s, osteopathy in California was thriving and the profession's college, the College of Osteopathic Physicians and Surgeons, had gained a high reputation of academic rigor and professional standards. Dr. Frank MacCracken's suggestion to formulate an osteopathic oath soon found support at the national level of the profession.

Under the auspices of the Associated Colleges of Osteopathy, a committee was formed that was chaired by Dr. Frank MacCracken and included Drs. R.C. McCaughan, Walter V. Goodfellow, and Edward T. Abbott. Their text of the oath was used until 1954, when the American Osteopathic Association(AOA) Bureau of Professional Education proposed minor amendments that were approved by the AOA House of Delegates. For half a century now, this version of the oath has been in use among osteopathic physicians and surgeons.

The osteopathic oath seems to aim at a wide scope of responsibilities, including the well-being of the community and the profession's organization. Professional conduct and loyalty, and upholding the profession's reputation were important issues for a relatively new profession that found itself in a minority position. As this volume will show, these high standards of not shaming the profession, proposed in 1938 by California's osteopathic doctors, haunted the profession in 1960 when the AOA Board of Trustees used this phrase of the oath to remove a California member from his position on the Board of AOA. In that crisis year of 1960, the AOA president provided a similar explanation for ousting the California Osteopathic Association.

Nearly 70 years after the inception of the osteopathic oath, the culture of medicine in California has matured to increasingly accept diversity in values and health beliefs. While discrimination against a minority medical profession might always be a propensity, there are many signs of mutual respect and collaboration, as the later chapters in this book will show.

The popularity of osteopathic medicine with its emphasis on whole-person care and belief in physiological self-healing properties has much increased in the past 10 years in California, similar to counter movements to medical care in the mid and late 1800s when osteopathy originated. Indeed, the founder of osteopathy, Andrew Taylor Still, M.D. was a physician disillusioned with his profession, as he felt helpless in saving the lives of his wife and three small children and many of his patients to an epidemic of meningitis.

Having studied many healing arts of his time, during the late 1800s, Dr. Still proposed to improve upon allopathic medicine by taking a different, scientific and anatomically based approach to diagnosis and treatment for the whole body. The alignment of the spine comprised an important aspect in assessing the patient's health, especially for patients presenting with a mechanical problem. He rejected blood letting and surgery, unless as a last resort, and the use of most of allopathy's pharmacology, at that time called *materia medica.*

He did not like using medications whose actions were unknown at his time, just because symptoms changed. He used certain chemical treatments for specific diseases, though, like poisonings, i.e. antidotes which he called "chemistry". By the time of the late 1880s, he had become a renowned doctor and was able to publicize his healing art as osteopathy. Not only osteopathy's philosophy and science were his discovery; also the name was coined by him. He wrote, "Osteopathy is compounded by two words, osteon, meaning bone, (and) pathos (or) pathine, to suffer. I reasoned that the bone, 'Osteon', was the starting point from which I was to ascertain the cause of pathological conditions, and so I combined the 'Osteo' with the 'pathy' and had as a result, Osteopathy."

Dr. Still often treated patients who were "cast-off" from M.D.s and mainly suffered from chronic ailments. Skillful, painstaking manipulation frequently helped patients and increased the reputation of osteopathy. By 1892, he had become so popular that he was able to open a school for osteopathy in order to train his family members as well as interested M.D.s and others. He called his school the American School of Osteopathy, still in existence in Kirksville, Missouri, today, though now called the A.T. Still University Kirksville College of Osteopathic Medicine.

Osteopathy in California: A brief historical review

As described in Chapter 2, the history of osteopathic physicians and surgeons in California began in 1896 with the founding of the Pacific Sanitarium and School of Osteopathy (PSSO) in Anaheim. By the turn of the 19th century California became the first state outside of Missouri to have a successful osteopathic medical school, now called Pacific School of Osteopathy and located in Los Angeles, its city of destiny.

Aubrey C. Moore, D.O., one of Dr. Still's students at his American School of Osteopathy in Kirksville, Missouri, moved to Southern California in 1895 upon the suggestion of a grateful patient who wanted this new medical art to be available also in his home state. In the late 1880s, California, especially Southern California, had started to advertise its Mediterranean climate for health promotion and healing. The historian Kevin Starr explains in *"California, a History"* (Modern Library, 2005) that the opening of the transcontinental railroad route into Southern California between 1885 and 1887 made possible a middle- and upper-middle class migration that was prompted significantly by hopes for better health and even healing of tuberculosis. Rest, alternating with movement in fresh air and sunshine were accepted modes of treatment for tuberculosis at that time.

Osteopathy with its emphasis on well-balanced musculoskeletal movement and nutrition was in a good position to meet the needs of the new health seekers. Indeed, two decades later, Frank MacCracken, D.O. saved many of his patients from succumbing to the flu epidemic in 1918 by opening all their windows to fresh, albeit cold, winter air. Frank MacCracken D.O. had tuberculosis and moved with his family from Nebraska to Southern California which must have kept its promises of healing the afflicted because Dr. MacCracken continued to practice and teach osteopathy for many more years in Southern California. His daughter, Betsy MacCracken, D.O. followed his foot steps in Los Angeles, as described in Chapter 3.

Returning to the historical roots of osteopathy in California, B. W. Scheurer, M.D., a German physician with subsequent medical training in America, was practicing allopathic medicine in Los Angeles in the 1890s. His wife was from Kirksville and thus he heard about osteopathy. He persuaded Aubrey Moore, D.O. to set up a school to teach him and other M.D.s and health professionals.

As they started the first osteopathic college outside of Missouri, the Pacific Sanitarium and School of Osteopathy (PSSO) in Anaheim in 1896, they patterned their two year (10 months per year) curriculum after Jefferson Medical College in Philadelphia, one of the finest medical colleges in the country at that time, and after the American School of Osteopathy in Kirksville. While the American School of Osteopathy in Kirksville led to a Diplomat of Osteopathy (D.O.) degree, the PSSO became the first osteopathic medical school to award the Doctor of Osteopathy degree and to add to the greatest number of D.O.s in the western states. In 1900, 73 D.O.s practiced in California, Oregon, Washington, Arizona, Nevada and Idaho; 40 of these practiced in California.

In spite of various tribulations, osteopathy in California continued to thrive, as described in Chapter 3. D.O.s were trained as interns at the Los Angeles County Hospital as early as 1916 and attended patients there and at the out-patient obstetrics clinic. They were given their own segregated "Unit II" of the Los Angeles County Hospital in 1928 which was expanded in 1958 by public vote as the Los Angeles County Osteopathic Hospital. This became the pre-eminent osteopathic training hospital in the country. From it sprang several osteopathic sub-specialty societies (i.e., in medicine, surgery, radiology, obstetrics and gynecology and pediatrics) and later, residency training programs developed.

Chapter 4 describes how from the early 1940s to 1961, political leaders of the California Osteopathic Association (COA) engaged in bargaining with the political leaders of the California Medical Association (CMA) to create a merging of the two professions. Part of the objectives for this merger was to remove the strongly felt discrimination by allopathic physicians. As part of the bargain, before the California M.D.s would accept the D.O.s into their hospitals, D.O.s had to give up their state association (COA), their college (COP&S), their distinctive degree (D.O.), their unique philosophy and principles, their use of osteopathic manipulative therapeutics, and their homage to A.T. Still as their founder. For most D.O.s, these compromises were acceptable in return for professional respect and social acceptance.

To accomplish these objectives it was necessary to reverse the provisions of the 1922 Osteopathic Initiative Act in order to restrict the Osteopathic Board of Examiners from issuing new licenses to D.O.s. As that initiative passed in 1962, the board could only regulate those that elected to maintain their D.O. degree and licensing, until there were less than 40 D.O.s in the state, at which time the osteopathic licensing board would cease to exist.

In compliance with these requirements, COP&S became the California College of Medicine (CCM) in 1962. As described in Chapter 5, CCM granted the M.D. degree to the former COP&S osteopathic faculty, alumni, and future graduates, as well as qualifying graduates from out-of-state osteopathic colleges. This was the first, and so far the only time a D.O. degree granting school abandoned its degree conferring power and transformed itself into an allopathic school. The rest of the osteopathic medical schools in America did not follow suit. To the contrary, like a catalyst, the California merger created a chain reaction of numerous osteopathic schools sprouting around the country thereafter.

Also in California, not all osteopathic physicians agreed with the merger. In 1961, they organized as the Osteopathic Physician and Surgeons of California (OPSC) to protect their rights. After a long series of court battles the California Supreme Court restored the power of the osteopathic medical board to grant new licenses to D.O.s in 1974, as a separate licensing board, the Osteopathic Medicine Board of California. As most states have composite boards made up of both M.D.s and D.O.s, there are currently only 13 other states besides California with separate licensing boards for osteopathic physicians.

Osteopathic education was in a drought in this state from 1962 until 1974 when the Supreme Court of California restored the licensing power of the osteopathic licensing board. This ruling made possible for osteopathic education to be resumed in California in 1977 with the founding of the College of Osteopathic Medicine of the Pacific (COMP) in Pomona. Over a decade ago the San Francisco Bay Area put another college on the map, the Touro University College of Osteopathic Medicine (TUCOM). It is housed in Vallejo now and graduated its first class in June 2001. California is once again amongst only a few states with two osteopathic colleges, joining Missouri, Pennsylvania, and Arizona. The two California programs will soon produce between 350 and 400 new D.O. graduates per year.

Osteopathy in California today: A separate yet equal medical profession

With the addition of a second osteopathic medical school in California the number of D.O.s lost in the amalgamation of 1962 has long been replaced. During the past forty years, educational opportunities in osteopathy have increased all over the United States. In 1968, there were just five colleges of osteopathic medicine in the U.S. In 2008, there are 25 colleges and three branch campuses nationwide.

In 1968, the five colleges enrolled 1,879 students and annually graduated 426 D.O.s. In 2006, enrollment totaled 14,435, more than a seven-fold increase, and the colleges graduated 2,713 D.O.s. By comparison, the numbers of allopathic medical students and graduates have not quite doubled in the same time frame (AACOM, Washington, D.C., e-newsletter

2/2007). While many reasons must have affected the increasing demand for education and training in osteopathic medicine, including more room to grow in this under-represented profession, California's renewed contribution to the profession's visibility and respect for serving community needs might have contributed significantly to the dramatic growth.

Chapter 6 provides historical narratives by M.D.s and D.O.s that address the effects of the re-establishment of osteopathy in California on their relationship as well as the effects of the merger on the professions' identities. Lessons learned from the past helped to shape the relationship between both medical professions who, after all that has been said and done in the past century, always wished to improve healthcare in California.

Occupational profile of osteopathic physicians in California today:

Today, osteopathic medicine is based on four principles which form the cornerstones of the osteopathic philosophy of comprehensive patient care:

1. The body is a unit; the person is a unit of body, mind, and spirit.
2. The body is capable of self-regulation, self-healing, and health maintenance.
3. Structure and function are reciprocally interrelated.
4. Rational treatment is based upon an understanding of the basic principles of body-unity, self-regulation, and the interrelationship of structure and function.

These tenets were developed in 1954 by the Kirksville multi-disciplinary D.O. and Ph.D. basic science faculty. The American Osteopathic Association (AOA) accepted the tenets nation-wide in 1997, with the publication of the *Foundations for Osteopathic Medicine* text book. The entire philosophy of that profession is expounded in that text, which is required reading for all osteopathic medical students.

Recently, as a requirement of the California Department of the Consumer Affairs, the California osteopathic profession conducted an occupational analysis of the 2,623 D.O.s licensed and residing in the state. Based on a scientifically acceptable response rate to questionnaires, the majority of respondents specialize in family/general practice (43%), eight percent in internal medicine, 7% in emergency medicine, and 6% in osteopathic manipulative medicine. More than half of respondents practice in southern California (59.9%); nearly half own their practices (41.1%); and the majority practice in metropolitan areas (87.4%).

Many of the tasks and knowledge base identified as "relevant, important and frequently utilized" are germane to the practice of medicine in general. They include medical chart and data analysis, communication skills, application of basic sciences, especially anatomy, physiology, biochemistry and pharmacology, utilization of technology, and understanding the legal aspects of medical practice. Even with the close collaboration with allopathic medicine, the knowledge of osteopathic principles and their application is rated as "moderately" to "highly important", and only 11.4% of D.O.s indicate that osteopathic principles have "no, or an insignificant, impact" on the way they currently practice medicine.

Thus, many people who study healthcare in California feel confident that osteopathy is here to stay. Others argue that osteopathy might have outlived its aim to improve upon allopathy, as osteopathy might be inclined to forego its distinctive characteristics. The following historical account of gaining and losing and re-gaining the osteopathic distinctiveness is thought to provide an improved understanding of the relationship between allopathic and osteopathic medicine in California.

Allopathy and osteopathy in California: Records of the relationship

Published as well as archival sources, together with other legal and historical documents, provided a structure for describing the historical relationship between the two unlimited licensed medical professions in California. Historical narratives of individuals who witnessed the developments of that relationship allowed us to add life to archival and legal documents. The narratives give meaning and significance to events and aid in our understanding of California's unique contributions to healthcare.

Contributors of historical narratives

One of the major endeavors in completing this volume has been the collection of personal interviews by Michael Seffinger, D.O. with key persons who affected the relationship between the osteopathic and allopathic professions. All interview participants have played a meaningful role in the history of medicine in California since the 1950s. Some were involved in facilitating the merger between the osteopathic and allopathic professions. These included physicians, legislators and their assistants, lawyers, public relations people and representatives of professional organizations, like the California Hospital Association. Others were individuals who vigorously fought against the merger and ultimately achieved, through the decisions of the court, the return of osteopathy's professional independence in California. This wide array of individuals signifies the broad swath of Californians who were involved with shaping the special events of the past fifty years. Through these people's eyes and retrospective lenses we can better interpret the documented historical events of California's recent past.

In retelling this saga, we are hopeful to help in the healing process of the wounds that were inflicted in the past, and to bring better understanding and cooperation between the two professions. As both professions are in pursuit of providing optimal care, they might gain from the other's science and art.

The relations between osteopathic and allopathic medicine are complex and multifaceted. To shed light on the complexity, we listened to the thoughts and concerns that shaped the decisions made by the members of each profession. The interviews have been able to capture their personal, social, economical, educational, political, and research aspirations.

Most interviews were audio-visually recorded and transcribed verbatim. For logistic reasons, a few interviews were conducted by obtaining written responses to the interview questions. All participants subsequently reviewed and edited, as needed, their transcripts. They agreed for their historical narratives to be quoted in this project. Most interviews were conducted at the participants' work settings or at their homes.

For this book we extracted sections of the interview narratives that spoke to events described in the following chapters. The Appendix provides brief professional biographies of our interview participants and of key historical persons.

The historical narratives of the following individuals served as a vital layer of evidence in describing the journey of the M.D.-D.O. relationship in California:

> **Ethan Allen, D.O., Paul Alloy, M.D., Stuart Chesky, D.O., J.D.,**
> **Donald Dilworth, D.O., Emery Dowell, M.S., Richard Eby, D.O.,**
> **Viola Frymann, D.O., Dolores Grunigen, B.A., Stanley Golanty, M.D.,**
> **Scott Haldeman, M.D., Ph.D., D.C., Seth Hufstedler, LLB,**
> **Steven Kamajian, D.O., Richard Kammerman, M.D, Mitchell Kasovac, D.O.,**
> **Allen Korneff, Donald Krpan, D.O., Betsy MacCracken, M.D., MPH,**
> **Alan Menkes, D.O., Jay Michael, M.S, Thomas Nelson, M.D.,**
> **Robert Norcross, M.D., Victor Passy, M.D., Philip Pumerantz, Ph.D.,**
> **William Ryan, D.O., Richard Ryder, M.D., Michael Seffinger, D.O.,**
> **Robert Steedman, M.D., Cynthia Stotts, D.O., James Taylor, M.D.,**
> **Jerome Tobis, M.D., Seymour Ulansey, M.D., Stanley van den Noort, M.D.,**
> **Norman Vinn, D.O., Matt Weyuker, and John Wykle, M.D.**

This book tries to give recognition to these individuals, as they witnessed and often shaped the historical events. To attempt to summarize the underlying themes expressed by the interview participants, one might consider the following groups:

- Those who actively brought about the merger
- Those D.O.s who were observers and felt to derive benefit from receiving the M.D. degree
- Those who fought vigorously to oppose the merger and participated in the recrudescence of osteopathy in California
- Those who joined after the merger and contributed to the M.D.—D.O. relationship.

The phenomenal expansion of osteopathic medical schools that followed the merger seems causally related to the efforts expended by some of the interview participants. This outcome was probably not anticipated by those who attempted the amalgamation of D.O.s and M.D.s into one profession, but legal endeavors have since protected osteopathy with equal rights to allopathy. Thus, the vision to create a friendly environment nationwide for side-by-side osteopathic and allopathic medical education seems to become a reality.

Chapter 2

Pioneering osteopathy:
The medical and social climate in early California

Education

Impart strength to feeble frames
Displace the pallor of disease with the rose-tints of health
Supplant the moans of pain with songs of gladness

Mission Statement, **Pacific School of Osteopathy and Infirmary**,
Los Angeles, Spring & Franklin Streets, June 1897 re-incorporated.

The early years of medicine in California were characterized by distinct differences in the fundamental practices and underlying philosophies that distinguished the education of D.O.s from M.D.s in California. The best source of information about the early years of osteopathy is contained in an unpublished manuscript by Dain Tasker, D.O. on the history of osteopathy in California, housed at the Special Collections and Archives at the University of California Irvine (UCI) libraries. The following section provides a synopsis of Dr. Tasker's chapters addressing education and training during the early years of osteopathy in California (1896 to 1906).

From Kirksville to Anaheim

As the news spread of Dr. Still's successful new approach to diagnosis and treatment, patients came to see him in Kirksville from far and wide. Needing help to treat so many patients, Dr. Still tried to train friends and colleagues in his new discipline informally but soon recognized that comprehensive education and training were required. Thus, A.T. Still, M.D. founded the American School of Osteopathy (ASO) in 1892 in Kirksville, Missouri.

Grateful patients wanted to facilitate new beginnings for osteopathy in their respective communities in other states. Aubrey C. Moore, D.O., one of Dr. Still's first graduates, initially moved to Illinois to practice osteopathy, where he was accused, and acquitted, of practicing medicine without a license. He then moved to California in **1896** to set up a practice.

California had no formal board yet for Dr. Moore to get licensed as an osteopath. Not to repeat the legal battles he had encountered in Illinois he practiced under B.W. Scheurer, M.D., a graduate of German and American schools who was a licentiate of California. Dr. Scheurer must have been impressed by his colleague's skills, because together they opened the **Pacific Sanitarium and School of Osteopathy** on June 1st, **1896** in the abandoned Del Campo Hotel in Anaheim. This was the first osteopathic school established in the U.S., other than Dr. Still's original school, the American School of Osteopathy, and some other short lived schools, one across the street from the American School by one of Dr. Still's graduates.

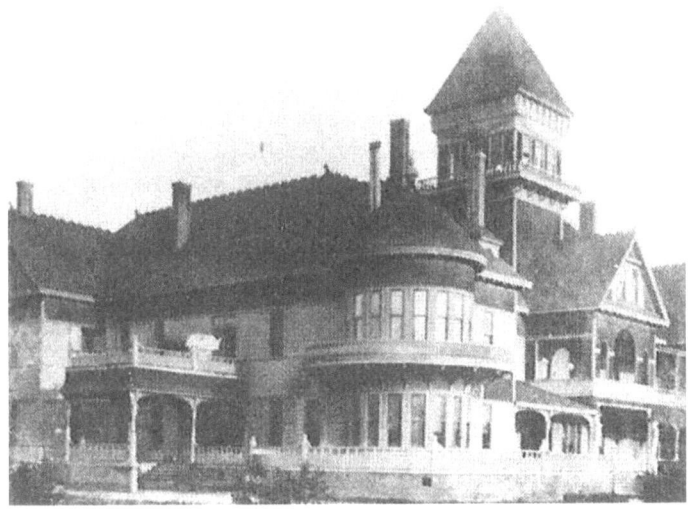

Figure 2a. "Pacific Sanitarium and School of Osteopathy in Anaheim, 1896"

In pursuit of highest educational standards

In September 1896, they had already started a second class which included two M.D.s, Dr. Smith and Dr. Henry. While still a student, Dr. Henry simultaneously served as faculty and in the following year became president of the school. C.E. Henry had a degree from Jefferson Medical College in Philadelphia and was especially well-liked. Prior to obtaining his medical education, Dr. Henry had been a pharmacist in Kirksville and was familiar with osteopathy as practiced in that town. He integrated this knowledge of osteopathy with his allopathic medical training obtained in Philadelphia. Thus, the school pursued the highest standards of education. In **1897**, a new name was used, **Pacific School of Osteopathy and Infirmary.**

By February 1897 their clinic already saw 20 patients per day. At the end of the year, course work was extended to 20 months. Thus, the school offered 2 years study even though Dr. Still's school in Kirksville did not yet require 2 years. In **1897** Dr. Moore became owner of the Anaheim school, while Dr. Scheurer was not mentioned further in Tasker's manuscript.

Soon there were not enough patients in Anaheim, a relatively small town, to provide sufficient clinical cases for student teaching. In June **1898** Dr. Moore decided to move the Pacific School to Los Angeles on Flower & 10th Street. Los Angeles at that time had a population of almost 100,000. The name at that point was **Pacific School of Osteopathy (PSO),** although an archival source at UCI ("Historical Outline, UCI-College of Medicine") continues to use the name Pacific School of Osteopathy and Infirmary until 1902 when the infirmary was closed.

On January 5, 1898 the first class of nine students graduated with the degree as Diplomate of Osteopathy. The valedictorian of the first class was **Dain Tasker**. Dain Tasker, D.O. became the major advocate for osteopathy in California as well as its invaluable historian. Drs. Smith and Henry received the Doctor of Osteopathy degree, since they already held an M.D. degree. The graduates of the **1899** class, however, each received the Doctor of Osteopathy degree. Kirksville followed suit with this degree in 1901, when it gave A.T. Still an honorary Doctor of Osteopathy degree. Subsequent graduates have received that degree since. However, osteopathic schools established abroad grant only the Diplomat of Osteopathy degree and prepare their graduates for limited, manipulation-based practices.

The second class of graduates included Dain's sister, **Anna E. Tasker, D.O.** from Wisconsin. Women were drawn to osteopathy at a time when medical schools were not supportive of women enrollment. Student diversity was embraced by osteopathy in California since its early days. The graduation motto of the second class was "*With brain and heart and hands to serve humanity*".

After another year, the nine-person faculty included three women, Amelia Brotherhood, Estelle Strasser, and Anna Tasker. Dr. Brotherhood had already 5 years teaching experience at the University of Utah. She had also published an article in the October 1899 issue of *The Osteopath*, entitled "An educator's view of osteopathy". In the conclusion of her article Dr. Brotherhood **argued for 3 years education** to raise standards and to require entrance qualifications of students.

By **1900,** a 3-year course became the requirement to obtain the Doctor of Science of Osteopathy in California—long before other osteopathic schools held such high standards. Entrance requirements included high school completion and exceptional character. In 1901, PSO also required a thesis for graduation.

In the same year, **Carle Phinney, D.O.** a former student at the Pacific School, became Professor of Anatomy and eventually president of the faculty.

Dr. Brotherhood introduced osteopathy to **Dr. Clement Whiting**, Professor of Biology at Utah State University. Dr. Whiting and his wife Lillian moved to Los Angeles in proximity of the college. Dr. Whiting taught basic science and lab techniques at the Pacific School and the quality of his courses was praised by Dr. Tasker: "*He had no ideologies to defend. His importance in osteopathic education increased year by year. He gave his all for osteopathy*". In 1902, Dr. Whiting assumed also a position in public sanitation, under the Board of Public Health. He facilitated D.O.s' interaction at the highest governmental level in California long before osteopaths in other states could do so. He worked hard to get D.O.s accepted in serving the Los Angeles County health care needs.

A decade later, Dr. Whiting also became a leader in uniting the two osteopathic schools that existed then in Los Angeles, the Pacific College of Osteopathy—the new name given in 1904 to the PSO—and the Los Angeles College of Osteopathy. Unfortunately, he was struck by a car on the way to the merger meeting between the two schools in 1913, bringing his life to an abrupt untimely end.

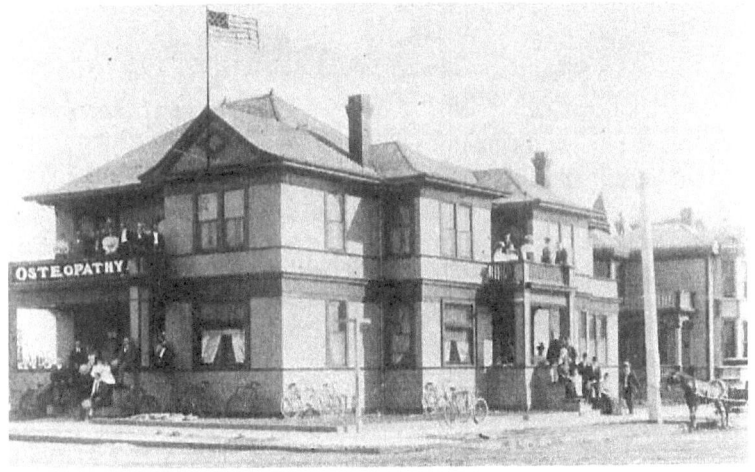

Figure 2b. "Pacific School of Osteopathy in Los Angeles, 1898"

The challenges of teaching osteopathy in California

The mechanical concept of a joint lesion as a primary cause of a functional disorder was the dominant teaching in all osteopathic schools and the reason for their existence. To get a true perspective of osteopathic teaching it must be recognized that the schools were conducted for profit and based on teaching a secret technique. Once students started new schools, the "secret" depreciated. The new generation focused on lab methods instead of didactic teaching, because demonstration is the best method of teaching manipulation.

Prior to 1901, anatomy at the Pacific School was taught by palpation because there were no other means. Students palpated bony landmarks and related these to deeper structures. Palpation increased their confidence and understanding. They were not allowed to dissect cadavers until the legal recognition of Osteopathy in 1901. But even then they could hardly obtain sufficient number of cadavers because the four medical colleges had priority claims. The D.O.s acquired an amendment to the State Statute that cadavers would be proportioned to student enrollment. The DO college had 400 students (a greater number than the medical schools) and they received their proportion. Every student had to dissect a whole body.

After his graduation in 1898, Dain Tasker was immediately recruited to teach theory and practice of osteopathy. This was quite a challenge as Dr. Moore and Dr. Burton, the initial teachers, had not put their lecture notes on paper and there were no publications by Dr. Still or the American School of Osteopathy available at that time. This frustration no doubt prompted Dr. Tasker to write his own book on osteopathic principles and practices, published in 1901.

Associated with a bankruptcy and yet another complete re-organization of PSO in 1904, the school changed its name again to **Pacific College of Osteopathy (PCO)**. The college expressed a commitment to the "development of the true science of health" and began to facilitate conducting research ("Historical Outline, UCI-College of Medicine"). Struggles for educational privileges, better standards and financial solvency continued.

In **1909,** PCO became the first osteopathic medical school to expand to a four year curriculum. The charter of PCO allowed to offer an M.D. degree, which it did from 1904-1910, to D.O. graduates who took an extra 6 months, or so, of course work in *materia medica* and other practices common to M.D.s of the time. In 1910, the AOA threatened the PCO with removal of accreditation if it continued to offer the M.D. degree and PCO withdrew the M.D. program thereafter.

A separate osteopathic licensing board had existed since 1901, but it was replaced by a composite licensing board in 1907 for the following reason: In 1907, the osteopathic licensing board did not allow the graduates of the new Los Angeles College of Osteopathy (founded in 1905) to sit for the osteopathic licensing exam, as their curriculum was not as long or inclusive as that offered by the Pacific College. The curriculum of the Los Angeles College of Osteopathy (LACO) included teaching *materia medica* and surgery and used mostly M.D. preceptors. The AOA did not accredit it. However, the LACO prevailed in court action in 1907.

In addition, the 1901 osteopathic practice act was repealed and replaced by legislation with a composite licensing board consisting of five allopaths, two eclectics, two homeopaths and two osteopaths. Education and training standards were determined for 1) a drugless and for 2) an unlimited physician and surgeon classification. Effie E. York of San Francisco reported in *JAOA* in 1907 in its June 1 issue that on March 4, 1907 the new medical practice act had been signed by Governor Gillett.

On April 27, 1907 Drs. Dain Tasker and Ernest Sisson were appointed to represent the osteopaths. All practitioners were to take the same examinations in anatomy, histology, gynecology, pathology, bacteriology, chemistry and toxicology, physiology, obstetrics, general diagnosis, and hygiene. *Materia medica* and mechanotherapy were relegated to the colleges to determine whether and to what extent they should be included in the curriculum. In order to sit for an unlimited license, *materia medica* courses were required. Mr. York remarked that the *"consensus of opinion is that osteopathy has been greatly benefited by this legislation."*

Dr. Tasker wrote in the *JAOA* July 1, 1907 edition, page 448:

> *"California is making an attempt to regulate the practice of the arts of healing on the basis of an examination in what is known about the body in health and disease rather than on the basis of what is believed to be the proper method of treatment. Any one who desires to practice any known or unknown form of healing in this state must pass this examination. It must be conceded that, so far as the state's safeguarding the public from the practice of charlatans and quacks is concerned, this examination is as far as it ought to go. Any further step is more or less an effort to favor a special form of therapy. I have always been an advocate of independent boards of examiners for osteopaths, but if our medical laws would all eliminate the question of definition [as to what constitutes medical practice vs osteopathic vs chiropractic practices], and examination in methods of therapy, there would be no good and sufficient reason why there should be more than one board of examiners for all schools."*

At PCO, a faculty of four taught 50 students. The curriculum comprised the same subjects as in allopathic medical schools except *materia medica*. Students saw patients in an infirmary on the 1st floor of the building. Needless to say, the famous Flexner Report of 1910 had little effect on the Pacific College of Osteopathy, as its standards were already amongst the top in the nation. However the California

47

state composite medical board insisted on increasing admission requirements and curricular hours in *materia medica* in order for graduates to be allowed to sit for the unlimited licensure examination.

At the turn of the 20th century one more osteopathic college, namely the California College of Osteopathy, existed in San Francisco, founded in 1898. Aubrey Moore, D.O. had moved to San Francisco around 1898 to help with this school's development. It suffered badly in the great San Francisco earthquake of 1906 and lasted only until 1912. There was no other osteopathic school in the San Francisco Bay area again until 1997, when the Touro University College of Osteopathic Medicine opened its doors, as described in Chapter 5.

The aim of osteopathy in California at the turn of the 20th century

To educate other health practitioners and the public on osteopathy, they started publication of a monthly journal, *The Osteopath,* as early as July 1896. The front page of volume 1, number 1 explained that the "*the object and aim of osteopathy are to improve and advance our present system of surgery, obstetrics, and treatments of general diseases to a more satisfactory position than they now are*". Publication of *The Osteopath* was discontinued in 1902.

Dr. Tasker based many of his historical accounts on documentations in *The Osteopath.* One issue featured an article by Dr. Still, entitled "Osteopathy defined". Still explained *"The human body is a machine run by the unseen force called life and that it may be run harmoniously it is necessary that there be liberty of blood, nerves, and arteries from generating point to destination"*. Dain Tasker explained that the social climate in California was favorable to Dr. Still's philosophy of osteopathy because of a general distrust of drugs among the public.

California's initiative to regulate education

In 1897 efforts started for osteopathic schools nationwide to form an organization to regulate osteopathic education and to standardize the curricula. In **January 1899,** first mention can be found of an *American Association for the Advancement of Osteopathy,* in *The Osteopath, 3* (6). This organization, founded in 1897, later became known as the American Osteopathic Association. While it was hoped that all osteopathic schools would become members, for the time being the list of colleges that joined included The Pacific School of Osteopathy, Los Angeles; the Northern School of Osteopathy, Minneapolis, Minnesota; the S.S.Still College of Osteopathy, Des Moines, Iowa; the Milwaukee Institute of Osteopathy, Milwaukee, Wisconsin; and the Western Institute of Osteopathy, Denver, Colorado.

First textbooks on osteopathy in California

Textbooks were vital in the beginning years of osteopathy in California to ensure uniformity and high quality education. In 1899 two authoritative text books appeared:

- "The Practice of Osteopathy", by C.P. McConnell, D.O., M.D.
- "Principles of Osteopathy", by Charles Hazzard, D.O. (Hazzard; 3d ed. rev edition (1899) ASIN: B00087D4M6)

Dr. Tasker quotes extensively from the book "The Practice of Osteopathy", by C.P. McConnell, D.O., M.D. while mentioning little about Hazzard's book: *"Osteopathy includes all that is reliable in the therapeutics of medicine . . . . Osteopathy is not exclusively a system of mechanical therapeutics, although manipulation enters very largely into the work. It is a system that includes all methods of healing, that have been found trustworthy and scientific, whether it be mechanical correction of the tissues, the giving of proper food, the use of antidotes, care and attention to hygienic rules, or nursing, and the various aides to prevent and relieve the ravages of disease. Osteopathy rests on a broad basis that in the liberal sense includes all that is good and in accord with natural laws of the human body, and that is not confined to narrow channels of thought of bigotry. Our students receive teaching in all branches of medicine save one, materia medica."*

The two books had authoritative backing from the American School in Kirksville and served to outline for the profession at large the work they were doing or attempting to do. "At long last there was something on paper that could be analyzed or altered as time indicated, connected with experience", Tasker stated, as he seemed to view osteopathy as unfolding and adapting.

Textbooks apparently played a big role in the beginning years of osteopathy in California where practitioners were so far removed geographically from the main educational resources in Kirksville. When in San Francisco the California College of Osteopathy did not survive the destruction of the earthquake in **1906,** osteopaths all over California donated textbooks to those who lost their libraries. This professional support and empathy apparently was important to Tasker, as he mentioned the event in his manuscript. Since he had worked so hard to promote the profession in California, practitioners donating their reference texts must have implied for him a strong group cohesiveness and identity among osteopaths in California.

With no major osteopathic college in northern California between 1912 and 1997, the center of osteopathic education in the West was in southern California.

Graduates from the Pacific School of Osteopathy were located from Sacramento to San Diego.

Osteopathic clinics for teaching and training:

In addition to textbooks, education in osteopathic medicine required clinics for education and training. The first clinic, for teaching purposes only, was established by the Pacific School of Osteopathy in July 1900 in a cottage at 10th and Flower Streets in Los Angeles. In 1908, PCO established a maternity hospital.

Through the efforts of Clement Whiting D.O. the Los Angeles County Hospital accepted students of PCO for clinical training in 1909, and in the following year PCO opened a clinic in downtown Los Angeles, in the Jones building on North Street.

Olive Clark, M.D. a graduate of Women's Medical College in Philadelphia took charge of the Department of Ob/Gyn. She was an inspiring leader for women students.

Financial controversies

During these thriving years, the S. S. Still College in Des Moines had bought 80% of the stock of the Pacific College in 1905 and announced that they had joined the Pacific College faculty. The Pacific College replied, stating that *"stockholders and faculty will not stand for commercialization"* of PCO ("Historical Outline, UCI-College of Medicine"). Differences in philosophy caused animosity with Drs. Shaw and Forbes of the Des Moines faculty and their students. Arrangements were made, though, and by **1905** two schools existed in Los Angeles, namely the **Los Angeles College of Osteopathy** and the **Pacific College of Osteopathy.**

The 37 graduates of the Los Angeles College of Osteopathy faced a hostile situation, though, as the State Board refused to recognize the Los Angeles College due to lower standards for admission and course work requirements. The Pacific College of Osteopathy continued with its 3 years and 10 months course. In addition, graduates at the Pacific College had observed osteopathic examinations in the clinic and learned to provide treatment.

While the Los Angeles College was a for-profit institution, the Pacific College had no apparent financial motive. Both were reviewed in 1906 by the AOA because tension between the two colleges created an acute problem not only in California but also within the AOA.

Some truce was established between the two schools to get favorable legislation. The Los Angeles College grew by obtaining labs and a more suitable building. The College's reapplication for AOA membership was accepted.

In 1909 the Carnegie Foundation reviewed both schools. The **Flexner report** in **1910** referred to the LA College as "a thriving business". In contrast, the Pacific College was described as teaching at a hospital, running a dispensary, and conducting research projects. The Los Angeles College tried a rebuttal to the report because of the commercial criticism.

By **1909** a four-year course as well as post-graduate courses were offered at both schools in Los Angeles. While the Pacific College offered the post-graduate courses for free, the LA College charged. By 1911 students of the Pacific College were allowed to be present at (allopathic) surgical clinics of the LA County General Hospital.

In **1913** the Pacific College reincorporated for the third time in order to be "free from sectarianism, and never be for private gain". Thus, the Pacific College enforced its purely educational, non-profit basis. Professor Whiting was still chair of the faculty.

In **1914**, after many years of conflict and competition, the two colleges were able to join and a new name, **College of Osteopathic Physicians & Surgeons (COP&S)**, was chosen. This name increasingly stood for a college of highest standards and remained the official name until the merger in 1961. In 1914 COP&S required a high-school diploma and offered a 4-year course. The D.O. degree stood for Doctor of Osteopathy.

Dr. Dain Tasker resigned from the Board of Trustees so he could continue representing the profession on the State Board of Medical Examiners. Dain's wife, Dr. Cora Tasker continued on the Board of Trustees.

In **1919** new State law requirements for graduates of medical and osteopathic colleges to be eligible to sit for the state licensing exam included for schools to cover *materia medica* and pharmacy. COP&S provided even more hours than required by State law for these and every other subject and pursued educational standards that were higher than those at any osteopathic college nationwide.

With about 500 students in attendance, the College had more students enrolled than each of the 10 medical colleges of the Western coast. The consolidated alumni and student body at this time included a working force in the field of more than 800 graduates.

Pioneering Research

In 1900 *The Osteopath* published the first reproduction of an X-ray of the pelvis of a young man who had been injured. The X-ray required 1 hour exposure! The injury was interpreted as subluxation of the right innominate.

In 1904 first research projects were conducted once the school, at that time called the Pacific College of Osteopathy, moved to larger facilities in Los Angeles. These projects addressed the effects of manipulation upon the body, and the ratio of urea excretion to purine bodies, as cited in a manuscript entitled "History of the California College of Medicine" (DeStefano, Lee and Schwartz, 1964, unpublished archival document at UCI).

Scientific experiments rather than faith in theory

Drs. Henry and Smith were especially interested in the lesion theory of diseases. With their broad educational background they stimulated students to conduct scientific experiments rather than to accept the theory on faith.

Clement Whiting was the first D.O. in California to conduct epidemiological and public health research. Louisa Burns, D.O. began her research endeavors in 1903.

Louisa Burns, D.O.

A summary by Myron Beal, D.O., F.A.A.O. in the 1994 yearbook of the American Academy of Osteopathy (AAO) describes vividly the personal investments, including personal financial contributions, that were needed to conduct research:

"Louisa Burns was motivated to enter the Pacific College of Osteopathy through her personal experience of the benefit of osteopathic treatment reversing the disabling effects from spinal meningitis. She began her laboratory research studies of osteopathic principles while she was a student. After she graduated in 1903 she served as a teacher and clinician at the college and in her spare time conducted research on the physiology of the nervous system.

"In 1914 she joined the A. T. Still Research Institute in Chicago. The research plans called for keeping experimental and control animals for long periods of time which required them to be in relatively good health. Conditions in Chicago at the Research Institute were found to be unsatisfactory for maintaining healthy animals. Therefore, it was decided to move the Institute to Sunny Slope in South

Pasadena, California where the climate was milder and the facilities were away from an urban area.

"The move to Sunny Slope was completed in 1917 by Dr. Burns as Institute Director. Sunny Slope was purchased by the Burns family in 1917 for $8,000 to provide a place for the work of the A. T. Still Research Institute. Interest payments, taxes and some improvements during the years 1917-1919 were made by the Burns family. Gifts from various persons were used to purchase equipment and retire part of the mortgage. In 1919 the A. T. Still Research Institute provided a loan of $4,500 to clear the mortgages. For several years the A. T. Still Research Institute paid $50 a month which was called rent and was just enough to pay taxes, interest, the cost of public utilities and building repairs. In 1931 the A. T. Still Research Institute could not carry on experimental work, nor continue payment for expenses. The property which had been deeded to the Western Osteopathic Research Laboratories in 1919 to facilitate the work of the Institute was returned to Louisa Burns.

"She undertook to carry on such research work that was possible under the limited financial circumstances. In 1935 the Sunny Slope property consisted of about 3.76 acres belonging to Louisa Burns, of which 2.5 were under cultivation. There were five living rooms which were occupied by Louisa Burns and her family who cared for the place. There were two work rooms, one containing records, books, files and x-rays. The other contained various items of equipment. There were a few hutches for animals used in the then current studies. A clinical laboratory at the Merrill Sanitarium in South Pasadena provided many patient records of interest and the income from the laboratory helped defray the expenses at Sunny Slope.

"Dr. Burns had been employed by the A. T. Still Osteopathic Foundation and Research Institute and paid $100 a month. This was continued when the American Osteopathic Association took over the management of the Institute in July 1936. The committee on research assigned additional funds for specific research activities and as of 1941-42 recommended an annual allowance of $1,200. In 1944 the research committee recommended an additional allowance of $50 a month for secretarial help and animal maintenance. In 1945, Dr. Burns allowance was increased to $200 a month."

In 1918, Dr. Burns formulated a thesis for research study. It was that *"the abnormal condition called a bony lesion exists and it may cause disease in distant parts of the body."* A corollary to this hypothesis was that if a bony lesion is a disturbance in the normal relation of bones, a similar condition could be produced in laboratory animals either as a disturbance in bony relations or some other pathological condition. Disease should occur in distant parts of the bodies of the affected animals. The correction of such bony lesions should result in at least partial recovery from the diseases so produced. If the above conditions can be met, study of the tissue changes during the pathogenesis and recovery should increase the understanding of the nature of bony lesions.

Based on this hypothesis, plans were made to produce bony lesions in animals and to study the tissues concerned in the lesion compared with similar animals that were without lesions serving as controls. In addition, methods of correction were to be studied as well as the results of correction. Dr. Burns' published work represents a wide interest in subject matter like the pathogenesis of bony lesions, their effect on total body economy and the specific effects on various organ systems of the body. She conducted animal experiments producing bony lesions and observing their effects on segmentally related visceral function and described the effects both grossly and microscopically. Dr. Burns attempted to correlate basic research with clinical phenomena. She also contributed to the development of osteopathic skills of palpatory diagnosis and manipulative treatment.

Her work has been criticized for the lack of specificity of some reports, a lack of details concerning the number of animals involved, and the lack of controls. Wilbur Cole, D.O. worked with Louisa Burns from 1949 to 1951. His Louisa Burns Memorial Address reproduced in the same yearbook represents the best critique of her research work and its importance.

"Louisa Burns was the first person in the osteopathic profession to establish and carry out a long term research program. She attempted to introduce new evidence in support of the osteopathic concept of the relationship of structure and function by correlating basic research with clinical phenomena. Her work focused the attention of the profession on the necessity of research and its importance to develop basic knowledge and understanding. Dr. Burns published work consists of experimental animal studies, observation of both animal and human behavior, and the application of osteopathic concepts to the understanding of disease and its treatment." Her work is summarized in the book *Pathogenesis of Visceral Disease Following Vertebral Lesions.* Selections from her published work are included in the 1970 AAO yearbook as well.

Dr. Beal cited the following references:

1. Cole, W. V.: Louisa Burns Memorial Lecture. JAOA 69:1005-17, Jan 1970.
2. American Osteopathic Association archives.
3. Northup, George W. ed.: Osteopathic Research: Growth and Development. Chicago, Illinois: AOA 1987.
4. Gevitz, Norman: *The D.O.s: Osteopathic Medicine in America,* The Johns Hopkins University Press, Baltimore, Maryland, 1982.

5. Burns, Louisa: Pathogenesis of Visceral Disease Following Vertebral Lesions. Chicago, Illinois: AOA 1948.

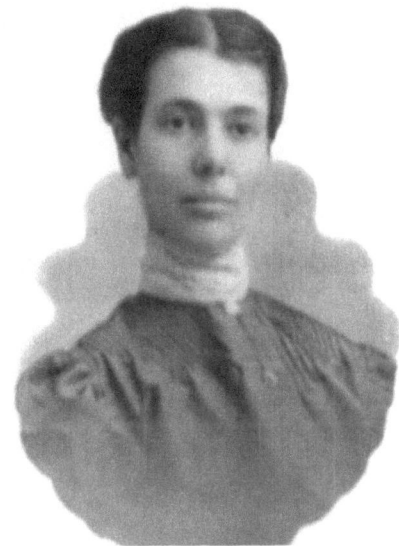

Dr. Louisa Burns is a graduate Bachelor of Science as well as a Doctor of Osteopathy. She is a thoroughly scholarly woman and has done and is doing much original work and investigation along the lines of neurology and experimental physiology.

She creditably occupied the chair of physiology in the Pacific College and now assumes her present duties in the laboratory department because of her deep interest in and adaptation for them. She enjoys the hearty support of all the students who have been taught by her.

Figure 3. "Louisa Burns, D.O."

Pioneering Professional Development and Socioeconomic Support

Defining Osteopathy

Although A.T. Still and his immediate students in Kirksville had defined osteopathy, Dain Tasker also offered his preference for the definition. Initially, he pointed out, osteopathy was defined as "*the science of treating the body, viewed from an anatomical and physiological standpoint, without the use of drugs*" (Dain Tasker, unpublished manuscript).

Another aspect of osteopathy suggested by a colleague as he was writing the history of osteopathy recommended: "The story of the development of osteopathy in California should stress the conservative, ethical and dignified administration of the first law. This approach created in the public an attitude of respect and confidence" (from an undated letter to Dain Tasker, D.O.).

Dain Tasker's recollections of professional development

Dain Tasker, D.O. looked at his half century of practicing and promoting osteopathy in California as the "Fifty golden years". His account provides an exemplar of osteopathic professional development during the beginning years of osteopathy in California. Since he spent most of his professional career to establish osteopathy in California, his brief summary is most illuminating about those pioneering years (chapter 66 of Dain Tasker's unpublished manuscript, "A History of Osteopathy in California").

Dain Tasker's mother was a practical nurse who later became an osteopathic physician herself. He briefly wrote about his adolescence and high school years, mainly to point out his interest in anatomy already in those early years.

For health reasons he moved to Riverside in California in 1892 and worked as a ranch hand, saving his money to become a doctor. A letter by his mother, describing osteopathy, influenced Dain Tasker deeply in that he changed his plans from becoming an M.D. to studying osteopathy. He graduated from the Pacific College in 1898 and immediately joined the faculty of that college. He did post-graduate work at the American School of Osteopathy in Kirksville where he also joined the faculty. He married Cora Newell, D.O. and they practiced together.

Dr. Dain Tasker was instrumental in organizing the California Osteopathic Association (see below). The purpose of the COA was to establish better practice rights. He wrote that "he finally succeeded in getting a law through that allowed for a State Board of Examiners". Dr. Tasker became president of the first Board of Osteopathic Examiners. In 1907 a composite Board was enacted and Dr. Tasker became its president in 1909.

For 21 years he served on various Boards of Osteopathic Medical Examiners in California. He also was President of COA in 1901 and 1907.

He taught Principles of Osteopathy at the Pacific College and published his lectures, with illustrations, in 1903. This book went through five editions and served as text book in all recognized colleges.

During WWI Dr. Tasker served on a national committee of the AOA to obtain recognition for D.O.s by the Army Medical Corps.

He realized the need for more osteopathic hospitals and served as a roentgenologist at Wilshire Hospital in Los Angeles from 1925 to 1947. His hobby was color photography. Many of his X-ray photos of flowers resembled delicate etchings.

Concluding his autobiography, Dr. Dain Tasker stated that he and his wife, Dr. Cora Tasker, retired to a beautiful ranch in Oceanside, raising avocados, taking pictures, and playing golf [probably around 1955].

The profession of osteopathy in California seems to owe its strong roots and almost unequaled high standards to Dain Tasker, D.O. He must have worked untiringly for 30 years of his career on promoting the profession, specifically in California. He then seemed to have worked mainly as a radiologist at a hospital in L.A. for 25 years until his retirement. In 1960, however, in his last entry about California, he criticized the AOA for its lax standards and publicly acknowledged support for the COA-CMA merger at the board meeting of the COA.

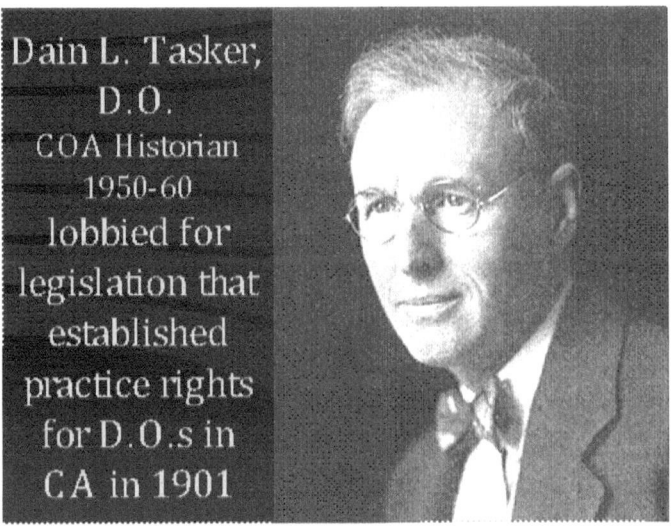

Figure 4. "Dain L. Tasker, D.O., COA Historian"

The California controversy at AOA, 1899

As early as the turn of the 20th century, California's osteopathic physicians raised controversies, as suggested by the following historical arguments about the extent of performing surgery:

The 2nd annual convention of **the *American Association for the Advancement of Osteopathy*** was held in Indianapolis in July 1899. Dr. Tasker was sent by the Pacific School of Osteopathy to present on courses of study. Dr. H.E. Goetz presented on the subject of "Degenerations of the spinal cord". Dr. Tasker advocated more extended study of surgery but others contradicted with the reminder "no drugs, no knife".

"Courses of Study" brought forth considerable discussion, as Dain Tasker recommended a more extended study of surgery "because it is scientific and a logical part of an osteopath's education. The necessary use and not abuse of surgery is what we advocated". He praised osteopaths for not being attached to the knife but warned at the same time to not mar its future progress by proclaiming liberalism and yet denying the necessity of emergency surgery. The moderator of the discussion did not believe in any need for adding surgery to the courses of study and a committee was formed to arrive at a resolution.

Tasker concluded that they "*had stirred so much controversy that many D.O.s from the parent school in Kirksville expressed doubt in the quality of teaching osteopathy in California. This doubt continued for nearly half a century*". Next to this paragraph is in pencil a check mark, underlined, together with a question mark, suggesting that Tasker pondered whether to retain this statement when he reviewed his manuscript in 1951. In support of the skeptical view of California's liberal approach in education it is worth noting that Dain Tasker mentioned "The officers of the California College of Osteopathy [in San Francisco] and the D.O.s in Kirksville were scarcely on speaking terms" (Chapter 4 of his "History of Osteopathy in California", unpublished manuscript).

Dr. Tasker quoted from his remarks at the graduation ceremony in June **1900** when he advised "to get away from the use of noxious drugs" and continued to explain "*Our theory is that the body is a machine and good health depends on the perfect adjustment of every tissue, perfect nerve force and perfect circulation*". He quoted Professor Whiting not to define osteopathy because it would be a hindrance. "*Let osteopathy be free to grow. Let every osteopath be an investigator and let him discover as much new truth as he can, and let osteopathy be broad enough to receive this new truth . . . . Accept new truth from without as well as from within*" (Chapter 4, pg. 8). He also stated to "*never seek the fatal help of past legislation. Encourage investigation in every direction*".

This quote again points out awareness in California of adaptation and change as necessary conditions for osteopathy to thrive, a foresight that seemed not present at that time at the parent school in Kirksville.

Establishing a D.O. practice during the pioneering years in California

From **"Medical Women of the Gold Rush Era"**: Interview with Sara Faustman, relative of Dr. Louise Heilbron:

"*Louise C. Heilbron, D.O. (1873-1933) was a member of a prominent pioneer family and the best known osteopath in the State. From time to time she lived in the Heilbron mansion still standing at 8th and O streets. She was born in Sacramento, the oldest of 10 children, but moved to San Diego at age 15. She always wanted to be a doctor, but the death of her father when her youngest sibling was an infant called upon her to stay close to home, so she opted to attend the California College of Osteopathy, graduating in 1900.*

"Dr. Heilbron's first practice was in San Diego where she is credited with organizing the PTA and becoming a charter member of the San Diego Business and Professional Women. She moved to San Francisco just in time for the earthquake to demolish her office and home. Upon returning to Sacramento she maintained a busy practice for over 20 years until her death following a ruptured appendix. She was co-founder of the Sacramento Soroptimist International and chair on public health matters for the California Osteopathic Association. She is buried in Sacramento's Old City Cemetery."

Irma West, M.D. obtained this information about Louise Heilbron D.O. through an interview she had with her relative, Sara Faustman, about 10 years ago and provided it to Dr. Seffinger per email in June 2005. Dr. West came upon Dr. Heilbron's grave at the Old City Cemetery when she was researching medical pioneers of Sacramento about 20 years ago.

Additional data obtained by Dr. West about Louise Heilbron, D.O. came from the obituary and records at the Sacramento's Old City Cemetery. Louise Heilbron appeared in a booklet, *Walking Tour of Medical Pioneer Grave Sites*, which Dr. West prepared for the Sacramento Sierra Valley Medical Society. As this booklet is out of print, the brief biography above was published in *Sacramento Sierra Valley Medicine,* March/April 2004, page 30, entitled *Early Medical Women.*

Recently, a historian in San Luis Obispo sent Dr. Seffinger information about a brother of Dr. Andrew Taylor Still, Thomas Chalmers Still, M.D., who also was a physician and had moved to California as early as 1863. This brother had studied manipulation with Dr. Still in the early 1890s in Kirksville and seemed to have practiced osteopathy in California as an osteopathic physician at a much earlier date than is commonly assumed as the beginning of osteopathy in California. He did not join the early efforts, though, to establish osteopathy in California.

Policy and Regulations

Efforts to regulate the practice of osteopathy in California

In **1899,** a bill to regulate the practice of osteopathy in the State of California to license D.O.s was proposed (Senate Bill # 477). Nothing happened in response to the bill.

Tasker suggested in his notes that the stalling of enactment might have resided with an M.D. chairing the committee who had no interest in promoting osteopathy.

The relationship between allopathic and osteopathic doctors was not the only source of conflict. Understandably for a new science and a new social movement, osteopathy showed professional strain even within the group. For example there was little communication between D.O.s in Northern and Southern California. Each osteopath was an individualist, for self-preservation.

The Osteopathic Association of the State of California

The personal efforts to obtain professional recognition and independence were astounding, as can be gleaned from a letter written by W.J. Hayden, D.O.

He described that on October 15, **1900** they decided to form an organization and representation by mail. Dr. Hayden approached Dr. Tasker with the idea who agreed. They invited all the D.O.s they knew to Dr. Hayden's office in Los Angeles. Dr. Tasker was chosen temporary chairman. He appointed a committee to frame a constitution and by-laws. Letters were sent to every D.O. in the State for the selection of officers. In November 1900 they met again in Dr. Hayden's office to count the ballot. Dr. D.L. Tasker was elected president, Dr. Effie Sisson first vice president, Dr. J.S. White second vice president, and Dr. Hayden secretary. Treasurer was R.D. Emery, D.O.

The purpose of the organization was to win professional independence in California. They decided that the first step was to present a bill to the Legislature and that Dr. Tasker was most qualified to take this bill to Sacramento. (Articles of Incorporation, Constitution, and Articles I through VI are provided in Tasker's unpublished manuscript in Chapter 5). This document is of interest in that, with only minor alterations, it became the articles of incorporation of the California Osteopathic Association from 1917-1962, and then the articles of incorporation of the 41st Medical Society from 1962-1997.

Of interest is the Pacific Coast Directory of Osteopathy, published in 1900 in the July issue of the *The Osteopath*. The directory included osteopaths in California, Oregon, Washington, Arizona, Nevada and Idaho. There were 73 D.O.s practicing in all these states. Dain Tasker listed 40 practitioners in the Osteopathic Association in 1900 (Tasker, chapter 4).

On November 3, 1900, the Osteopathic Association of the State of California convened. Dr. Tasker was chosen to get a bill passed to recognize osteopathy in

California. He traveled extensively and tried to convince strategically important persons.

In support of his efforts he quoted from his letter, written in February **1901** to Dr. Still, *"Osteopathy has scored a victory in California. Last fall the D.O.s in California formed the Osteopathy Association of the State of California with a membership of about 40"*. Dain Tasker was the first President of the Association. The Association subsequently changed its name to **California Osteopathic Association (COA)** in 1917, which remained in effect until 1962.

The first Board of Osteopathic Examiners

In his letter to A.T. Still, Dr. Tasker also described his campaign to pass AB 230 to obtain a separate Board of Osteopathic Examiners. He mentioned the poor odds of 4,500 M.D.s in California who would not look favorably at such separate boards, compared to 50 D.O.s who were hoping for professional independence with the establishment of an osteopathic board. Dr. Tasker visited 40 Senators and 80 Assemblymen to secure their support. He even contacted the local newspapers to gain publicity for the profession's efforts.

The bill passed the Senate on 2-19-1901. *"It gives us a Board of Osteopathic Examiners and makes us independent of the M.D.s. We are not prohibited from performing minor surgery. The Osteopathic Association of the State of California is incorporated and a legally organized body. This is the best bill osteopathy has had"*. Honorable Judge Grove L. Johnson of Sacramento was very helpful in this fight because Doctor C.A. Haines, D.O. had helped his daughter with diabetes, after 12 M.D.s before him had been unsuccessful.

AB 230 became a law by the Statute of Limitation without the Governor's signature on March **1901**. Tasker proudly emphasized that no money was spent on dinners or cigars. The whole campaign was clean and honorable. *"Success was due to our patients and their friends and to the united strength of all D.O.s in the state"*. Tasker concluded his letter to Dr. Still by assuring him of *"the continued love and respect of all D.O.s"*.

At the election of the Board of Osteopathic Examiners Dain Tasker received 40 votes, Ernest Sisson 39, C.A. Haines 30, J.S. White 26, and A.H. Potter 22. Dr. Tasker quotes from a letter he wrote *"The burden of proof of fitness to practice is on the individual colleges"*. Practitioners had to have a diploma from an accredited college.

The Composite Board of Medical Examiners

This assurance of professional independence lasted until **1907** when the Medical and Osteopathic Acts were repealed. Instead, a **Composite Medical Board** was established in the same year, comprising five allopaths, two osteopaths, two homeopaths, and two eclectics. The Composite Board of Medical Examiners existed until 1922 when the osteopathic profession established its own separate licensing board. In 1919, the medical board arbitrarily refused to examine more osteopaths for licensure. A three day investigation was followed by a trial. The minutes from the trial noted that the educational standards at COP&S were higher than those required by law for medical licensure. Thus, the Board was ordered to administer the examination to osteopaths. Distrust remained, though, that the situation might not mean a long-term relief from antagonism. The California Osteopathic Association started to secure legislation for a separate Osteopathic Board ("Historical Outline, UC Irvine, College of Medicine").

The Osteopathic Initiative Act

In 1913, the Medical Practice Act of California was passed by the legislature. It established detailed educational and training requirements needed for eligibility to take the two types of state licensing exams, the drugless practitioner and the unlimited physician and surgeon. At that time in the state, the "drugless" practitioners consisted of osteopaths, chiropractors, naturopaths, herbalists and homeopaths. The eclectics injected medications and were typically M.D.s. Some clinicians of that time period had several degrees. Some doctors with one degree also helped other professions develop. For example, a couple of graduates from the osteopathic profession helped the chiropractic school in Los Angeles to build that drugless profession in the state.

Some M.D.s helped to train D.O.s to become unlimited licensed physicians and surgeons. From 1916 to 1921, D.O. graduates of COP&S were accepted as interns at the Los Angeles County Hospital under the tutelage of M.D.s (see *History of Los Angeles County Hospital(1878-1968) and the Los Angeles County—University of Southern California Medical Center (1968-1978)*, by Helen Eastman Martin, M.D., pg. 59; Los Angeles, USC Press 1979). However, this opportunity did not continue beyond 1921, partly because of the possibility that the hospital might lose its accreditation if the association with D.O.s persisted. Thus, the county M.D.s were forced to discontinue the training or working alongside D.O.s.

The state licensing board, the majority of which consisted of M.D.s, also decided not to allow D.O.s to sit for the licensing exam in 1919, likely for the same reason, though they stated that it was because the COP&S did not meet the requirements for accreditation by the licensing board. The County used the excuse that since the licensing board no longer accredited the COP&S, then it should no longer accept its graduates as interns. The faculty of the COP&S filed suit against the State Medical Licensing Board in 1919; it took 2 years to settle. The D.O.s prevailed and the licensing board was ordered by the courts to accept applications for licensure as physicians and surgeons from D.O. graduates from COP&S. However, the D.O.s felt betrayed and lost trust in the M.D.s on the composite licensing board. They felt they needed their own licensing board to regulate the practice of D.O.s in the state by themselves.

In **1922**, the State measure No. 20, entitled "Osteopathic Initiative Act", was placed on the ballot for California voters. Osteopathic physicians in California raised funds and campaigned vigorously against the opposition of the majority of allopathic medical doctors as well as from some osteopathic doctors in the state. The California Medical Association (CMA), the state's major newspaper, and the AOA opposed the measure as well. The CMA simply did not want two separate licensing boards for physicians and surgeons. The reason the AOA opposed it is that it adopted the 1913 Medical Practice Act, which from the AOA national standpoint, required too stringent educational training to sit for the physician and surgeon license and would be difficult for D.O.s from the other osteopathic colleges to qualify to sit for that examination.

Yet, the Osteopathic Initiative Act passed by over a 100,000 vote margin. Thus, in 1922 a separate Board was established, the **California Board of Osteopathic Examiners**. The Board was given the power to approve colleges and hospitals, to examine applicants for osteopathic licensure, and to provide jurisdiction over all osteopathic physicians and surgeons with California certificates.

This Board, established by public vote, was of great importance to the profession. Although D.O.s had been legally considered as an equal and distinct medical profession, with unlimited practice rights available to members, including use of surgery and drugs since 1907, the establishment of their own licensing board strengthened their position and preserved their future. They could build and staff their own hospitals. Empowered by this new law, COP&S moved its clinic to the Luckenbach building on South Hill Street where it occupied four floors. About 2,500 patients were seen there annually.

Improved licensure conditions attracted an increased number of students to enroll at COP&S. The increased revenues made possible a new science building and laboratories for the study of anatomy and physiology, bacteriology, chemistry, pathology and histology.

The California Board of Osteopathic Examiners established in 1922 still exists, though it is now called the Osteopathic Medical Board of California, residing alongside the Medical Board of California under the auspices of the state Department of Consumer Affairs. Although between 1962 and 1974 the osteopathic licensing board was temporarily unable to grant new licenses, it has always maintained its activities in overseeing and renewing the licenses of D.O.s in the state. These events will be described in Chapter 5 of this monograph.

While the profession was protected through its own regulatory authority, it expanded through increased opportunities for education and training, and through increased political activities at the state and national level. Chapters 3 and 4 will address osteopathy's growth and its effect on the relationship between the osteopathic and allopathic professional organizations from the late 1920s to the late 1950s.

Chapter 3

M.D.s and D.O.s in the 1930s to 1950s

Dain Tasker, D.O., serving as the profession's historian, provided information about events at the College of Osteopathic Physicians and Surgeons (COP&S) until the 1950s in his archival manuscript "The History of Osteopathy in California", chapters 66 to 70. The professional journal at that time on clinical education and professional news, *Clinical Osteopathy*, provided papers discussing clinical skills, educational opportunities, and professional organization issues from the mid 1930s to the late 1950s. A document, identified as *"Historical outline—UCI, CCM"* at the archives at the University of California, Irvine (UCI), provided further details about events in this time period.

The *Louis Chandler, D.O.* collection at the archives of the Pumerantz Library at Western University documented detailed information regarding relations with the allopathic profession. Dr. Chandler who was a graduate of the College of Osteopathic Physicians & Surgeons (COP&S) in 1913 and president of COP&S from 1922 to 1924, maintained thorough files with documentation about his professional activities. By examining this wide array of archival material, this chapter describes how events in osteopathic and allopathic medicine unfolded in California from the late 1920s to the late 1950s.

The crowning event for the osteopathic profession in 1922 had been the establishment of a separate Board of Osteopathic Examiners, as described in Chapter 2. With rising confidence in the profession's status as equal to allopathy, student enrollment at COP&S increased and required more training opportunities for the greater number of graduates. Also more beds were needed at hospitals to care for the increasing number of patients seen by osteopathic physicians, especially in densely populated areas like Los Angeles County. Thus, the Los Angeles Board of Supervisors was asked to expand the Los Angeles County Hospital, with a separate building for the osteopathic profession.

Patient care

In California generally, D.O.s were not allowed to train or see patients in hospitals controlled or owned by allopathic physicians. Especially relatively large facilities adhered to this regulation, while smaller hospitals quite often had dual staff privileges. "Dual staff" entailed an M.D. staff and a separate D.O. staff working side by side. Privileges were granted by each staff for their own members. In large M.D.-operated facilities, D.O.s were usually not permitted to practice. Warren Bostick M.D. documented in his recollections of the allopathic attitude toward osteopathy: *"If the Medical Staff processed the osteopath's application consistently and rejected his membership primarily on the basis of quality of care, education and scientific practice, its decisions were undisturbed legally."*

This segregation of the two equally licensed medical professions lasted until the Hill Burton Act in 1945 required open access for licensed services at hospitals built with federal funds. Since many hospitals in California were not built with federal funds, hospital segregation continued to be a major barrier to professional growth and practice.

The Los Angeles County Hospital

As the Los Angeles Board of Supervisors approved an expansion of the Los Angeles County Hospital, a new building was added in 1928 and the old building, known then as Unit II, was given to the osteopathic profession. The greater part of the hospital was called Unit I and was operated by allopathic medicine. USC Medical School provided training at Unit I.

Dr. Golanty:

"L.A. County had two divisions or two units of county hospital system at that time located in East Los Angeles; this is apart from the Harbor Hospitals that came later and the hospitals out in San Bernardino Valley, but on the main campus of the L.A. County system there were two units, Unit I and Unit II. Unit II was the uniquely osteopathic hospital and out-patient clinics. It was separate from the Unit I complex which was run and housed by the University of Southern California and at that time when I started, shared by a school called the College of Medical Evangelists which today is Loma Linda University.

"There were two training programs in one house, much as Arrowhead Medical Center right now. They shared several training programs from different universities in one building, but we were a separate and distinct unit. Patients were assigned to either the two units on some system that the County had developed. Once you were a patient in one unit you were a patient in that unit forever. You were transferred from one unit to another if you happened to arrive at the wrong one by mistake and if you were transferable. The County had funded this for years."

Dr. Ulansey:

"I started off at PCO [Philadelphia College of Osteopathy]. *This was my entrée into the medical field. I completed three years at PCO. Having heard of the greater opportunities afforded the students in California, both students and graduates in Los Angeles, California, I said, 'That's for me, that's where I*

want to go' . . . I served a clerkship or externship and some class work in Los Angeles [starting 1945]. I was most impressed by my experience in California at the County General Hospital which was a marvelous institution. It was such a revelation to me as compared to the clerkship that I served in my junior year in Philadelphia . . . . The revelation at Los Angeles was that I found myself as a clerk extern doing work that the residents at PCO did.

"The faculty and the attending physician staff were willing to impart what experiences and knowledge that they had gained to us, the students, the young aspiring physicians coming up. It was a revelation. It really was something that, as I said, for the rest of my life I will never forget the experiences I had at the L.A. County General Hospital . . . . The L.A. County Hospital had 4,000 beds, 500 of which were osteopathic [in 1958] . . . I did my internship, my residency, a fellowship, and then I became a voluntary assistant in anesthesia for a couple of years.

"And from there I became a junior attending physician. I've remained on the staff, the teaching staff at the County Hospital, and at COP&S, teaching students as they came up, interns, and new residents. I was in that department for something like 25 years, and gave up one day a week to go to the County. I say gave up, it was a two way street, I learned from it; and I gave something in return for learning. We did everything. We saw everything; things that you didn't see in private hospitals. It was just a marvelous exposure. The beautiful part about L. A. County was patient care; directed by either interns or residents. We were the doctors. Yes, we were overseen by residents more senior to us and they in turn were overseen by attending staff. It was a ladder effect. It was a good exposure . . . I lived and breathed County Hospital."

Immediately "Unit II" started to thrive. Senior students at COP&S spent one trimester at Unit II. They also learned at Monte Sano Hospital and at City Maternity Services. Unit II existed until the 1950s when the osteopathic physicians were able to have their own hospital, called the Los Angeles County Osteopathic Hospital.

The first prospective, randomized study on treatment effectiveness

A valuable opportunity occurred in 1932 at the Los Angeles County Hospital for a natural, prospective experiment to be conducted. This study was able to compare osteopathic and allopathic care during a poliomyelitis epidemic in the Los Angeles area. Unit II of the L.A. County Hospital provided osteopathic medicine, while Unit I provided allopathic care, each Unit following their respective protocol. Unit I was reserved for M.D.s only and had 3,574 beds, while Unit II was reserved for D.O.s and had 196 beds.

Because of a mandate in 1928, each Unit of the L.A. County Hospital was a separate facility, including segregated staff and maintenance. Incoming patients were allocated to either Unit I or Unit II by using a ratio to accommodate the difference in bed availability. Louis Bartosh, D.O. reported a 6:1 ratio being used, meaning 5 patients went to Unit I

67

and the 6th patient to Unit II, whereas Louis Chandler, D.O. and the "*Historical Outline UCI-College of Medicine*" reported a 10:1 ratio for patient allocation.

Documents in the Chandler files at Western University state that, in addition to the random allocation, patients could choose to go to Unit I or to Unit II. Because of this provision for self-selection, Unit II saw one-seventh of the total number of patients instead of the allocated one of every ten. He cited as example for the public's interest in osteopathic care that in 1928 Unit II delivered one third of the obstetrics patients, had 6,000 hospital inpatients per year and 200 ambulatory clinic patients per day.

In 1933, the combined records of the Los Angeles County General Hospital showed 46,464 inpatients and 518,377 outpatients, making the L.A. County Hospital the third largest hospital in the country. Records separated for Unit II only, the osteopathic Unit, showed daily 2,352 inpatients and 1,695 ambulatory outpatients. Monthly, there were 4,849 admissions and 415 babies were delivered.

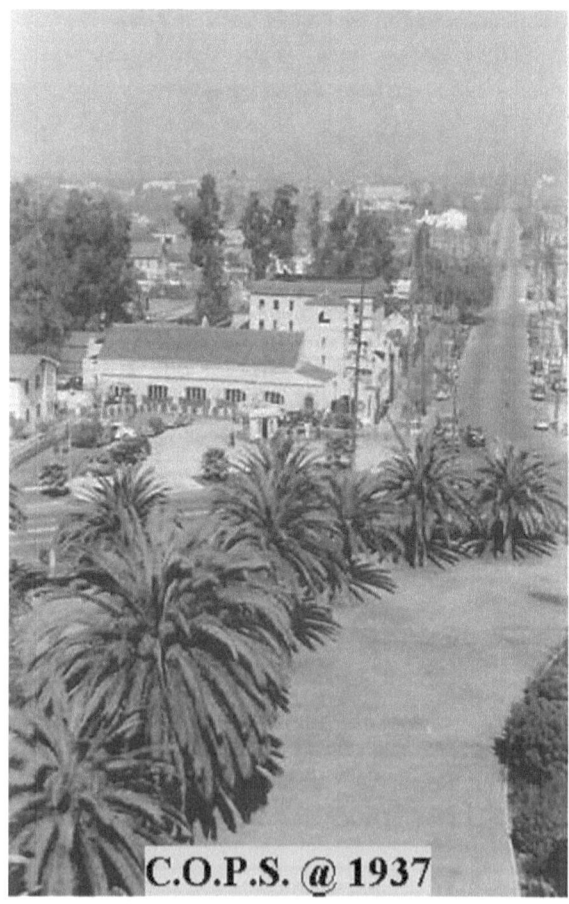

Figure 5a: "College of Osteopathic Physicians & Surgeons, Los Angeles, 1937"

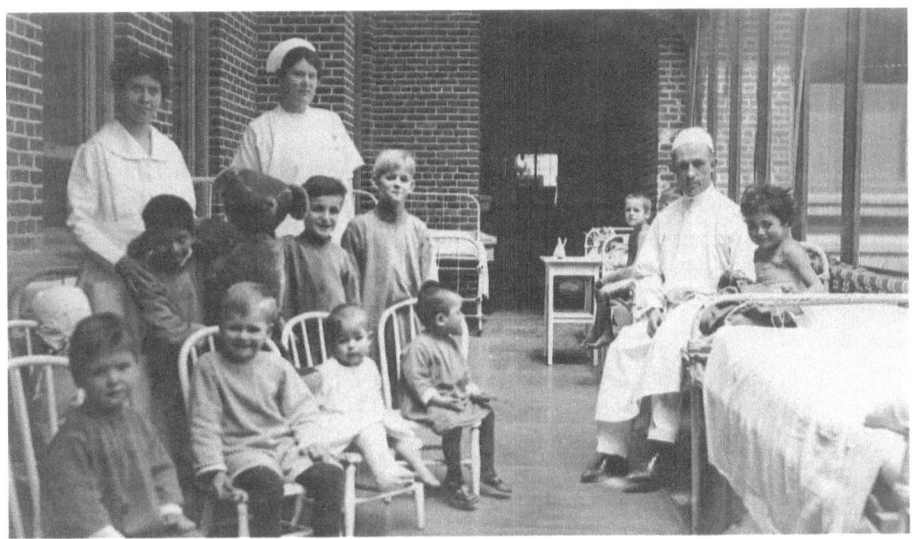

Figure 5b. "Glen Cayler, D.O., children's ward,
Los Angeles County Hospital, Unit II"

The table below summarizes the morbidity and mortality statistics for the LA County Hospital from 1930-1933:

Statistic	M.D. Unit I + D.O. Unit II	D.O. Unit II	The D.O. Difference
Mortality	9.7%	5.5%	(-) 4.2%
Average Length Of Stay in the Hospital	16 days	9.7 days	(-) 6.3 days
Coroner's cases for total hospital	14%	14%	same

Louis Chandler, D.O reported these data in the *Journal of the American Osteopathic Association.* He compared the morbidity and mortality statistics from 1930-1933 of the Los Angeles County Osteopathic Hospital with the entire Los Angeles County Hospital (inclusive of Units I and II). The osteopathic unit had less average mortality and less hospital days per patient while caring for the same percent of unexpected deaths (coroner's cases). This was the time period in which one in every ten patients was randomly admitted to the osteopathic unit.

There were several caveats to such a comparison: While it was reported that fewer patients transferred out of Unit II once admitted there, and more than 10% were actually admitted to it, it is unknown what results would have shown if those patients were removed from the analysis. It is also unknown whether patients were discharged earlier from Unit II due to a lack of adequate numbers of beds available in Unit II. In spite of these limitations, Dr. Chandler interpreted the data to mean that the care given at the osteopathic unit was superior to that provided in Unit I.

Understandably, M.D.s locally and nationally were upset about Dr. Chandler's interpretation of the records. After 1933, the randomization of patients was discontinued and no further comparisons were conducted. The osteopathic Unit easily filled its number of beds and provided patient care without such allocation. Possibly both professions came to the realization that each had qualities that were appreciated by the public.

In 1938, Unit II of the L.A. County Hospital celebrated the 10th anniversary of having opened its doors in February 1928. The March issue in 1938 of the journal *Clinical Osteopathy* wrote: *"This was the climax of a hard fight by the profession in California for recognition and the opportunity to demonstrate to the public what osteopathy can do for human ills"*.

Osteopathic hospitals

While Unit II at the L.A. County Hospital helped to serve the needs of patients who were poor and underserved, osteopathic physicians in the surrounding communities needed access to hospital beds for their patients with healthcare resources. In 1940, four of 27 nation-wide osteopathic hospitals approved by AOA were located in California: Doctors Hospital in Los Angeles, Unit II of the Los Angeles County Hospital, Magnolia Hospital in Long Beach, and Monte Sano Hospital in Los Angeles. In addition, there were several other osteopathic hospitals, albeit not AOA approved at that time.

Dr. Ulansey:

"[Regarding] *hospitals, the osteopathic profession in the Los Angeles area consisted of about . . . Well, I can name them: Doctors Hospital, Monte Sano Hospital, the Wilshire Hospital, which was the pride and joy of the city, the Burbank Hospital; there were a number of these smaller institutions which were typical of California at that time. But they were D.O. hospitals, varying in size from 30 to 75 beds, while the allopathic hospitals also were growing; they were 100, 150 bed hospitals. We didn't have too many of the larger institutions so typical of the well established east coast large cities or eastern United States."*

Several osteopathic hospitals were founded by graduates of COP&S in this time period. Howard Norcross, D.O., a graduate of COP&S in 1936, founded and owned *Doctors Hospital* in 1939. Howard's brother was a chiropractor and wanted to have a hospital for referring his patients and those of his colleagues, if needed. *Doctors Hospital* had an internship and residency training program for D.O.s until 1960.

Dr. Howard Norcross' nephew, Robert Norcross, D.O., graduated from COP&S in 1951 and had just completed his surgical residency at *Doctors Hospital* in 1954, when he was drafted into the army as a private to go to the Korean War. The *L.A. Times* was made aware of the situation and published an article about the absurdity of a surgeon being drafted as a private foot soldier. Robert Norcross, D.O. was given an honorable discharge. Although past American presidents, including Theodore Roosevelt, had supported D.O.s inducted as military medical officers, allopathic physicians and nurses usually refused to work with their osteopathic colleagues in this capacity, until required by law.

Being spared the draft, Dr. Robert Norcross practiced at the newly founded **Bay Harbor Hospital** in Lomita, California, in 1955. Parenthetically noted, the contributions by the Norcross family to osteopathic medicine continued when James Norcross, D.O. and Tim Norcross, D.O. graduated from the College of Osteopathic Medicine of the Pacific in Pomona, California, in 1982 and 2004 respectively.

James Taylor, M.D. and a graduate of COP&S in 1958, practiced at *Bay Harbor Hospital* for 30 years.

Dr. Taylor recalls*:*

> *"At the time of the change in the D.O. license to a M.D. license statewide, I practiced at Bay Harbor Hospital, a new D.O. hospital. I helped establish* **Bay Harbor Hospital** *in Torrance with George Wall, M.D. and DO from 1958 to 1959. While I was at Bay Harbor Hospital, I opened a pain clinic. I studied and used neurolinguistic programming, hypnosis, thiamine, osteopathic manipulative treatment, and epidural injections."*

In 1943, **Burbank Community Hospital** was located in the city of Burbank. Dr. Betsy MacCracken recalls it as *"one of our finest hospitals"*. After the merger it became Thompson Memorial Hospital. The facility no longer exists, though.

The **Merrill Sanitarium** was a psychiatric hospital that employed the uniquely osteopathic approach to the care of the mentally ill. Merrill Sanitarium provided a combination of environmental, cognitive and osteopathic manipulative therapies to patients. Edward Merrill, D.O. also practiced at *Monte Sano Hospital* in the Los Angeles area, together with Louis Chandler, D.O.

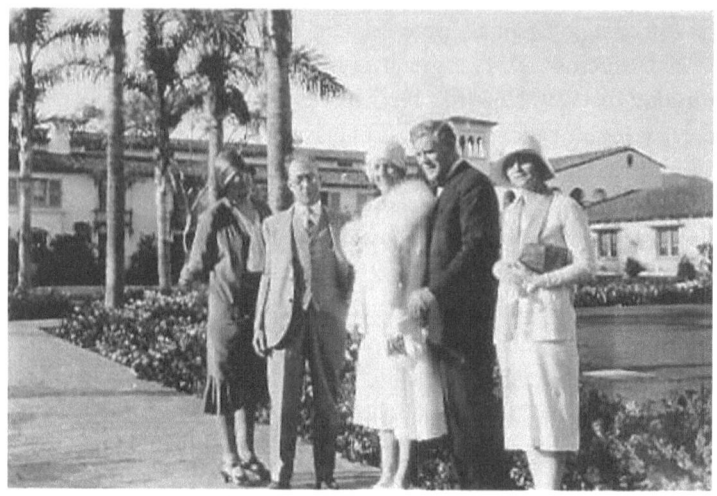

Figure 6. "Merrill Sanitarium: Myrtle and Carle Phinney;
Kappy and Edward Merrill, 1930s"

Monte Sano Hospital and Sanitarium served as an osteopathic institution for nearly 50 years. Built in 1923 on a hillside at the corner of Glendale Avenue and Waverly Drive in Los Angeles, the three-story Spanish-style hospital, with terraces for each room, provided its 50 patients with a mind-expanding panoramic view of the San Gabriel Mountains. As the first modern osteopathic hospital in Southern California, it was envisioned as a "perfect health recuperation resort" on its "hill of health". It outlasted the merger between M.D.s and D.O.s in the 1960s and only closed down in the 1970s.

Dr. Betsy MacCracken*:*

> *"I interned at **Monte Sano Hospital** which was a hospital owned by the Los Angeles Clinical Group. This was a group of nine specialists. It was unusual for a clinical group to exist in those days, meaning a group of physicians. We banded together that way."*

Dr. Ryder proudly recalls that he was born at Monte Sano Hospital, initiating his experience with osteopathic medicine at the earliest age. In September 1956 he matriculated into the College of Osteopathic Physicians and Surgeons and graduated in 1960 with a D.O. degree.

Dr. Ryder:

> *"I was born at the **Monte Sano Sanitarium and Hospital** in Los Angeles on July 12, 1931. It was located above Riverside Drive near the intersection of*

Glendale Blvd. At the time I understand it was one of few if not the only Osteopathic Hospitals in Los Angeles outside of Los Angeles County General Hospital Unit II. It has since been torn down. Milton Kranz, DO attended my birth. My family went to osteopathic doctors connected with the Los Angeles Clinical Group, an early group practice. My mother said it was a very hot summer day, but the sanitarium was located above Riverside Drive next to the Los Angeles River where it got a cool afternoon breeze. Remember this was before air-conditioning."

Glendale Community Hospital was located in Glendale and well-known as an osteopathic hospital. Dr. Marsh and Dr. Dieudonne practiced there. Several members of the Board of Trustees of COP&S became active Directors of Glendale Hospital. Like Unit II of the Los Angeles County Hospital, Glendale Hospital served as an important teaching and residency training resource of COP&S.

Dr. Betsy MacCracken:

*"Windsor Hospital became **Glendale Community Hospital**. For many years, Dr. Edward Abbott practiced there. He later became Dean of the graduate school at the College* [COP&S]. *"*

Park View Hospital was primarily an osteopathic hospital, located in Los Angeles at Hoover Street near Santa Monica Boulevard. There were several owners in the early 1950s, in particular two brothers, Joe Farber, D.O. whom **Dr. Alloy** recalls as "*an excellent surgeon and also a very good teacher, and Mannie Farber, D.O. who did some surgery and also a fair amount of anesthesia*". Dr. Alloy was able to "*work out a preceptorship/residency program that continued for a number of years with additional residents, primarily involving Dr. George W. D. Robbins. The hospital was approved for five internships.*" Thus, osteopathic physicians even at these relatively small hospitals were able to provide specialty training.

Rio Hondo Memorial Hospital was located in Downey and was a strictly osteopathic hospital. Stanley Kaplan, D.O. had been instrumental with 10 or 11 additional D.O.s to develop this hospital which by the late 1950s had become extremely busy,

Dr. Alloy:

*"**Rio Hondo** had an active intern and residency program in general surgery from 1957 to 1962. There were 5 interns from COP&S and other osteopathic colleagues per year, and three residents completed their training there".*

La Mirada Hospital was located close to Norwalk. Several D.O.s from Whittier and Norwalk built this hospital. According to Dr. Allen, it was most pleasant to use and flourished.

At **Whittier Hospital**, M.D.s as well as D.O.s provided services. A grateful patient had donated funds with the stipulation that Whittier Hospital would be an open-staff hospital.

St. Helen's was located in Artesia. This osteopathic hospital was privately owned by Dr. Richards.

Magnolia Hospital in Long Beach was established in 1938. COP&S had an intern training program at Magnolia. Donald Dilworth, D.O., for example, completed his internship there in 1945. Within less than a decade, osteopathic physicians outgrew this hospital and founded the **Pacific Hospital** of Long Beach. The popular internship program continued throughout the 1950s until 1962. A residency program in Internal Medicine was offered in 1956. The internship for D.O.s re-opened in 1980 due to the efforts of Janice Chin and Stanley Golanty, M.D. who had graduated from COP&S in 1959 and obtained the M.D. degree from CCM in 1962.

San Diego had an osteopathic hospital in **Hillside** which provided intern training. Dr. Frymann practiced there.

Osteopathic physicians were also quite prominent in the **public health system** of California.

Dr. Golanty recalls:

> *"I think in our third or fourth year we went to a public health clinic in East Los Angeles and one in Watts. A Dr. Robert Kolts, Chairman of the Dept. of Public Health and Preventive Medicine was the head of the Watts Public Health Clinic. So, we were all feeling good about the fact that it* [the Watts Public Health Clinic] *and the one in East Los Angeles, I believe, were directed, or at least housed then, by many D.O.s in our public health system here in Los Angeles, including Betsy MacCracken, D.O."*

These recollections show that, while the osteopathic profession was relatively small in the mid 20th century, it had a certain culture. California D.O.s were proud to build and own their hospitals where they were free to practice medicine according to their principles and philosophy. Even though the profession was centrally controlled by the AOA, housed in Chicago, California D.O.s were able to establish and maintain their unique professional culture largely by way of their highly respected college and their own hospitals.

Dr. Krpan:

> [The profession] *"was small. We had, I think, there were, when I was in school, 17,000 osteopathic physicians in the country. We had five schools* [in the whole country]. *We had an advantage at that time over what we have at this time and that is that we were able to train all of our graduates in osteopathic hospitals. At that time there were over 200 osteopathic hospitals*

[nationwide]. *We had approximately, and I don't know the exact number, but we had approximately 500 graduates from osteopathic colleges each year and they trained in osteopathic hospitals. They had to train in osteopathic hospitals, as there were no slots available in allopathic hospitals. And there was an abundance, a surplus of training slots at that time".*

Hospitals with dual medical services

In the early 1950s, ***Santa Ana Hospital*** was a prominent example in Southern California for hospitals comprising two complete medical staff, one comprising osteopathic physicians and surgeons, the other allopathic physicians. Initially known as Santa Ana Valley Hospital, it had been an allopathic facility, but in 1935 its doors opened for osteopathic physicians as well. Dain Tasker, D.O., in his *"History of Osteopathy in California"*, explained the opening of Santa Ana Valley Hospital to patients cared by osteopathic physicians as a way to rescue the hospital from its impending economic demise as a strictly allopathic hospital. Dr. Tasker observed that shortly after opening the hospital's doors to osteopathic services, census improved 100% and the hospital was thriving. To promote continued visibility of osteopathic services, the hospital hosted continuing education programs taught by W.W.W. Pritchard, D.O. and offered by the Orange County chapter of COA. The course had 100% attendance throughout the series of classes.

Santa Ana Community Hospital, as it became known in the 1950s, celebrated its 48th year by adding a north wing to the 2-story structure, at a cost of $ 500,000 (no year is cited by Dr. Tasker in the archival document but the context suggests 1950). The 39 COA members of its staff included Forest J. Grunigen, D.O. (Tasker, chapter 26).

Dr. Kammerman:

*"I will try to piece out the details of the development of the old **Santa Ana Community Hospital** as I have heard. It seems that James Irvine of Orange County became sufficiently ill that he required to be in the hospital. Santa Ana Hospital was the only facility available in Orange County at the time, to my knowledge. When he was apprised that his personal physician, Dr. Horace Leecing, could not attend to him because he was a D.O., James Irvine called his attorney and had him come to the hospital. After a short conference, the attorney left and about one hour later he returned and informed the administrator of the hospital that James Irvine owned the hospital and could have any doctor he chose. Dr. Leecing came to the hospital and provided the care that James Irvine needed and began to organize the osteopathic staff. The existing M.D. doctors refused to have anything to do with the osteopaths and desired to maintain their staff also.*

"Therefore the hospital developed a dual staff, each one responsible for its own members. A board of directors was appointed by Mr. Irvine and eventually

he donated the hospital to the community [and Santa Ana Hospital changed its name to Santa Ana Community Hospital]. *Dr. Leecing was a graduate of COP&S in about 1928 and passed away in the 70's. At first, osteopathic specialists and surgeons came to the hospital to provide care for their patients from Los Angeles. I also think that the transfer was easy because the hospital was about to become bankrupt. Eventually M.D. specialists began to work with the D.O.s and harmony was very easy after the merger."*

Mark Twain Hospital was located in San Andreas, a small town in the Sierra foothills.

Dr. Wykle:

"I opened up an osteopathic general practice in San Andreas in 1948. There was a bond measure passed the day I arrived in San Andreas for a new hospital in San Andreas, called Mark Twain Hospital. Senator Teale wrote into the bond measure that there will be no discrimination of D.O.s who wanted to admit and care for patients there . . . but the hospital wasn't built until 1950. There were other hospitals that would not accept our patients, like in Redding. So, other than the Vannousse Hospital, which was a D.O. hospital in Stockton, we didn't have any alternatives until the Mark Twain Hospital was completed.

"After that, Steve and Barbara [Teale, both osteopathic physicians] *and I decided we didn't have to work together. So, we separated and I took the patients in San Andreas and they stayed in West Point. We did our own surgeries at Mark Twain* [Hospital], *like hysterectomies, hernia repairs, appendectomies, tonsillectomies.* [For] *anything complicated, we called over Joseph Cosentino, D.O., who was a fine surgeon, to help us. I was the only person that was any good at anesthesia, so I did anesthesia for both the M.D.s and D.O.s at Mark Twain Hospital. The former discrimination against D.O.s was wiped out at that hospital.*

"The M.D.s surgical skills were less than ours, and Cosentino was better than anyone in the region. For example, we did total hysterectomies, whereas the M.D.s still did classic sub-total hysterectomies. Also, we were used to giving our patients IVs afterwards to restore electrolytes and water; the M.D.s were using catheters up the rectum to replace fluids. So, we finally got them to let us put in the IVs for them."

Palomar Memorial Hospital was located (and still is) in Escondido:

Dr. Dilworth:

" . . . the question is about our hospital privileges in Escondido and fortunately, way back as early as 1919, there were two D.O.s who were in

Escondido from the old school. One of them was especially proficient in obstetrics. So, when they first opened the first hospital, she was granted the obstetrics permission. As a result, she made a good establishment for the D.O.s—so much that the hospital in Escondido then from its very beginning had been willing to accept both the M.D. and the D.O. degree.

"Our hospital is known as the **Palomar Memorial Hospital**. It has some 250 beds, so it is pretty large now . . . . Well, of course, in those early years it wasn't a full-fledged established hospital, hardly, but it got its start and from that very start it had had a couple of D.O.s along with the M.D.s."

Hollywood Leland Hospital was located in the heart of Hollywood, one block off Sunset and Vine. It was later renamed Hollywood Community Hospital.

Dr. Ulansey:

"Quite by chance I became very friendly with the owner of that hospital; it was privately owned. He was getting along in years and he presented me with a proposition, "Why don't you buy my hospital?" I was newly out of school, that was in the mid 1950s, and in practice a couple of years . . . . I did put together a group of doctors, both D.O.s and M.D.s. We put up, which was for me, a lot of money. We did purchase that hospital with 16 of us . . . .

"We operated that hospital very successfully and expanded it to 125 beds. A six story structure came out of a one story structure. We were very proud of it. We had students and interns until the amalgamation took place, until the AOA cut us off . . . We had students, interns, externs and residents from Pomona at our hospital when the Pomona College [College of Osteopathic Medicine of the Pacific] began in 1978. They had their first students come out to clerkships around 1981 or 1982. We had a resident in surgery and one in family medicine. Then with the growth of the Medicare and the MediCal, particularly the MediCal situation, it was no longer feasible to operate the hospital. We had to sell it around 1983 or '84."

Osteopathic care in patients' homes

Given the difficulties in obtaining staff privileges at hospitals, patient care in the home presented a welcome alternative for osteopathic physicians, especially in obstetrics. The Los Angeles County maternity service provided care at obstetrical clinics and in patients' homes in the 1940s and '50s, meeting the needs of the indigent and teaching whole-person care to junior medical students. **Dr. Riedell** was Chief Obstetrical Resident at that time. He delivered "babies by the dozen" in a 474 square mile area, as he later vividly described in his memoirs "**Babies by the Dozen: Free Home Delivery, 1941**" (Fithian Press, 1998). He taught junior medical students at COP&S the full spectrum of maternity service, as they witnessed Dr. Riedell making life and death decisions without outside help for as long as he was needed.

Edwin Riedell, D.O. (later to become M.D.) was a graduate of COP&S in Los Angeles and an intern and resident at Unit II of the Los Angeles County Hospital in the 1940s. For his postgraduate training Dr. Riedell was one of the rare osteopathic physicians who was afforded the opportunity to receive postgraduate training from M.D.s locally in the Los Angeles area. When in the 1950s Dr. Riedell was asked to submit case studies from his residency training to partially fulfill the requirements for his Board certification, he remarked on the cover page of his case reports that he wished other D.O.s could have also had the opportunity to train with experienced M.D. surgeons in Los Angeles (instead of having to go abroad to get surgical specialty training). In his experience, M.D.s were more attentive to details and oversaw every part of his training, compared to the osteopathic surgical training where he felt that he received less direct oversight. His cases document conventional medical care as was typically offered by the M.D.s at that time.

Dr. Seffinger:

> *"I visited Dr. Riedell's daughters in Berkeley a couple of years ago, a few months after his passing. They shared with me some of the papers in his files, now in boxes in the garage. I received copies of his book, **"Babies by the Dozen"** [Fithian Press, Santa Barbara, 1998] which is a unique historic account of the life as an obstetrical intern delivering babies at the homes of the poor and uninsured in Los Angeles in the 1940s.*
>
> *"Dr. Riedell later went on to be active in the merger of the COA and CMA and obtained his M.D. degree in 1962 from the California College of Medicine, to become UC Irvine School of Medicine in 1968. As they were still in mourning, Dr. Riedell's daughters did not wish to be interviewed for this project, but let me have a copy of his case studies and the book he authored during his retirement."*

Dolores Grunigen:

> *"Ed Riedell and Fory [Dr. Forest Grunigen] were very good friends, and when Ed was looking for some help with his book I steered him toward the Santa Barbara Writers Conference which I attend yearly in Santa Barbara. He always said he couldn't have published without this help.*
>
> *"**Dr. Riedell** truly was an exceptional individual as well as a hands-on physician whose first instincts were for the patient. His support for the merger was most useful, as he had many contacts in the allopathic community, unlike other D.O.s who were not taken into many practices because of their degrees. At that time, a D.O. was looked upon as a "second-class" practitioner due to*

the allopathic definition of his [or her] practices, i.e., manipulation, which was scoffed at regularly. In particular, in his [Dr. Riedell's] *obstetrics practice, manipulation of the back and legs of pregnant patients was welcomed. In his early days of practice, manipulation was often the only treatment available for easing of pain and suffering, as medication was often either not available or inadequate. Dr. Riedell's long active practice is a testimony to his methods of practice.*

"As an aside, he was never sued for malpractice or even accused of wrongful practice during those years. He was truly an excellent example of the quality of care given by a majority of the ex-D.O.s who merged into the mainstream of medicine."

Education

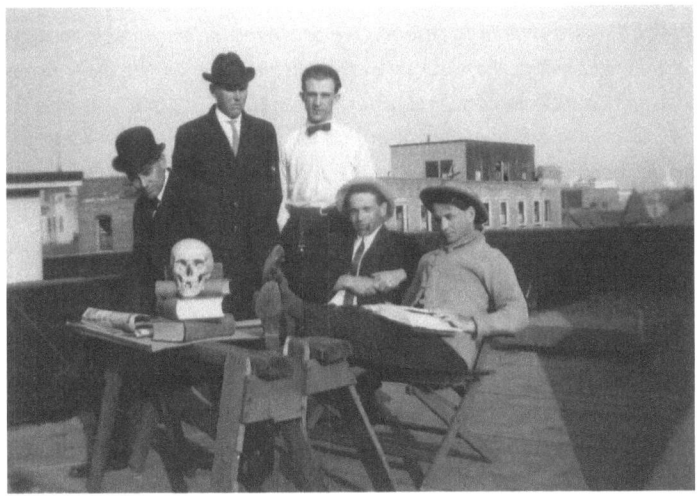

Figure 7. "Studying osteopathy:
Glen Cayler and students at COP&S, 1920s"

COP&S was the only osteopathic college that had included teaching ***materia medica*** in its curriculum since 1914. The AOA took much longer to adapt osteopathic practices to include the use of medicines and did not mandate teaching pharmacology in all osteopathic colleges until 1929. Thus, in the 1930s the difference between osteopathic and allopathic medical education nationwide narrowed quite a bit because the barrier against pharmacology was no longer an issue.

The scope of practice of osteopathic physicians had been unlimited in California since the earliest years of the 20th century, but in some other states, such as Illinois, D.O.s had a limited scope of practice and were not allowed to prescribe medications, in spite

79

of offering this education in the osteopathic medical curriculum. This gave California an image of leadership in terms of professional advancement and collaboration, if not competition, with allopathic medicine. Obtaining an added M.D. degree was one option toward collaboration and recognition as equal to allopathy.

Dr. Golanty:

> "In our first year in school we were told that osteopathic physicians who practiced south of the Mason Dixon line in the United States had restricted licenses. They could practice osteopathic medicine, but they could not prescribe medicine, nor could they perform surgery. If they even wanted to practice in Texas or Maryland or Florida, they would not be able to prescribe or to perform surgery, even though that was taught in the schools. And in fact, the year that I applied for medical school (1953-54) in the state of Illinois where there was a school, the Chicago Osteopathic School, the state still had a limited license for the graduates of osteopathic medicine and they couldn't perform surgery or medicine either in Illinois. I believe it was the year I entered school or just before (1954) that we were told that that had been overturned the law in Illinois, and now that was the first year that this could happen (1955). So, we were left with just the Southern states that had limited licenses."

Educational leaders with dual degrees

There were several osteopathic leaders that had both M.D. and D.O. degrees. **Lynn van Horn Gerdine, M.D., D.O.** was president of COP&S from1924 to 1935. Under his leadership COP&S expanded its student body, faculty and research and developed a post graduate school which offered a masters degree in basic science. **Carter Downing, M.D., D.O.** was President of San Francisco Osteopathic Medical Association. He expanded his unique textbook, ***Osteopathic Principles in Disease***, published in 1935, by integrating osteopathic principles and manipulative treatment with conventional medicine in the care of patients with a wide variety of illnesses. **Carl P. McConnell, M.D., D.O.** wrote a standard osteopathic text at the turn of the 20th century and moved to California in the 1920s. In 1928, he helped to further the development of research in osteopathic manipulation that Louisa Burns, D.O. had begun as early as 1903. In 1937, he founded the nationwide Academy of Applied Manipulative Therapeutics which evolved in 1943 into the American Academy of Applied Osteopathy. Currently this organization is called the *American Academy of Osteopathy.*

There were influential allopathic physicians in California that had a significant impact on osteopathic education throughout this time period as well. **F. M. Pottenger, M.D.** established a pulmonary clinic in Southern California and authored a remarkable textbook, entitled *Symptoms of Visceral Disease*, that became a required standard text in all osteopathic medical schools, including COP&S from the 1920s to 1960.

The dual degree issue

A letter to the editor of *Clinical Osteopathy* in 1935 (October issue) described a D.O. student at an osteopathic college who had asked about obtaining an additional M.D. degree by which to attract patients and then to *"sell them osteopathy"* while they were coming for allopathic care. Why would he want to do that, the letter writer replied; only 35 out of 8,500 D.O.s had an additional M.D. degree, i.e. 99.5% of D.O.s had no problem getting patients who were seeking osteopathic care.

Apparently this reply minimized the problem, because five years later *Clinical Osteopathy* published another letter, now urging to offer ways to obtain an M.D. degree. The letter explained the *"reason for dissatisfaction in the profession is the fundamental disparity between increased training and license compared to low political, social and postgraduate opportunity."* The letter also stated *"Many D.O.s are non-members* [in COA] *because they want an M.D. degree and the enlarged horizon it implies. If we do not settle the latter problem, it will settle us."*

Another 5 years later, in the 1940s, COP&S received numerous requests from alumni to provide courses that would qualify to apply for the M.D. degree. Many D.O.s were tired of the barriers against practicing their profession, and the option of a dual degree had become apparent as a way to be provided with the same opportunities and privileges available to their M.D. colleagues.

A few osteopathic physicians had started an M.D.-granting university, **Metropolitan University**, in the mid-1940s. It was not an accredited institution and soon was closed.

Dr. Ulansey:

"During this difficult time there was a group formed who secured a charter and became known as the **Metropolitan University**. *This was really a non-status medical school but they had the right to grant an M.D. degree that had no legal status for licensure to practice. To secure this degree, we had to attend lectures for one year, were given credit for our previous osteopathic education and our one year of graduate study. This was prior to the amalgamation and purely to gain admittance to educational and clinical opportunities. All osteopathic physicians who participated in this program were members of the AOA, the California Osteopathic Association, and the Los Angeles Osteopathic Association. The trustees of the COA became aware of this program and started discussions with the Metropolitan University in order to understand the reasoning behind this program and whether or not the participating D.O.s wanted to become*

M.D.s. The answer was simple. These D.O.s just wanted graduate study made available to them."

Since D.O.s did not want to take chances of getting an M.D. degree that did not afford them the respect they hoped for by their allopathic colleagues, they urged COP&S to offer an added M.D. program.

In the 1940s a special commission, the *Evaluation Commission*, was set up by the COA House of Delegates to investigate this request for the M.D. degree further. **Louis Chandler, D.O.** was Chairman of the commission. Members included **Drs. Cayler, Dieudonne, Dooley, and Walden**. **Glen Cayler, D.O**. was a mentor to Forest Grunigen, D.O. who two decades later successfully contributed to the merger between the osteopathic and allopathic profession (see Chapter 4). The Evaluation Commission existed in addition to the COA Fact Finding Committee. Both committees were appointed by the *House of Delegates* and both had to report directly to the *House of Delegates.*

Meetings were held by the *Evaluation Commission* in September 1948 and February 1949. Apparently the *Evaluation Commission* was concerned about duplicating efforts pursued by the *Fact Finding Committee*. They invited Forest Grunigen, D.O., Chairman of the Fact Finding Committee of the COA. Dr. Grunigen emphasized that the *Fact Finding Committee* of the COA and the counterpart of the CMA, *the Committee on Other Professions*, required from its members not to release any information until it had been acted upon by the official bodies.

From these minutes it becomes apparent that at that time the objective among COP&S alumni was not to abandon the D.O. degree. Rather, they wanted to be provided by COP&S with the opportunity to obtain a dual, M.D.-D.O. degree. The alumni requested a course that offered additional studies for the MD degree. They thought the course should be taught by M.D.s to make sure it would be recognized by allopathy.

The Commission members discussed whether this change should be started at the state or national level. Because the COP&S alumni so urgently requested this course, the Commission recommended a poll to be conducted on economic and social aspects of the dual degree. They thought it important to ascertain whether educational, socioeconomic and political conditions would improve if osteopathic physicians held a dual degree.

The discussion, as documented in the ***Chandler*** files in 1948 at the archival collection of Western University, concluded with the consensus that an official objective to issue a dual degree would weaken amalgamation (merger) chances. This realization put the *Evaluation Committee* in a dilemma because, as Howard Willis, D.O. explained, *"definitely 51% have decided that they would desire this particular kind of degree. If they are being rubbed off by continuing policies which ignore their desires without representation, that's not going to strengthen the College . . . . The human factor is still there, and they are becoming quite a bit discouraged because it is becoming evident throughout the profession we are not getting anywhere."*

Disagreements on osteopathic theory: W.G. Sutherland, D.O.

There were controversial osteopathic physicians in California during this period as well. W.G. Sutherland, D.O developed a theory on osteopathy in the cranial field and proposed a "primary respiratory mechanism". He theorized a cranial bone motion that was related to inherent brain motion and linked to cellular respiration and cerebral spinal fluid fluctuation.

He was a journalist by trade and began writing his case presentations and techniques based on the understanding of osteopathic principles and anatomy and physiology beginning in 1916. He called himself *"Blunt Bones Bill"* and wrote primarily about techniques related to the body, not the cranium, in newsletters and small circulated local publications in Minnesota, where he lived. He first began writing short articles about the cranium in the late 1920s, but not his full theory. He began discussing his ideas to single D.O.s who were interested and then to small groups, and presented his ideas to the AOA, the JAOA (the *Journal of the American Osteopathic Association*) and to D.O.s who were well respected for their OMT skills, in the mid 1930s.

No professional journal or group welcomed his theories. When he tried to publish his theory, both the *Journal of the American Osteopathic Association* and *Journal of Osteopathy* turned down his manuscripts. The only publisher that was willing to publish this theory of cranial bone mobility and its relationship to cellular respiration was *The Western Osteopath* in 1939. *"Our editorial board is headed by a man who believes it is better to print an original article, even if he disagrees with it, than it is to print something which is nothing more than a rehash of medical literature"* (Dr. C.B. Rowlingson, editor, *The Western Osteopath*, 1939). The *Western Osteopath* published Dr. Sutherland's booklet, *The Cranial Bowl*, in 1939. The *Western Osteopath* was a peer reviewed publication, not a research journal, nor a nationally renowned journal, but, nevertheless, a professional journal.

Dr. Sutherland lived in Minnesota at that time but moved to the Monterey Peninsula sometime in the 1940s. He settled in Pacific Grove near Carmel on the Monterey Bay and died there in 1954. His wife compiled his publications and speeches into a book to show the progression of his thoughts, but his theories were considered by California's osteopathic physicians, like Dain Tasker, D.O., quackery that debased the osteopathic image. They frowned upon Dr. Sutherland establishing the *Cranial Academy* which became a component society of the Academy of Applied Osteopathy (now the *American Academy of Osteopathy-AAO*) because of their link to the AOA.

Dr. Tasker and others had tried to portray to the public and to the AMA and CMA an image of osteopathy as scientific medicine. Sutherland's ideas were based on anatomy, physiology and applications of a philosophy, but not on laboratory science. There was talk of (Divine) Breath of Life as well, which belonged to the vitalistic philosophical period of medicine. Such concepts really concerned the California D.O.s who feared the M.D.s would not accept them as long as they had philosophical and religious minded proponents in their midst, even if licensed by their licensing board.

They were upset with their professional organization, the AOA, for not taking initiative to regulate the promulgation of outlying theories. Led by the articulate writings and arguments of Dain Tasker, D.O., COA leaders and others used examples such as Sutherland's cranial concepts to sway the COA membership towards merging with the CMA. They called for disbanding of the AOA and promoted merging with the AMA. (Dain Tasker, chapters 77 to 79 in the COA files).

As described in the following chapter, the merger between the COA and the CMA did occur, and Dr. Sutherland's theory is still respected. In 2006, COMP offered a 40-hour course in osteopathic approaches to the cranium using Sutherland's model. This course has been required of all 2nd year students since Dr. Frymann developed the course in 1980. **Dr. Frymann** was one of Dr. Sutherland's last students to have taken a course from him, several months before he passed away in his 80s.

Also the ***Cranial Academy*** is still in existence, as is a "*Sutherland Cranial Teaching Foundation*" which preserves his teachings. There are numerous books on derivatives, including craniosacral therapy, that are used by massage and physical therapists. While his concepts still create controversy within the profession and among basic scientists, clinicians find his techniques to be highly effective in many patients, often more so than other accepted approaches.

Dr. Frymann:

> "... when I first became involved in doing cranial work, as I had been so inspired by Dr. Sutherland and his treatment of babies, I went to the Hillside Hospital in San Diego and I asked for permission to treat their newborn babies. Well, what they had to say to people who do cranial work was that they were the 'head shrinkers'. They had no use for these crazy people. But there was a man who was an anesthesiologist and he said: 'I was treated by one of those head shrinkers when I had a really bad headache—you give them permission'. And that was how I got the opportunity to examine newborn babies over an eight year period and they didn't have any use for it. Not once in all those years that I was doing it, did the obstetrician ever come to see what I did to his babies. Not once. But anyhow, that's how I got started doing research."

Most of Dr. Sutherland's theories have withstood the test of time, as they have shown to provide clinically applicable and effective techniques. Also basic science is catching up to his understanding of the relationship between the cranial bones and the functions of the brain and the cranial nerves. Covering a span of 80 years, over 500 scientific articles have been published concerning this relationship. Cohesive rigorous research effort is lacking, though, and only bits and pieces of the puzzle are supplied by various unrelated research endeavors at different institutions.

Dr. Seffinger:

> *"In 1984, Dr. Frymann came to teach at Michigan State* [University] *a course called 'osteopathy in the cranial field'. The dean there did not allow her to teach during regular school hours; so we had to have her come during vacation only. At that time still, within the D.O. profession as well as the M.D. profession, the concept of cranial manipulation was very controversial. Anybody who taught that was pretty much banned from the schools. Right now, in contrast, here we are 20 years later and every school teaches it and it's on the* [osteopathic] *licensing exams. You know the research has built up quite a bit. So, it's accepted more so now than it certainly was back then."*

Research

Osteopathic research in California has a proud legacy. ***The A. T. Still Research Institute*** was founded in 1909 as a research lab, independent of the labs in osteopathic colleges. As described in Chapter 2, the Institute initially held offices in Chicago for a few years. When research did not progress sufficiently, **Louisa Burns, D.O.**, as the Institute's director, moved the research program in 1915 to Sunny Slope Labs in Pasadena, California.

Even with this new start, the first five bulletins published clinical applications of osteopathic theory, rather than experimental investigations. Osteopathic research was as under-funded then as it is in the 21st century.

A long-term vision for osteopathic research

The Pacific College of Osteopathy (PCO) was one of the first colleges nationwide to develop a proposal for a long-term research program, as prepared by Louisa Burns, D.O. Her aim was to obtain evidence on osteopathic concepts in several different fields. She had started to conduct laboratory studies while still a student at PCO, investigating the physiology of the nervous system as taught at PCO.

In Pasadena she carried out animal and clinical research studies from 1915-1955. Her work stimulated the profession to pursue scientific inquiries that tested the theories of the osteopathic concept. She suggested that it was especially important to show the integral role of the neuromusculoskeletal system in the cause and effect of pathophysiologic processes. *Western University* in Pomona, California, has a collection of her numerous books and research data, as well as her personally signed physiology textbook by J. Martin Littlejohn, D.O., M.D., a professor at the American School of Osteopathy in Kirksville, who later went on to establish the Chicago College of Osteopathy and the British School of Osteopathy.

In 1939, patient charts at Unit II of the L.A. County Osteopathic Hospital showed that pneumonia recovery in children cared for at that osteopathic institution had a significantly higher recovery rate than that at a similar sized county hospital in New

York. These research results provided a great boost to osteopathic physicians and their acceptance by the public.

Dr. Golanty:

> *"We also had a textbook that we were to read in osteopathic medicine. Everyone was kind of thirsty to want to know about the science of it and we were hoping to see information about it. The text's name I've forgotten; it was written by **Louisa Burns**. The book had a lot of information in it, dealing with rabbits. She would create osteopathic lesions in these rabbits and sacrifice them and try to demonstrate the somato-visceral reflexes culminating in disease. There was a little research laboratory that was on the campus that's located behind our classrooms. I don't think any of us ever really got to go inside the place where she was working. I believe she died just about the time that I entered the school so we hardly got to see her."*

Medical research at COP&S

Dr. Tasker, in his unpublished manuscript on the *History of Osteopathy in California* mentioned for the year 1948 that the medical research department at COP&S included an outgrowth of cancer research begun by Dr. Davis at the University of Chicago. *"Cancer research is now included in the broader medical research program. That program will also include new research problems of graduate students who wish to make such research a major contribution to the degree of Medical Science"* (Tasker, chapters 66 to 70).

Osteopathic physicians and students donated significantly to a *Louisa Burns Research Fund,* according to Dr. Tasker's notes, in 1948 and '49. He cited that a sum of $612 was collected for Dr. Burns' research. She said she'd buy a card sorting machine for her study on the correlation between pathological conditions and special lesions (pg. 10 of the Tasker document). She had accumulated more than 1,000 case records. The sorting machine would save her 6 years hand labor. She encouraged all osteopaths in California to contribute cases for this research. While the card sorting machine was helpful, Dr. Burns would have also needed a new typewriter and microscope.

Wilbur Cole, D.O. moved to California from the Kirksville College of Osteopathy (formerly the ASO) in Kirksville, MO in order to learn Dr. Burns' methods and become familiar with her research. He wanted to carry her studies further upon her retirement and indeed pursued the studies when he moved back to Missouri.

Socio-economic conditions

The *Clinical Osteopathy* journal in 1934 provided economic information, including a comparison of incomes among M.D.s, D.O.s and dentists in 1933, based on a survey with a 49% response rate for D.O.s and a 34% response rate by M.D.s and dentists. A summary of the survey showed that 50% of M.D.s made $2,999, compared to $1,999 for D.O.s and dentists. Clearly there were economic advantages of having the M.D. letters after one's name.

In 1936, the Los Angeles area was reported to have the greatest concentration of osteopathic physicians anywhere, as one sixth of D.O.s worldwide practiced in California (*Clinical Osteopathy*, 1936, May issue). For September 1936, the journal quoted 1,487 D.O.s in California, a stunning growth from the pioneering 40 D.O.s in 1900. By the end of 1937, the California Board of Osteopathic Examiners reported 1,718 licentiates in California.

The California Health Survey in the 1950s

The California Health Survey was conducted between May 1954 and May 1955 by the U.S. Bureau of the Census for the State Department of Public Health. The survey included personal interviews with members of 10,000 representative California households. About 30,000 persons provided information about their illness episodes or illness among family members in the 4 weeks prior to the interviews. The survey then asked for name and address of the treating doctor. As part of a secondary data analysis project with one-half of the state survey sample, the Stanford Research Institute ascertained the type of doctor, i.e. doctor of medicine (M.D.), osteopathy (D.O.), or chiropractic (D.C.) who provided the treatment (*Chiropractic in California*, 1960).

M.D.s attended 88 % of the conditions, compared to 8.5% attended by D.O.s and 3.5% by D.C.s. Most D.O.s (96.4%) saw their patients in private practice or a private clinic. Among patients with Spanish surnames, 17.5% used the service of osteopaths. Over 90% of patients attended by M.D.s were white, non-Hispanic, compared to 82% of those attended by D.O.s. Two-thirds of all persons attended by osteopaths resided in Los Angeles County, while the Bay Area counties showed virtually no patients attended by osteopaths.

Among the conditions attended by D.O.s, hypertension, menstruation and menopause, anemia, arthritis and rheumatism, overweight, and back conditions were the most frequent. In 1953, D.O.s in the Los Angeles Metropolitan Area attended 13,989 live births, compared to 102,978 live births attended by M.D.s. The San Diego Area had 525 births attended by D.O.s and 19,692 by M.D.s.

The public often sought osteopathic services in the care of children. Sixteen percent of the patients cared for by D.O.s in California were children age 9 years or younger, and 5.6% were teenagers, compared to 20% children and 9% teens cared for by M.D.s. As described in Chapter 6, osteopathic services for children continue to be sought in the 21st century at the Osteopathic Center for Children in San Diego by parents from near and far. Viola M. Frymann, D.O., F.A.A.O., F.C.A. serves as its medical director (see Appendix).

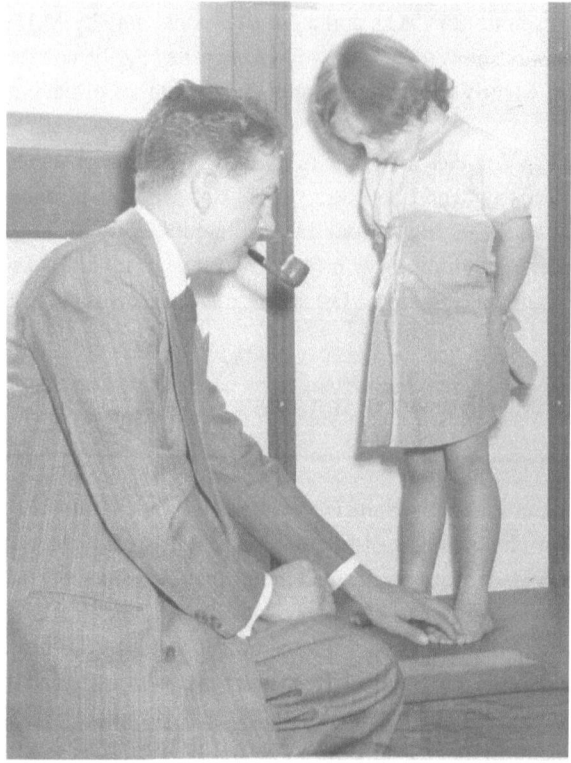

Figure 8. "Dr. Miller, Orthopedics, 1951"

A comparative analysis of selected osteopathic and medical schools was included in the California Health Survey as well. Osteopathy was represented by the only school in California, COP&S, founded in 1914. Allopathic Medicine was represented by two schools in Southern California, University of California Los Angeles Medical School (UCLA), founded in 1950, and the College of Medical Evangelists (CME), established in 1910. COP&S and CME were approved by their respective national professional associations. UCLA Medical School was approved after its first class had been graduated in 1955.

In 1957, the total income of COP&S was $752,041, compared to $2,900,000 for UCLA Medical School. COP&S received 42% of its income through tuition and fees, and CME received 34%. COP&S received 32% from gifts and endowments, and CME received 62% in this manner.

At COP&S, each full-time faculty had 4.7 students, CME had 3.6, and UCLA had 1.3 students to instruct and guide. The vast majority of osteopathic and medical school faculty volunteered. At COP&S, 54% of the faculty had academic degrees, compared to only 3% of the CME faculty and 24% of the UCLA Medical School faculty. Faculty members at COP&S spent about 40% of their 40 hour week in the classroom or the teaching laboratories which was a similar ratio to the medical school faculty. The number of publications per full-time faculty member in 1957 was 0.76 at COP&S, 1.7 at CME, and 4.1 at UCLA Medical School. Student characteristics at COP&S compared to those at CME and UCLA did not differ in age and pre-professional college background.

The California Osteopathic Association (COA)

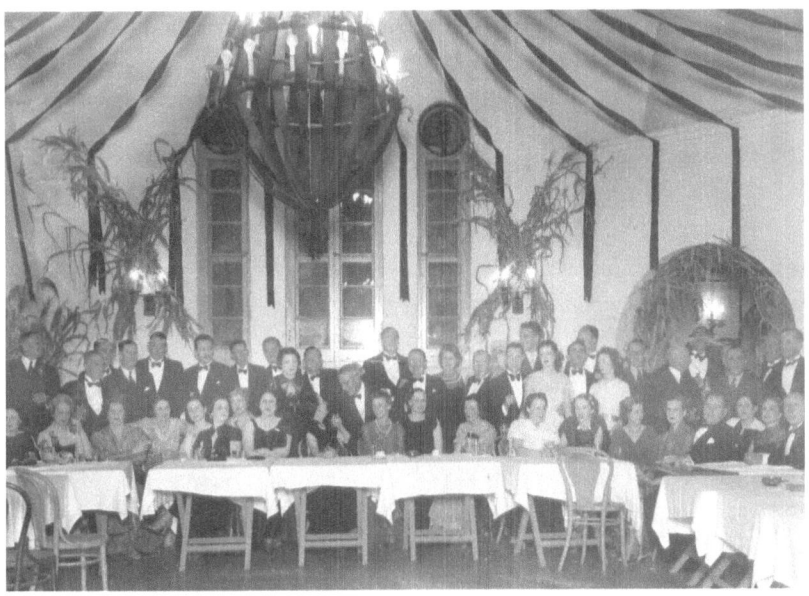

Figure 9. "COA convention, Coronado, 1930s"

More than half of California's osteopaths in 1936 were members of COA, while only one third held a membership in their national organization, the AOA. Osteopathic physicians at that time apparently felt insufficiently supported by the national organization. This argument was made 25 years later by Dorothy Marsh, D.O. As the president of the COA in 1961, she referred to a long-standing lack of trust and sensitivity to California's needs for financial and political support at the national level.

In October 1940, the membership roster of the COA included Betsy, Daisy and Frank E. MacCracken, R.E. Eby, Cora and Dain Tasker, and Glen Cayler, prominent osteopathic physicians in California. COP&S provided space for the COA's central office in the 1940s until more representative offices were found on Wilshire and then on Santa Monica Boulevard in Los Angeles.

Osteopathic physicians often practiced geographically separated from their colleagues. To overcome a sense of disconnect, divisional societies were organized throughout the state in the 1930s and '40s. The L.A. County Osteopathic Society was the first to be formed, followed by Southside and Westside societies, and many others. Each divisional society sent delegates to the COA conventions and was given political duties as well as privileges.

Alumni Association of COP&S

Another important association was that of the COP&S Alumni. In the 1940s they had become visibly active by conducting educational events throughout the state. Their college journal was called the *Cortex*. Issues can be traced back to 1913. The full set is held in the archives of the Pumerantz Library at Western University. *Cortex* issues provided photographs and membership rosters, in addition to professional and social news.

Dr. Steedman:

> *"The alumni at that time would support the students and have special alumni meetings and social get-togethers to invite the students and to help them along. They had a student loan organization. The Alumni were there to act as big brothers as well. If certain students were having problems in a certain specialty in studying, they could get together with these alumni and they would meet with them and go over certain things and help them in the courses. They were there also to help with the annual class parties by donating certain amounts of money. We would collect money from all the students in the class and then the Alumni Association would help us or even allow us to have our parties at their homes or other places. So they were always contributing to the education and to support the maintenance of students . . . . the alumni were always so supportive. We were active with that Alumni Association so we knew what was going on with the school and potential amalgamation and purchase of and construction of County* [Los Angeles County Hospital] *Unit II."*

Nationwide visibility and honors for California D.O.s

In 1940, the July issue of *Clinical Osteopathy* published news from the AOA convention. All 14 representatives of the California House of Delegates were present, including Glen Cayler, D.O. Alternates included Frank MacCracken, D.O.

For the year 1947, Dr. Tasker's manuscript provided a list of various honors and awards given at that time, including a plaque to Frank MacCracken, D.O. for having raised $31,855 for the Andrew Taylor Still Memorial Building, making California a greater contributor to the project than any other state.

For that year Dr. Tasker wrote about his own honors: "Dr. Tasker was honored as the founder of the osteopathic profession in California." He continued to list others who received honors as well, including members of the California Osteopathic Surgical Society who obtained two war surplus buildings for animal surgery and surgical photo labs (Tasker, chapter 66).

Visibility and honors continued with succeeding years. In the 1950s (Dr. Tasker cited no year but the context suggested early '50s) Dr. Don Littlefield, a Long Beach psychiatrist and senior psychiatrist at Los Angeles County Osteopathic Hospital was chosen as president-elect of the American College of Neuropsychology at its annual meeting in

Missouri. Dr. Thomas Meyers, Professor of Psychiatry and head of the Department of Neurology and Psychiatry at COP&S was elected Fellow of the American Association on Mental Health Deficiency in 1950. The Association was founded in 1876 and was one of the oldest of American Medical Societies. Dr. Meyers was the first osteopathic physician honored in this manner (Tasker, chapter 26).

Antagonism

Dr. Ulansey:

> *"And another thing that was very bad at that time: there was a rise in malpractice. We found that the allopaths would testify against the osteopaths and the osteopaths would testify against the allopaths, but they wouldn't testify against their own kind. So that was a major friction and had a strong influence in the future of the two professions."*

On August 19, 1940 LIFE magazine published an informative, three-page article on osteopathy, including photographs of osteopathic manipulation and statistics on the number of states (33 at that time) where qualified doctors of osteopathy were permitted to practice on equal footing with doctors of (allopathic) medicine. This prompted Dr. Fishbein to write prejudiced and uncivil comments about osteopathy in JAMA and to deny the facts about the licensing status of D.O.s. Apparently he did not expect having to prove his statements in court, and indeed no one seemed to have held Dr. Fishbein accountable for his behavior.

Fortunately, a reprint of a letter to the editor by Mark Twain appeared in the December 1940 issue of *Clinical Osteopathy,* defending osteopathy enthusiastically. Mark Twain wrote the letter in the 1800s, as a contemporary of A.T. Still, M.D., D.O. He also publicly defended osteopathy in court. Claiming his right and liberty to choose who treated him, he preferred doctors of osteopathic medicine. Fittingly, his name was chosen for a hospital that provided dual services in the Sacramento area.

Antagonism and discrimination against D.O.s were of course nationwide problems and not just frustrating to California's D.O.s. Politically engaged D.O.s in California apparently were the only ones, though, to seek a way out from discrimination through merging with the mainstream medical profession.

Serving in the Armed Forces

As noted earlier in this chapter, osteopathic physicians and surgeons could only be drafted as soldiers, not officers. The Armed Forces did not allow D.O.s to serve as medical officers until 1966.

In a brochure entitled *"An appeal to reason"*, published by the California Osteopathic Association in 1942, D.O.s were given a discouraging picture of their professional future. The apparent goal was to promote the idea of obtaining an M.D.

degree. Questions were raised about their obligation to the war (WWII) and their draft prospects. *"You don't have to face the prospect of being drafted as a private in the army . . . ."* A plan called for *"the granting by the Surgeons General of the Army and Navy temporary commissions to osteopathic physicians and surgeons while taking further work in military medicine at government schools, being graduated with commissions in the Army or Navy medical corps."* An appeal was made to General Magee of the Army and Admiral McIntyre of the Navy to *" . . . realize while we are only a relative few in numbers, we stand willing and able to do our part if you but give us a chance."*

The brochure was signed by the Committee for the Standardization of Medical Education and Practice in California, Emerson Hutchinson, D.O., Chairman, Charles Nicholas, D.O., Vice-Chairman, and Jack Stein, D.O., Secretary-Treasurer.

Dr. Wykle:

> *"During World War II, as a D.O. I was not requisitioned to the army because D.O.s were told we were more valuable taking care of the public at home. Actually, the armed services were discriminatory to D.O.s then, and did not allow D.O.s to be medical officers, which actually worked to our advantage. The M.D.s found out about that when they returned from service and found all their patients happily cared for by D.O.s."*

Dr. Eby:

> *"[In 1941] when I learned that Pearl Harbor had [been attacked], I wrote to the president of the California Osteopathic Association and told him by whatever means he found available to send a letter to the Surgeon General of the United States—he was the one conscripting all doctors into the army, navy and air corps—telling him that the California COP&S would all as a unit go into the armed services as our contribution to the American war effort. Consequently, we got a letter back saying 'no'. Only M.D.s could go because 'they're the only doctors that are trained'. He said he had no authority to hire a D.O. anywhere, 'but I suggest to you, Dr. Eby, that you tell all your members, however many you got, 5, 10, 100, that you are deferred from serving in the war effort as physicians'. He didn't know that we had D.O.s in Washington DC making recommendations on public health policy; he didn't know who would be in charge of civilian health during the absence of the M.D.s when they went into the services. Within the 4 years of the war the word had gotten out to all America that these guys are not 'little m.d.s'. They're doing a better job than their former doctors in most cases and we did so simply because we had to, to be sure."*

Dr. Golanty:

"We were told we couldn't serve [as medical staff] *in the military. They would not take us into the army. I believe that it is rather common knowledge that that is part of what caused the growth of the osteopathic profession during World War II to begin with, the strength in those states like California that had lots of D.O.s that was because they were taking care of patients while the M.D.s were off to war. We had heard that one of the senators from the state of Missouri, I think it was Stuart Symington, I may be wrong on the name, but he had indicated that if his son were dying on a battlefield he would not allow a D.O. take care of him. That's in the Congressional Record, and I saw it personally. I went to the UCLA library and found the citation and I read it. So I may have the person wrong, but I know the citation was right."*

Dr. Betsy MacCracken:

" . . . then the war broke out and I joined the Navy. In the navy I was always in administrative positions and as such began to know that particularly middle management was where my strengths lay."

Dr. Seffinger:

"Did it bother you that you were not allowed to be a physician or medical officer?"

Dr. Betsy MacCracken:

"No it didn't bother me. I was assigned over as an administrator in the Bureau of Medicine and Surgery. It didn't bother me."

Dr. Seffinger:

"Some of the people have commented that it bothered them, so . . ."

Dr. Betsy MacCracken:

"It didn't bother me at all . . . The only thing I can say is that it taught me my love for administration. They were writing the medical history of the war in our office and the men that were writing the history would take me to some of the interviews on account of my medical knowledge that I could pass some notes and tell them what it meant, but that was the only time that my medical experience counted."

The Second World War affected osteopathic medical education.

Dr. Alloy:

"I then came out to Los Angeles in February of 1947 and began my internship at the County Hospital. This was all during and immediately after the Second World War years; and during that period of time our education was compressed from the standpoint of time. We had no summer vacations. We had several weeks off and were able to accomplish four years worth of normal education within three. The same thing applied with my internship—a twelve month internship was condensed to nine months."

Dr. Dilworth:

"The Second World War was well established; all of the students were being drafted; and it was my opportunity to receive from President Roosevelt the letter that exempted us from the draft, if we would be faithful to the osteopathic profession, which meant—going to the school and passing all of the classes. And so, that was very successful in giving me the opportunity of becoming a D.O.. When I went to intern in Long Beach, we finally celebrated the big VE day and the war was over.

"There was a slight movement on foot to see if they could get recognition to cross over to the medical profession directly. Most of it was just talk in those early years and some of it was because 'none of the osteopathic doctors were being accepted into any of the armed services' and they would have liked to have had that privilege, but since it wasn't granted to them, it led to an attempt to try to find how to get equal recognition for the two different professions."

Dr. Ulansey:

"This deferment [of D.O.s] resulted in their staying home and building substantial and lucrative practices while the M.D.s were drafted into the military.

"The patients had now become accustomed to a different approach to medical practice. The osteopaths listened more attentively to the patients. They spent more time with the patients. This was very good public relations for them. It paid off. They built their practices. They didn't lose them when the allopaths returned, which made a lot of allopaths very, very unhappy. This fomented further friction between the two groups. This is one of the reasons why we started talking about a merger. It was an attempt to standardize education, examination, and licensure in the issuance of one degree for the practice of medicine in California."

Dr. van den Noort:

"As I view that past time from my perspective, I think what was happening in California towards the end of the Korean War and that era was that a lot of the M.D.s in California had been off to wars such as World War II, the Korean War and that the osteopaths didn't go off to war. It made them more powerful in the organization of medical care in California."

In 1956, public law 84-763 provided for the appointment of D.O.s as full physicians in the Medical Corps of the Armed Services. This law was not implemented, though, by the Department of Defense until 5-31-1966.

Policy and regulations

Training opportunities

As described in the beginning of this chapter, the L.A. County General Hospital provided M.D. and D.O. services, in Unit I and Unit II respectively since 1928. The visible success of Unit II was key to making the D.O.s proud of their work.

Dr. Ulansey:

"The younger generation was always eager to learn more. They wanted to do more; to see more; to hear more; and they were eager to be better doctors. The opportunities were there, but we couldn't take advantage of them because of the friction between the allopathic and the osteopathic professions. The allopaths had an unwritten rule—a code that they should not mingle with 'we who were less pure.' Some of them were unofficially very friendly, very cooperative and helped us immensely. They would lecture to us in small gatherings. They would work with us in some hospitals, not in the major hospitals, but in some of the smaller hospitals; some of the hospitals which were operated as osteopathic hospitals, or mixed staff, such as Hollywood Community Hospital or other D.O. owned institutions.

"The White Memorial Hospital was a little more friendly than most of the allopathic hospitals, and so their people were friendly. I formed a group of D.O. anesthesiologists known as the Los Angeles Society of Anesthesiologists. The doctors that I mentioned, allopathic F. Leffingwell, M.D., John Rupp, M.D., and John Dillon, M.D., would come and lecture to us; give us some good tidbits from what they had learned through their vast experiences. Few were friendly and helpful, but that was not the prevalent situation across

the county—meaning the Los Angeles County or State of California. We couldn't get into graduate schools. University of California at Los Angeles didn't yet exist as a medical school. In the larger medical hospitals, since we were not admitted to their staff, we could not attend their meetings or their educational programs. We so much wanted graduate level education and officially they would not admit us to allopathic programs given at the various medical schools. This was a bone of contention causing friction between the two professions."

Given the tensions with traditional medicine, how did the public perceive osteopathic medicine? Who were these D.O.s in the 1930s?

Dr. Eby:

"That is a good question, who were these guys? Even the people in California weren't quite sure who they were because they were called 'little M.D.s' by the real ones. We discovered we were called 'little M.D.s' by the public mostly in those days because the real M.D.s had said 'there's a bunch of quacks coming in from Kirksville and 4 or 5 eastern osteopathic colleges'. Of course, we were not excited about that, so we decided that we as a group, at this particular college called COP&S, under fine administration, we'd make it the best. So, what I got into was the class that wanted to make it better than it'd ever been and succeeded. [Participation in] politics, however, was of course available to anybody that asked, because that's the way kept by the medics. Now, I'm not putting down the M.D.s. They were in their business because they wanted to be M.D.s, and nobody should stop them in my opinion. But what they wanted to do was to stop everyone else."

Dr. Betsy MacCracken recalls:

"I was on attending staff over at the County Hospital. Somewhere along the line I developed a flair for infectious diseases. I loved the work on the communicable disease ward more than on the straight ward . . . . The big area was in the treatment of polio and the use of hot packs and passive motion of the affected areas; of particular interest, though, was the protection of the house-staff and the house-staff were limited in the number of hours they could work. They were kept living at the hospital and they were made to take a mid-morning break and have something to eat and they were well protected health wise. There were three hundred nurses at the medical unit that developed polio."

Dr. Seffinger:

" . . . and nobody developed polio in Unit Two? "

Dr. Betsy MacCracken:

"No. In later years one of our interns did develop polio."

Dr. Golanty:

"That third year, we had a new clinic building that had been built on the campus, today it's Norris Cancer Institute that belongs to the USC complex, but it was built adjacent to a clinic building that was already there . . . . The adjacent building was a rehabilitation building. So much of what we did that was osteopathic in the way of manipulation was done in the rehabilitation center. There was still poliomyelitis at that time and so a lot of polio patients, post-polio were there and we were doing a lot of strengthening exercises and treatments at that time for the polio patients. I recall that I had one young kid around 13 with a lot of disease that I'd take care of as his doctor for his manipulation and treatments that we gave to him.

"There was a clinic on the campus at the same location where the medical school itself (the first two years undergraduate portion) was. That clinic was particularly run by the medical students under a few full-time faculty, Dr. Charles Dieudonne who was an OB-GYN doctor, Dr. Ernest Stebbens who was an internal medicine physician, Dr. Jack Scoles, a surgeon, and Dr. Merlin Brubaker, an internist—those are the names I remember."

At that time of professional confidence, Dr. Forest Grunigen graduated at COP&S, in 1931. That pride led to his and others' feelings of frustration when they could not get into larger, allopathic hospitals in the L.A. area to train or to work. The available internships and residencies at Unit II of the L.A. County Hospital and at additional, smaller osteopathic facilities were insufficient to meet the needs of the COP&S graduates. Dr. Grunigen, like many of his colleagues, sought residency training at M.D. hospitals in Europe, as he was barred from receiving advanced training from MDs in the United States.

In the 1950s efforts were made throughout the greater Los Angeles community to obtain funds for an updated and larger osteopathic hospital instead of the small Unit II buildings they were using for the past 20 years. The success of Unit II helped convince people that a bigger and separate osteopathic hospital building was needed to meet the needs of the Los Angeles population.

Even students went to senators and legislators to develop finance for a County Hospital that would be osteopathic.

Dr. Steedman:

"We had been hearing for a long period of time that there was a big move to develop finance to be able to build a County Hospital that would be osteopathic and that County Hospital would be sponsored by certain of the senators. Even as students we went out and talked to individuals and to various legislators and discussed the need for a new osteopathic hospital and how we could better serve the community. That building was built for a little under $10 million and the COA did contribute some finances. As students we campaigned to get individuals to vote for the bonds that would pay for that hospital."

Dr. Kammerman:

"I went out talking to service clubs about getting that passed. I spoke to probably two or three service clubs. Doctors would be members of service clubs so I'd get up and come out and give them about a five minute presentation as to the benefits of putting that new hospital in. It was going to be an issue on the ballot. It was going to cost 9.22 million dollars to build it."

Dr. Taylor recalls:

"As students, we walked on the streets with pamphlets promoting the Los Angeles people's referendum to commit funds to build a new D.O. facility/hospital, [called] Los Angeles County Osteopathic Hospital (LACOH). The county referendum won and the hospital was built, in 1956 to '59."

Senator Teale was instrumental with legislative decisions, and Drs. Dorothy Marsh and Forest Grunigen helped with the campaign to get public support. The bills were passed in 1954 and 1955 and a bond was issued for funding the hospital project with tax money. The 500-bed facility was built and the old building eventually was torn down. The Norris Cancer Institute now stands in its place.

The new L.A. County Osteopathic Hospital was ready for services in 1959. The expansion into a 500-bed facility and a research laboratory had cost $ 10 million. It was one of the largest osteopathic hospitals nationwide at that time. It was unique, because it was largely paid for by tax dollars of the people of California, specifically for the osteopathic profession, largely due to student and alumni campaign and legislative support. Drs. Passy, Golanty, and Steedman were part of the first intern class that entered when the new Osteopathic Hospital had just opened its doors.

Dr. Golanty:

"The citizens of the County of Los Angeles had had a referendum, somewhere around the time of my third year of medical school, and passed a referendum for the building of a new osteopathic hospital . . . for just the D.O.s. So, we now had a new facility. It was opened just before I left as a med student. When I came back from residency, of course it was there and the old buildings that I was talking about that were there, most of them were torn down. I believe there are still a few vestiges of a few of them left, but the majority of it has gone. The new L.A. County Osteopathic Hospital had a cornerstone on the left hand side of the building as you face the front door, and a time capsule lay inside the cornerstone to be opened 100 years from the time that it was laid, containing the history of the osteopathic profession."

Residency and intern training hospitals

In the early 1950s two osteopathic hospitals were approved as residency and intern training hospitals. Doctors Hospital in Los Angeles offered one residency in surgery.

The L.A. County Osteopathic Hospital offered the following number in residencies: two in Anesthesiology, six in Internal Medicine, and one or two in Neurology, Obstetrics and Gynecology, Ophthalmology and Otolaryngology, Orthopedic surgery, Pathology, Pediatrics, Radiology, Surgery and Urological Surgery.

In 1952, the following osteopathic hospitals were approved for training interns in California: Doctors Hospital in Los Angeles, Glendale Community Hospital in Glendale, Hillside Hospital in San Diego, Los Angeles County Osteopathic Hospital, Magnolia Hospital in Long Beach, Los Cerritos Hospital in Long Beach, Maywood Hospital in Maywood, Monte Sano Foundation in Los Angeles, Park View Hospital in Los Angeles, and San Gabriel Valley Hospital in San Gabriel.

In addition, the following institutions were also registered osteopathic hospitals in California: Civic Center Hospital in Oakland, Cottage Hospital in Pomona, Glendale Emergency Hospital in Glendale, Thomas Ince Memorial Hospital in 29 Palms, Riverside Osteopathic Hospital in Riverside, and Wallace Memorial Hospital in Fresno.

Student education and training in the 1950s

Dr. Betsy MacCracken, in her manuscript on the history of the Pediatrics Department of the California College of Medicine, described that *" . . . on the Hospital side of Mission Road there was much activity in the late 1950s. A new Hospital was being built which was dedicated in 1959. By 1957 there were two Pediatrics Residencies. In 1958 Dr. Jane*

Hamilton was named Head Physician, Pediatrics. By the time the new hospital opened in 1959 there were three residencies in Pediatrics . . . .

"An integral part of student training in Obstetrics and Pediatrics was the Los Angeles City Maternity Services. For many years students spent a minimum of two weeks assigned to this service. For their obstetrical training they assisted with home deliveries, ante-partum and post-partum care. In the field of Pediatrics they handled the immediate care of the infant following delivery, made post-partum home visits and assisted the clinicians in the Child Health Conferences."

Dr. Nelson made an interesting discovery about the first Resident in the Pediatrics Department, going back to the 1940s.

Dr. Nelson:

"I discovered that the first Pediatric Resident at Unit II was appointed during the tenure of the first Department Chair . . . (they had the title of Department Executive in the old school) who was in place in the 1940s. I traced this ex-resident and found he had become the Public Health Officer for Placer County. I went to Auburn, California, and interviewed him there. We were about the same age and had been a resident at about the same time in the 1940s. One of the fascinating things I learned in the interview was that his Department Chair at the time was in contact with the Pediatric Chairman at UCSF at the time I was a resident there. These two men were meeting with each other fairly regularly discussing mutual problems. Although the UCSF chair was in place during the time I was a resident, and I was his first fellow, and a faculty member and I used to cover his practice when out-of-town, I never heard about these contacts from him. I found this a very interesting story."

The Osteopathic Physiatrist Program

In the June issue of *Clinical Osteopathy*, 1952, W.W.W. Pritchard, D.O. described the Osteopathic Physiatrist Program. For many years COP&S and L.A. County Osteopathic Hospital taught osteopathic manipulation as part of general medicine. In 1946 a committee was established to improve the efficiency of teaching manipulation. Basic principles were applied:

1. The human body is like a machine
2. Adequate circulation is necessary for health
3. The body contains the power to cure, provided manipulation makes intelligent use of the knowledge of the body
4. Mechanical adjustments include manipulation of various joints

5. Osteopathy considers the body as a whole
6. Osteopathy makes use of mechanical devices like levers, the pivot, and screws
7. Three general types of structure can be found, each type has an inherent tendency to disease
8. There are three important physiological pronouncements: Head's law, Hilton's law, and Wolff's law
9. Knowledge of the autonomic nervous system is of prime importance
10. There is a relationship between structure and function

At that time, the AMA had established a separate section of Physical Medicine & Rehabilitation and created a Specialty Board for Certification of Specialists in PM&R. These specialists were called physiatrists. Thirty-seven medical schools had departments of Physical Medicine and Rehabilitation as well as some hundred residents at medical centers and in the Veterans Administration. Dr. Pritchard urged to establish such a Board for Osteopathic Physiatrists as well, in order to supply to the public the certified service of osteopathic physiatrists.

With this goal in mind, Dr. Pritchard, in consultation with Wm. T. Sechrist, D.O., John Andrews, D.O., Robert Ruenitz, D.O., and colleagues, compiled a 30-page set of Standing Orders, in effect at COP&S and at the Los Angeles County Osteopathic Hospital in 1952. Complimentary copies were sent to every osteopathic hospital listed in the AOA directory.

Dr. Golanty:

> *"In the second year, we started having further introductions to osteopathic medicine at this point, with W.W.W. Pritchard, D.O., but this was when we began to see OMT being taught in a classroom and also in laboratories. Now, in my day, words such as muscle energy and fascial release, those terms were not used among ourselves. We learned something called soft tissue massage as a preparation to manipulation. What we learned as manipulation is what, I believe, people today call high velocity and that is what we were taught and did."*

By 1951, the L.A. County Osteopathic Hospital combined the Department of Physical Therapy and the Department of Osteopathic Manipulation into the Department of Osteopathic Therapeutics and Rehabilitation [stationary letterhead at that time included the term "and Rehabilitation", while text sources often did not include the term]. By 1952, the Department included already 30 osteopathic physicians, a physical therapist and an occupational therapist. The clinic was called the Rehab Center building. The 2nd floor was used for physical diagnosis and osteopathic technique courses. The 1st floor was used for rehab therapy with a variety of equipment.

The newly funded rehab center at Unit II seemed to have resulted in the unintended effect of reducing the visibility of OMT. Louis Bartosh, D.O. recalled in 1978 that in the late 1950s the new Unit II, the L.A. County Osteopathic Hospital, had a large, well-equipped PT department with only a single manipulation table in the background. "The last and only instructor in manipulation technique was phased out in 1957. The new instructor put great emphasis on physiotherapy and the word osteopathy was less in evidence," Dr. Bartosh recalled. He also felt that COP&S had a "disoriented program until its demise in 1962" (Bartosh, 1978).

Dr. Kammerman remembers, though, that *"in 1952 at COP&S Dr. John Andrews was strong in manipulation. He brought the manipulation program up to standards with a well organized program. Students were provided with 100 hours learning techniques. To obtain hands-on training they manipulated each other—and had no aches then!"*

In support of Dr. Kammerman's recollection, *Clinical Osteopathy,* January 1952, published an article by John M. Andrews, D.O., Director of Clinical Practice, General Osteopathic Clinic at COP&S, entitled "Clinical Osteopathy at the College".

In this article **Dr. Andrews** described the teaching protocol as follows:

> *"The Clinic sets up training programs for students, providing opportunities to observe and care for every possible type of case under the supervision of a licensed attending physician . . . . Another group observes at the LA County Osteopathic Hospital . . . . The Osteopathic Therapeutics Staff physician handles the case assigned to him as a general practitioner would. He will recommend a consult whenever indicated.*
>
> *"During the past few months there has been a renewed interest in posture studies and structural problems in relation to health. A definite effort is made to evaluate the relevance of structural problems . . . . They complete a structural exam status, identical to those used in the LA County Osteopathic Hospital . . . . Throughout the year, the Didactic Staff holds meetings and is teaching various techniques . . . . always keeping in mind the relationship between structure and function . . . The effect of lesions may be local or remote . . ."*

Dr. Andrew's program might have been implemented in response to criticism of insufficient training in osteopathic manipulation in the late 1940's. Dr. Viola Frymann, who had been a licensed allopathic physician in England, sought further osteopathic training at COP&S in 1947.

Dr. Frymann:

> *"Up to this point, my experience with osteopathy was people who used their hands to manipulate their patients. I didn't have to be at COP&S very*

long to find out nobody did that! Nobody! And I think if I hadn't been too proud to admit to my father that I had made a terrible mistake, I would have packed up and gone home. But there was a man there who was getting his license in California from Hawaii and he had to put in a thousand hours there and so in the afternoons when students were in the clinic he and I would get in the treatment room and he would teach me manipulation. That was really the main source whereby I learned the use of my hands.

"However, during this time, what was then the Academy of Applied Osteopathy in those days, announced an essay contest for students which was the significance of osteopathy in heart disease. I didn't know anything about it so I went to the library. I searched the books what literature there was and I wrote the essay and surprising enough they awarded me the prize. Next year it was the same topic only it was kidney disease and so I searched kidney disease. So this was another way in which I got education about clinical application of osteopathy but it wasn't through what they were teaching at school."

Dr. Frymann's two award-winning papers were published around 1948 and 1949, and republished in her collected works published by the Academy of Osteopathy in 2002.

Dr. Frymann was spared the first two years at COP&S because of her Bachelor of Medicine degree that she had earned in England. Thus, she missed the osteopathic manipulation courses taught in the first two years at COP&S but she completed the manipulation lab courses and practiced manipulation during her third and fourth year rotations. Her recollection seems to imply, though, a disappointing lack of general visibility of the value of osteopathic manipulation. She also realized that the mechanics of manipulation were not specified until the Academy offered the first course on mechanics in 1952. A survey of the COP&S Alumni in 1954 supports her perspective, however: only 16% of COP&S alumni used OMT in practice, compared to 53% of Kirksville graduates.

Dr. Frymann explained in her interview with Dr. Seffinger:

[The way] *"they taught manipulation* [at COP&S was that] *the instructor would show 'this is what you do, now go and do that.' You imitated what the instructor did. That was how it was taught. And sometimes it was somewhat traumatic. In trying to imitate they didn't give you a clue as to how much force you were supposed to put on. And so for years I had recurrent rib problems because of those courses on manipulation."*

Dr. Seffinger:

"Was it primarily the high velocity low amplitude?"

Dr. Frymann:

> *"That was all. There was nothing else. Nobody knew anything else. Well, the president of the school, Henley, he was troubled by the fact that these rumors kept coming back to him that his graduates couldn't do osteopathic manipulation. And so in onset of this he decided every student would give him an osteopathic manipulation before they graduate. He started at the beginning of the alphabet. Before he got through B's, he's given up that one. He didn't think he was going to survive the core class. But that was his token effort to prove that his students could do manipulation."*

Still much later, at the "Hearings on Restoration of Osteopathic Licensure" held in Santa Barbara on December 2, 1966, Dr. Frymann recalled that prior to the merger in 1962 *"there were many osteopathic physicians who were not using osteopathic manipulation. That was perhaps one of the reasons why the merger was able to take place . . . ."* Again on page 26 of that document, Dr. Frymann stated *"at the L.A. County Osteopathic Hospital it specifically stated in the standing orders that patients who had been delivered of a baby should receive an osteopathic treatment every day while in the hospital. This was not done . . . then it took the turn that COP&S did not teach osteopathic manipulation and that's why many D.O.s did not feel different from M.D.s and thus took the M.D. degree."*

Recollecting specialty training during the 1950s

The oral histories emphasize the importance of teachers and leaders in the various specialties who served as mentors to aspiring osteopaths in the 1950s. Especially COP&S alumni were supporting the students, be it with loans, or individual tutoring on difficult course content, or psychosocial nurturing. There were at least 30 alumni in the 1950s who as osteopathic specialists mentored students interested in their respective field.

The following persons were mentioned by this study's oral historians for their teaching and mentoring activities in their respective specialties:

Orthopedics: ***Dr. M. Henry*** *was a great teacher, later followed by Dr. Hopps.*

Ear, Nose, and Throat: ***Dr. T.J. Ruddy*** *was a co-founder of the Los Angeles College of Osteopathy in 1905, had a modern office in a tall office building on Wilshire and Western, taught lunch seminars in the Hollywood area and was seen as a prime mover in education.*

Dr. Ulansey:

> *"**Dr. T. J. Ruddy** was one of my professors in ears, nose and throat. A little story goes with him. T. J. Ruddy developed a procedure which we called the Ruddy finger treatment. This consisted of putting the operator's finger into the fossa of Rosenmuller through the mouth and manipulating that fossa.*

Actually what we did I think was to stretch and tear adhesions that existed there. It had a very profound affect. It seemed to help hearing. It helped a number of headache syndromes, head and neck problems, perhaps even more general than that, body problems. It was a very interesting experience learning from him who loved to teach, imparting his knowledge and experiences."

Obstetrics: ***"Dr. Dooley*** *was excellent and* ***Dr. Dorothy Marsh*** *was an outstanding teacher with her contributions to students."*

Dr. Golanty:

"I recall one doctor in particular, ***Richard Eby, D.O.****, an OB/GYN specialist, who taught a terrific class in obstetrics. He owned a hospital in Pomona. He was the advisor to the Psi Sigma Alpha honor society. I even went to his home for dinner when I was elected to it. At that time we had no idea that he would be involved with bringing osteopathic medicine and education back to California after the merger."*

Surgery: *"In the early years* **Dr. J. Willoughby Howe** *performed chest and heart surgery before anyone else. Then came* **Dr. McDowell** *in Norwalk who was a senior surgeon and on call as trainer."* Dr. Frymann was impressed by **Gordon Hatfield, D.O.**, a surgeon who taught her to look at the whole person.

Pediatrics: *"**Dr. Betsy MacCracken** and **Dr.Trendle** were excellent".*

Dr. Grace Bell was Dean in 1960. She was professor of biochemistry and provided extra opportunities for students to learn. She made students aware of the importance of nutrition in whole person care and published several papers on nutrition starting in the January issue of 1935 of *Clinical Osteopathy.* She was also an important role model for female students. In spite of the non-discriminating student enrollment policy and co-ed faculty at COP&S, Dr. Bell was the first and only female dean. When COP&S became an M.D. granting institution, the California College of Medicine, Dr. Bell became the first female Interim Dean of an American Medical School as well.

Dr. Golanty:

"Chemistry was taught by a fantastic individual. She was the Dean of the school, Grace Bell, D.O., and Grace Bell was an unbelievable professor of biochemistry. After having biochemistry in undergrad school taught by non-physicians, this was a real interesting class to me because I was learning biochemistry as it applied toward patients that we cared for in medicine and she, being the physician to teach it that way, was a fantastic individual. Dr. Bell subsequently was known as the first female Dean of an American allopathic medical school; this was a result of the amalgamation that occurred in 1962.

And if I'm not mistaken there is a chair and/or some edifice left behind at UC—Irvine right now in Grace Bell's name. I'm not sure, you'd have to check out what the honor is to her, but the school clearly recognizes her at Irvine as a medical school Dean."

Once osteopathy was recognized as fully licensed and equal to allopathy, enthusiasm and leadership became the hallmarks of the osteopathic profession in California. Counter forces from traditional medicine arose, lest the allopathic dominance might become impaired. Barriers against the practice of osteopathy, such as denying staff privileges and residency training opportunities, became increasingly frustrating to D.O.s. While many, if not most D.O.s tried to work within the confinement, efforts were made to set antagonism aside and to join forces under one umbrella for healthcare.

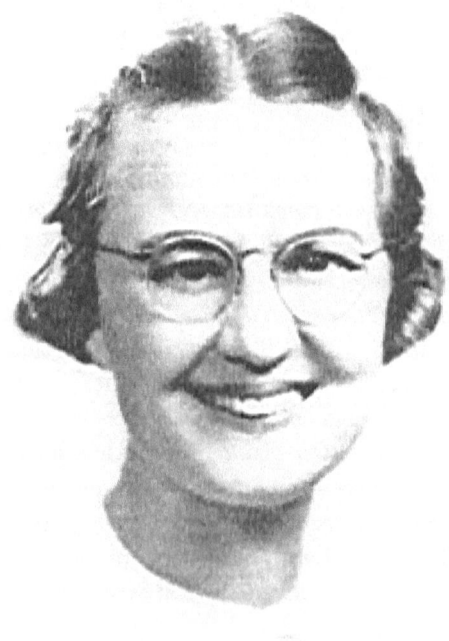

Figure 10. "Dean Grace Bell, D.O., early 1950s"

Chapter 4

Leading to a merger

After 50 years of segregated—with occasional side-by-side—practice of allopathic and osteopathic medicine in California, the leaders of the state osteopathic association seemed willing to forego its separate and self-proclaimed unique contributions to the healing arts in order to be acknowledged and respected by allopathy. Even though osteopathy had obtained the legal recognition of a fully licensed medical profession, the facts that many D.O.s were barred from consulting with M.D. specialists in hospitals and from admitting their patients to hospitals with specialized care, led some members in the osteopathic leadership to suggest a merger with the state allopathic profession. They saw this as a way to improve access of practice affiliation which would ultimately lead to *improved healthcare* for patients.

Given the constant barriers against the practice and growth of the osteopathic profession, the best solution seemed to be to join forces with allopathy under one professional umbrella. The allopathic profession suggested that since they could not regulate the osteopathic educational system or their hospitals, there were likely two standards of patient care being provided. They argued that a unification would create a single standard of education and patient care.

This potential solution to easing the professional tensions found increasing support when one of the pioneers of osteopathy in California unexpectedly died in 1938. Carle Phinney, D.O. died in office as president of COP&S. As will be shown in this chapter, Dr. Phinney was the last president of COP&S who was an osteopathic physician and supporter of the profession's ideal to function "separate but equal", expressed at the helm of this institution.

Administrative changes at COP&S

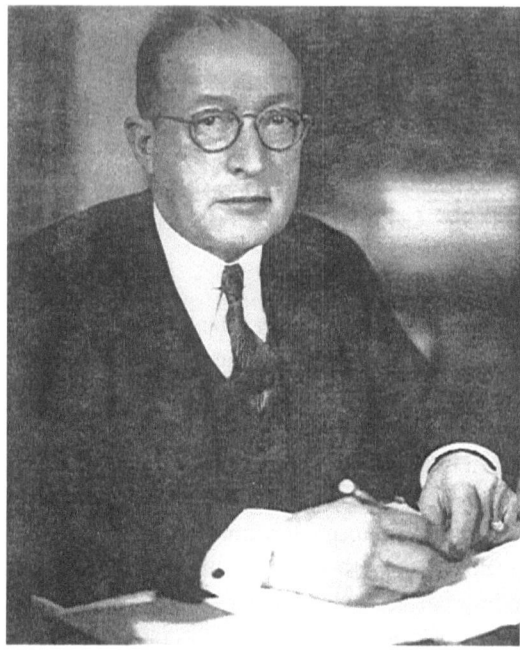

Figure 11. "Carle Phinney, D.O., 1938"

Carle H. Phinney, D.O., president of COP&S from 1936 to 1938, passed away in office at the age of 61. A Los Angeles local newspaper, the *Eagle Rock Sentinel,* reported that hundreds of his friends and acquaintances paid their last tribute to his memory. Pall bearers included many a renowned osteopathic physician in the profession's history: Earnest Bashor, Louis Chandler, Dain Tasker, L. van H. Gerdine, and W.W. Pritchard.

The College newspaper *Tenaculum* praised Dr. Phinney for his untiring and invaluable service to his profession for 37 years, despite the handicap of a serious heart ailment. Dr. Phinney and his wife, Myrtle Phinney, D.O. had been among the pioneers who helped to establish osteopathy in California. Carle Phinney came from Illinois to Los Angeles in 1899 to study osteopathy at PSO. In those early years, PSO offered a 2-year curriculum and Dr. Phinney obtained his D.O. degree in 1901. His wife to be, Myrtle Hemstreet, graduated a year later. PSO also conferred the degrees of D.Sc.O. and M.D. on Carle Phinney for his extra work and study—an example of the College's authority in the early 1900s to confer the M.D. degree.

Dr. Willoughby Howe, in his eulogy at the funeral services at the College Auditorium, expressed the mourners' feelings about Carle Phinney when he said *"Dr. Hopps, his son-in-law, told me that his little 6-year old grandson said what has been in all minds, "He was too young to die ".* It was this grandson, Dr. Harvey Hopps, a chemist, who maintained for the family a collection of newspaper clips about Dr. Phinney's passing as well as notes about the Phinney family tree, going back to 1631 when "Mother Finney" arrived at Plymouth Rock. These documents were donated recently to the Archival Collection at the library of the University of California, Irvine, through the facilitation of Dolores Grunigen.

Finding a new president for COP&S

In looking for a replacement in the office of the president, various options were debated both at the school, among the alumni and at the California Osteopathic Association. It was the function of the Board of Trustees, though, to elect the school's president.

Like most medical schools in the early 1900s, COP&S until 1919 had a Board of Trustees. The Board of COP&S was composed of osteopathic physicians. To avoid conflict of interest with the not-for-profit policy of the college, physicians on the Board of Trustees were replaced over the years by non-medical citizens. The president, thus, not only had to connect well with the academic expectations of the college but also with those of the lay community. The Board of Trustees had an advisory committee that provided a medical perspective. Several members of the advisory committee were also members of the COA, meaning they were osteopathic physicians. Forest Grunigen, D.O. was one of these advisory committee members in 1939 when the Board of Trustees searched for a new president.

As potential candidates from nearby institutions were considered, the idea was expressed, by Dr. Grunigen and others, to merge COP&S with the medical school of the University of Southern California (USC), whose faculty ran Unit I at the Los Angeles County Hospital. Improved relations between M.D.s and D.O.s by way of merging the two schools would have helped greatly with potential opportunities for internship and residency training of COP&S graduates at Unit I of the Los Angeles County Hospital. As mentioned earlier, segregated hospitals and the concomitant exclusion of D.O.s from staff privileges at larger facilities, like Unit I, caused ever increasing feelings of frustration among members of the osteopathic leadership and practicing osteopathic physicians.

USC medical school had been closed for a decade until 1928, but since then, faculty and students began once again to care for the impoverished Los Angeles community in Unit I. Although COP&S graduates were accepted as interns alongside USC graduates between 1916 and 1921 at the Los Angeles County Hospital, the American College of Surgeons withheld accreditation of the USC residency programs at Los Angeles County Hospital in 1928 when it learned that the osteopathic unit was connected by an underground tunnel, used by housekeeping staff. Accreditation was not restored until 1936 when a separate, more up to date and much larger building was built, with sufficient distance from Unit II to prevent any possible connection with the osteopathic physicians and no possibility of sharing patient care. It had to be clearly demonstrated that there was no collusion between the two professions at the county facility to receive accreditation (USC archives, *History of Los Angeles County Hospital(1878-1968) and the Los Angeles County—University of Southern California Medical Center (1968-1978)*, by Helen Eastman Martin, M.D.; Los Angeles, USC Press, 1979).

Relations between USC and COP&S were not close as a result of this imposed sanction but had become firmly re-established when the possibility of a merger between the allopathic and osteopathic colleges was discussed in 1939. The school also liked the idea of granting the M.D. degree and had scholars from other universities evaluate the school to compare it to other M.D. schools (Dain Tasker, chapter 55). This would, of course, increase competition with USC medical school. Given the close proximity between COP&S, the Los Angeles County General Hospital, and USC medical school, collaboration rather than competition in medical education and training prompted merger initiatives. While the negotiations eventually lost momentum, the Board of Trustees of COP&S recruited Ballentine Henley, JD from the cabinet of the President at USC as their new president in 1940, thus keeping a link to the idea of merging with allopathy.

W. Ballentine Henley, JD was the first President of the school who was not an osteopathic physician. Instead, he was recognized for his skills in public relations. He had been a member of the Dean's cabinet of USC and on the staff of the President, Dr. von Kleinschmidt. According to the recollections of Warren Bostick, M.D., President Henley provided strong links to the world of finance, industry, education and the professions in Los Angeles. He was a member of the Los Angeles downtown club of Rotary International whose membership included many local key leaders. His term in office was to extend for longer than any of his predecessors, from 1940 to 1964, and as provost until 1968.

The added M.D. degree as a venue to recognition

The Alumni Association of COP&S provided further strengthening of the liaison between COP&S and the Los Angeles community with the goal to be recognized as equal partner in meeting people's healthcare needs. In 1940, the Association had about 500 members (membership fee per year was $1!). Their publication was *The Western Alumnus*, *"a recognized organ of news merit by the profession"* (Editor's notes, 6-14-1940). In a section, called "The Field", all members were invited to submit thoughts and ideas regarding any subject of interest to the Alumni Association.

In June 1940, **Paul McCracken, D.O.**, President of the COP&S Alumni Association at that time (and no relation to Frank or Betsy MacCracken), submitted a piece entitled *"The old order changeth"* in which he stated *"The original stimulus responsible for our birth and growth is no longer present."* He suggested that allopathic physicians at their better institutions, especially in the orthopedic and physical therapy divisions, had recognized the role of structural therapy. Osteopathic physicians had expanded their teachings and actions to include all modern therapeutic measures. *"Thus, the combination of Allopathy and Osteopathy makes the complete physician"*, he stated. Yet, government had not continued to be supportive of osteopathic medicine. The government provided subsidy of allopathic medical practice and control of institutions, threatening the welfare of osteopathic physicians. As an example he cited the unwillingness of the War Department to recognize the D.O. degree in the Armed Forces.

Dr. McCracken reminded his colleagues of the late 19th century when allopathic medicine was unaware that medicine needed to change to a newer understanding of the healing arts. Similarly, osteopathy needed to become aware of the threats to its economic survival. He presented five urgent reasons for COP&S to provide an additional M.D. degree. He pointed out:

1. COP&S graduates have met the requirements of the Medical Practice Act of the state of California which has been accepted by the Federal Government.
2. COP&S was chartered to not only issue the D.O. but also the M.D. degree.
3. The additional M.D. degree would improve eligibility for Government Armed Forces requirements; he recognized that the AMA might not recognize the added M.D. degree but thought that resistance a lesser hurdle.
4. Business through private practice was rapidly being strangled through government controlled business.
5. The added M.D. degree would open doors to many hospitals that at that time only accepted M.D.s.

Professor of Biochemistry, Grace Bell, D.O., President-elect of the Alumni Association in 1939, replied by providing a detailed response that listed the barriers to obtaining equality:

1. An amendment would be required to the Medical Practice Act in order to use the M.D. degree.
2. COP&S would need to be approved by the respective allopathic agency.
3. Further studies might have to be offered to meet allopathy's requirements (she reminded her colleagues that COP&S required 2 years of further study for M.D.s who wanted to obtain the D.O. degree; surely, allopathy would have similar if not more stringent requirements).
4. Allopathy might not respect the osteopathic specialty training and allopathically controlled hospitals might continue to refuse staff privileges even to physicians with a dual degree.
5. This degree-granting process might have to be specific to California, as osteopathic colleges in other states in the U.S. might not want to provide the M.D. degree.
6. COA's relationship with the AOA would be affected; might the COA have to secede from the AOA?
7. Would COP&S have to be transformed into an allopathic and osteopathic college? Would the Medical Board of California and the AMA recognize a converted college?
8. Would the AMA permit that teaching osteopathic principles and methods be continued?

Dr. Bell thus recognized the limitations of an added M.D. degree and listed with astounding foresight the steps to be taken for an M.D. degree that would be recognized.

Preparing for a merger with allopathy

Forest Grunigen, D.O. saw the situation similarly. In **1941** Dr. Grunigen, by now a member of the Board of Trustees of the COA, announced that he would run for presidency of the COA, with the objective to organize an official committee to effect a merger. Dr. Grunigen was elected president of the COA and served from **1943 to 1944**.

In **1943**, the **Fact Finding Committee** of the COA was established, with Dr. Grunigen as chair. Once he completed his presidency, Dr. Grunigen continued his work toward a merger. The Fact Finding Committee met with a special committee of the medical profession chaired by Burrell O. Raulston, MD, Professor of Medicine and Dean of the University of Southern California Medical School. Dr. Raultson and Dr. Grunigen were successful at obtaining consensus about steps to be taken by the deans of the three medical schools in California and the osteopathic college and the COA.

Dr. Raulston reported the conclusions of his committee to the AMA Council of Education and Hospitals and to the Association of American Medical Colleges. Both organizations approved the recommendations of the Raulston committee for merger. (*Doctors of Medicine and Doctors of Osteopathy in California,* by Kisch and Viseltear, 1967, page15). They were not accepted, though, by either of the national associations, the AMA or the AOA. Thus, for the time being, merger negotiations were discouraged at the national level.

The COA House of Delegates recommended that "the constituted authorities of the COA and the COP&S be instructed to direct their efforts in a vigorous, aggressive manner toward qualifying the D.O. degree for full and complete recognition on a par with the holders of any other degree". Many students and California D.O.s agitated, though, for the M.D. degree. In November 1947, the AOA was made aware that the senior class of COP&S wrote a letter demanding a change in the name of their college and the M.D. degree to be granted instead of the D.O. degree. They argued that it was no longer a college of osteopathy and that osteopathy was only an adjunct in the curriculum.

The osteopathic physicians in general practice continued to suggest the added M.D. degree as a venue to gain staff privileges in all hospitals and admission to the Armed Forces as physicians. As described in Chapter 3, several Los Angeles D.O.s had developed a college, called Metropolitan University, which granted the M.D. degree to D.O.s.

A commission was established by the COA House of Delegates under the leadership of **Louis Chandler, D.O**. to promote communication on this topic. It was made up of four D.O.s from both sides of the issue, and was to "weigh, study, and explore all phases, causes, effects, and results of the granting of the dual degrees, M.D., D.O., by the COP&S to all past, present and future graduates thereof and then to transmit its findings and recommendations to the House of Delegates and to the Board of Trustees of the COP&S at the earliest possible moment . . . ."

Files maintained by Dr. Chandler (presently preserved in the archives of Western University) provide documentation of one of its meetings in February 1949. Commission members had invited representatives from the Fact Finding Committee of the COA, including Dr. Grunigen and Dr. Jenney. They were asked about a statement in the **CMA bulletin, July 1948** that mentioned an active committee of the COA to study the possibility of a merger of medicine and osteopathy in California. Dr. Grunigen described that it had been their first meeting to clarify how to conduct themselves and what methods to follow. Dr. Grunigen and Dr. Atkins had been invited to meet with the CMA Executive Council where Dr. Grunigen had explained that they were not wishing to talk amalgamation but to talk about mutual interests. At the next meeting Dr. Grunigen questioned the publication of discussions about a merger. Dr. Aleson took responsibility and admitted that he did it on his own.

Dr. Jenney pointed out that *"there has never been a meeting in which the definite undercurrent was not amalgamation"*. In each case, the committee's approach was not to forward the question of amalgamation and not to sell the CMA committee on the idea. Dr. Jenney explained that his committee was *"interested only in an M.D. degree which contains all of the necessary and proper ingredients toward the proper respect and carrying on and practicing of our profession."*

Dr. Jenney recalled that comments about amalgamation had always been initiated by the medical members of the committee. He likened the situation to *"the old deal of horse-trading. If we want to buy, we can get amalgamation with them. But it's at a price none of us will pay . . . . on the other hand, if we are not too eager, they'll get to a point where finally we can accept this, with all the glories of battle."*

Also discussed briefly at that meeting was the concern about Metropolitan University and the granting of an M.D. degree to D.O.s. This issue was detailed in the minutes of the AOA House of Delegates held in July 1948. Drs. Grunigen, Cayler, Carroll and Marsh represented the COA as California Delegates and asked the AOA to somehow sanction the D.O.s who took the M.D. degree from that institution. This M.D. degree did not make the holders eligible to sit for state medical licensing exams or enter medical specialty societies. The Metropolitan M.D. degree did enable them, though, to be admitted into post-graduate lectures given by M.D.s. The Metropolitan University M.D.s also incorporated and organized a Pacific Medical Association in order to improve their social, economic, political and educational opportunities.

Dr. Cayler, chair of the COA legislative committee, stated, "It seems to me that the only way to bring this to a conclusion is wherever and whenever any minority group or majority group starts discussions of this kind off the record, that the thing to do is to bring it into the Association and put it on the record and let the various State and National Associations determine what the policy is to be. If, after determining the policy, we find certain members of the profession, as we surely will find, violating these policies, then it seems to me that there is only one thing to do and this is for the specialty boards, the hospital boards, the Associated Colleges, the State Associations, the National Association, all to get tough and take proper disciplinary action. I think we should all be getting mighty tired of seeing members of our profession enjoying all of the rights and privileges which organized osteopathy has fought for and obtained for them, and then see that same group dealing unofficially with members of the old school of practice in an attempt to sabotage the organization which made them. The only way we are going to stop individuals doing things of that kind is to have policies established and regulation established for instituting disciplinary action and then having the courage to take such disciplinary action."

The AOA House of Delegates passed the following resolutions proposed by the California delegates:

"It is unethical for an osteopathic physician to hold forth or to indicate possession of any degree recognized as a basis for licensure to practice the healing art unless the osteopathic physician is actually licensed in the state in which he practices on the basis of that degree or could have been licensed at the time he received the degree or subsequently on the basis of that degree in the state where he now is in practice."

"It is unethical from this date for an osteopathic physician to seek to acquire or to receive a degree from a school or college of the healing arts which degree is not approved by the national professional organization recognized by the Unites States Office of Education as representative of that school or college of the healing arts."

"Every member of the House of Delegates is instructed to file charges against anyone violating this Code of Ethics and instruct the Committee on Ethics and Censorship to file charges before the Board of Trustees."

In light of this national pressure, the Metropolitan University was soon thereafter dissolved.

Wayne Pollock, M.D., who served as chair of the CMA's Committee on Other Professions from the early 1950s through and beyond the merger in 1961, was introduced to the D.O.-M.D. problems on a practical level in 1951 when he was called in as a consultant to the Sacramento Medical Society. He was asked to advise the Society how to cope with a difficult D.O.-M.D. situation in Amador County Hospital. The Amador County Hospital served patients in the vicinity of Amador, CA, a small community 40 miles southeast of Sacramento. When Joseph Cosentino, D.O., a well-respected surgeon in the region since 1946, was admitted to the staff of the Amador County Hospital, two M.D. staff physicians boycotted the hospital and sent their patients to hospitals in Stockton or Sacramento. To fill the void, three other D.O.s joined the staff.

In meeting with the citizens in the region, Dr. Pollock discovered that citizens were perplexed why M.D.s would boycott the hospital when the Hill-Burton Laws specifically stated that such hospitals were to be open to all licensed practitioners (Kisch and Viseltear, 1967, pp.22-23). In response to the insurgence of D.O.s onto staffs at county and federal hospitals, the CMA urged its members to build hospitals with private funds. Ten years later, Drs. Pollock and Cosentino worked together to garner support from CMA and COA members, respectively, in favor of the merger in 1961 and of Proposition 22 in 1962.

Taking the merger concept to the national level

Dr. Grunigen and Vincent Carroll, D.O. from Laguna Beach became active in national osteopathic politics and served on the AOA Board of Trustees through the 1940s.

Dr. Grunigen was first vice president of the Board from 1948-1950 and a member of the Board of Trustees from 1951-1957.

Dr. Carroll was a highly respected physician in southern California and active in community affairs. He was a mentor to many osteopathic physicians, including Dr. Grunigen. He was president of the AOA from 1950-1951 and past-president from 1951-1952. With his leadership he facilitated the U.S. Department of Education's decision to recognize AOA accreditation of medical colleges. This recognition contributed to the profession's increasing reputation and status as an equal partner in healthcare.

Dain Tasker, D.O., the profession's historian, noted that "*Dr. Vincent Carroll of Laguna Beach was elevated to the office of the president of AOA at its 54th Annual Convention in Chicago*". A native of Kirksville in 1904, Dr. Carroll conducted for 18 years a general practice of osteopathic medicine and surgery in Laguna Beach, specializing in general surgery (and he continued his private practice in Laguna Beach as an M.D. after the merger in 1962 until his retirement in 1986). He was past-president of the Orange County Osteopathic Society, past president and member of the osteopathic staff at Santa Ana Community Hospital, a member of the faculty of COP&S in Los Angeles, and past-president of the California State Board of Osteopathic Examiners. By his colleagues Dr. Carroll was perceived as having "*very honestly felt that most of medicine's problems could be solved by these organizations*" (L. E. Potvin, M.D., as quoted in the OCMA Bulletin, February 1987).

Tragically, Dr. Carroll's son, Vincent P. Carroll, was killed as a fourth year medical student in 1962. He had been on his way to present a research paper. To this day, the Committee on Promotions and Honors at the School of Medicine of the University of California Irvine recognizes each year medical student research accomplishments through the Vincent P. Carroll award.

Favoring the merger idea, **John Cline, M.D.** from the California Medical Association became president of the AMA in 1951. Dr. Cline had been a consultant during the COA-CMA merger talks in 1943. He was favorably inclined toward the osteopathic professional organization. Drs. Grunigen, Carroll and Cline continued to promote the idea of a merger at the national level, i.e. between the AMA and the AOA, but the AMA viewed osteopathy as a "cult" that could not be accepted into the folds of the AMA.

Mrs. Dolores Grunigen recalls:

> *"One aspect of the history* [of the M.D.—D.O. relationship] *is the use and rejection of the term "cultist." Dr. Cline's report of 1952 by the AMA stated in part: 'The sole fundamental difference in the teaching of medicine in schools of osteopathy and schools of medicine lies in the degree of emphasis placed on the study of the musculoskeletal system and the application of manipulative therapy . . . . The committee is of the opinion that application of the term 'cultist' to the teaching in the five colleges of osteopathy visited is not justified.' It seems to me that this term was one of the major thorns in the side for osteopaths as it became a part of the report to this national organization."*

Once Dr. Cline had completed his AMA presidency, he chaired a task force to survey the six osteopathic colleges in the U.S. with the objective to investigate signs of the "cult" notion. His group inspected five osteopathic colleges between 1953 and 1955 and reported to the AMA on the status of osteopathic education and whether there was indeed evidence of "cultist" practices. Only one osteopathic college declined to have site visits by Dr. Cline's committee, the Philadelphia College of Osteopathy.

Dr. Taylor recalls:

> *"In 1954 or '55, the Cline committee came to COP&S and one interviewer questioned at random a student in the hall. He said, 'recite the Krebs cycle' and she did. The school passed the grade. Geraldine Dyer was the student. She married Ralph Young, D.O., a pulmonologist, and became a pediatrician."*

Dr. Golanty recalls being informed about the report of the Cline Committee to the AMA:

> *"In my freshman year, we were also told that the American Medical Association had gone through the existing six schools at the time. The six schools were, as you know, Kirksville, Philadelphia, Chicago, Kansas City, Des Moines and California. They published an article based on some research that had been done by some people; I don't know who they were, probably AMA, who had gone to the six schools to look at the curriculums and teaching and said that cultism was not being taught in the school, that the first two years were rather comparable to what they thought were allopathic medical school training, but that the third and fourth year were weak and that they felt that that's where strength was needed to improve the schools. But they did not consider this to be cultism and it was good education otherwise."*

In summary, the **Cline Report to the AMA in 1955** recommended removing the "cult" label that the AMA had imposed upon the osteopathic profession since its inception. The committee had obtained evidence that the curricula of osteopathic colleges were just as science-based as those taught at the M.D. institutions, just with greater emphasis on anatomy and osteopathic manipulation. He recommended that the AMA should allow M.D.s to teach at osteopathic colleges and that the state medical societies should be allowed to determine their own protocol on ethical relations between M.D. and D.O. physicians.

The opinion of a small group won the vote, however. This opinion essentially required for the AOA, COA and COP&S to remove all statements in their literature that related their institutions, philosophy and practices to their founder, Andrew Taylor Still, M.D., D.O. They were asked to disband the term "osteopathy" and "osteopathic" from their courses and statements, before the AMA would consider removing the "cult" label, allow M.D.s to teach at

D.O. schools, or allow D.O.s to share patient care with M.D.s. COP&S and the COA complied with these requirements. COA delegates to the AOA influenced the AOA to do the same.

The Osteopathic Therapeutics Department in COP&S department had already changed its name to the Department of Physical Medicine and Rehabilitation. The desire of the osteopathic profession to have the cult label removed was so strong that even its founding college, then called the Kirksville College of Osteopathy and Surgery in Kirksville, MO, apparently buried a statue of A.T. Still on its campus. Several more years of debate ensued within the AMA until in 1959 the AMA Judicial Council proposed to accept D.O.s as separate and equal in status, because the AOA had changed its constitution, bylaws and policies and had expressed willingness to remove reference to Andrew Taylor Still and "the osteopathic concept" in their literature.

Dr. Golanty:

> "At an AOA meeting in Washington, D.C. at the end of the 1950s that I attended as an honor student, the California Osteopathic Association had put through a resolution asking for the removal of Andrew Taylor Still being the major thing about the osteopathic profession. In essence, the M.D. profession, as we had heard earlier when we were freshman students, felt that the osteopathic profession were cultists. We were cultists because we supposedly, quote unquote, "prayed to the teaching of one man." That's how they defined cultism. So, by saying that we were, in a sense, following everything backed on principles of one person, that was cultism.
>
> By taking out of the preamble of the AOA references like that, it allowed, as I understand it, that the profession was no longer considered "cultist" and therefore the stage was being set for the continuum of what I didn't know what was going on exactly, an amalgamation. I must say retrospectively, before I started the school, there was a lot of rumor going around that something like this was going to happen, an amalgamation of professions. And in our first couple years a lot of the students thought that it was. Many of the students that entered in, as I became a third and fourth year student and an intern, were banking on that idea that they had heard that it was coming."

Warren Bostick, M.D., a delegate from the California Medical Association, did not agree with this proposal and recommended an amendment based on the fact that California D.O.s were willing to give up their identity, their degrees, their school and their state association in exchange for freedom to practice with the same social status and privileges as physicians with an M.D. degree. Dr. Bostick announced that the CMA was in negotiations to amalgamate with the COA and to effect a take-over of COP&S, converting it to an M.D. school. This was the first public statement that such serious talks were occurring, and the AOA was immediately alerted.

Dr. Bostick further argued that the CMA would lose any leverage to get what they wanted if the AMA accepted D.O.s unconditionally. He recommended that M.D.s should be allowed to teach osteopathic students only if that college was in the process of being converted into an approved medical school. He proposed that M.D.s should only associate with those D.O.s who practiced under the same scientific principles as M.D.s and had unlimited licensure. Dr. Bostick's amendment was accepted.

In California, the COA removed language that said "we are a separate, complete and distinctive school of practice" and eliminated the tenets of Andrew Taylor Still as the "things that we follow forever".

Activities at the state level: Senator Stephen Teale, D.O.

Senator Teale of California significantly affected the M.D.-D.O. relationship in his state.

Dr. Steedman recalls that *"Senator Teale was instrumental in getting the L.A. County Osteopathic Hospital built [in 1956-59]"*. Yet, only a few years later Senator Teale supported the merger between California's osteopathic and allopathic professions. Since sparse official records are available on his merger-related activities, the recollections by Jay Michael, M.S. make a great difference in our understanding of Senator Teale.

Jay Michael recalls:

"I was a lobbyist for an organization of California cities when I met Senator Teale in 1957. The office of the League of Cities regularly had a cocktail party for invited people, including Senator Teale. Senators represented three counties. Senator Steven Teale represented El Dorado, Alpine and Mariposa. These were very small but Teale was powerful. Teale was a living God in that part of California. He was a D.O. in Railroad Flat, a small town. There was a very small hospital but it was critical to those people who lived harsh lives, in the mountains and so on.

"Senator Teale had a gigantic sense of civic responsibility. He could make things better. At times it was a great inconvenience to people but he did it anyway. In those days there was "cross-filing" (i.e. file both, for Democrat and Republican). Steven Teale always got cross-filed and was always re-elected by a wide margin.

"The League of California Cities had a "white hat", meaning no stigma. Most were honest legislators, very bright and articulate.

Steven Teale was Chair of the Joint Budget Committee as long as I can remember. It was a critical position. That committee hired and fired positions like a legislative analyst. Alan Post held that position for 35 years. He was an icon, an honest man. Steven Teale and Alan Post were close friends.

"In 1957 I was 25, Steven Teale was about 35, and we got along well. Steven Teale had two drinks at the League and then drove home for 35 minutes, on a winding road into the foothills. The population of his town was about

100. His home and hospital were adjacent. He was on call at night and on the weekends while his wife did the practice during the day. They were the only healthcare resource in the Foothills.

"At that time there was no lobbying arm of the CMA. The Public Health League provided the lobbying. The Public Health League consisted of doctors, nurses and health administrators. The general counsel for that group was 'Hap' Hassard.

"The CMA did not like the idea of the merger but Steven Teale was passionate about the merger. He did not feel so passionate about osteopathy. Steve's passion was to get rid of that distinction. He wanted osteopathy to go away and it was a disappointment to him that not all D.O.s were in favor of the merger.

"Steven Teale went to the CMA to convince them to grant the M.D. degree to the D.O.s. He went to the Public Health League and to the council, the governor, and the CMA. They were not buying it.

"About 1958, Steven Teale decided being 'no more Mr. Nice Guy' and proceeded. He had a proposal that was reasonable to both sides. As Chair of the Budget Committee he told the Regents there would be no UCI unless UCI took the soon to be converted osteopathic medical college and that he had the votes for that decision.

"Steven used his position as Budget Chair, and he had a close relationship with the legislative analyst and with Randolph Collier, Senate Finance Committee chairman . . .

"The healthcare advocacy system broke up between 1961 to '63. Ben Reede who had run the Public Health League was fired and the Public Health League broke up. Until then it had been so powerful that nothing happened unless the Public Health League signed off. In spite of Steven Teale's passion the Public Health League probably would have prevailed with its opposition. But because it broke up Steven Teale was able to succeed.

"The key for it all happening was Teale's high integrity and the respect he was given. His official address was Westpoint, near Railroad Flat. There was a Grange hall and on Saturday nights he played the violin, a fiddle. They played blue grass and Country Western, by ear."

Counselor Hufstedler recalls:

"He [Senator Teale] was a powerful man in the Senate, being the Chairman of the Ways and Means Committee. We had, I think eight legislative measures that had to be passed, a couple of constitution amendments, we had an initiative measure, and then we had several statutory measures. Steve took on the responsibility of dealing with all the folks you needed to, to get the matters organized so it could go through, eventually they all went through by a large majority (you know 90% yes and maybe a vote no here or there) and that was *about it. So he was the guy really responsible for making it easy where it could have been difficult to get all the legislative measures passed to get them on the ballots, and then of course the initiatives and other matters were adopted by the general vote. But he was a very strong man. A great believer in osteopathy and he thought this was good for the profession."*

Dr. Betsy MacCracken recalls about Steven Teale, who she knew even before they went to osteopathic medical school:

" . . . he was a classmate at Fresno State . . . . he walked into class wearing bib overalls, striped blue and white bib overalls . . . and a stalk of unruly blond hair. Well, he came from up there in the mountains . . . I was trying to think actually where he came from . . . I know that his family had been amongst the old timers that came in . . . not with the Donner Party, but I mean that came into that northern area. I knew his wife very well because we had been in school together and she lived in the same house that I lived in, so I knew Barbara very well."

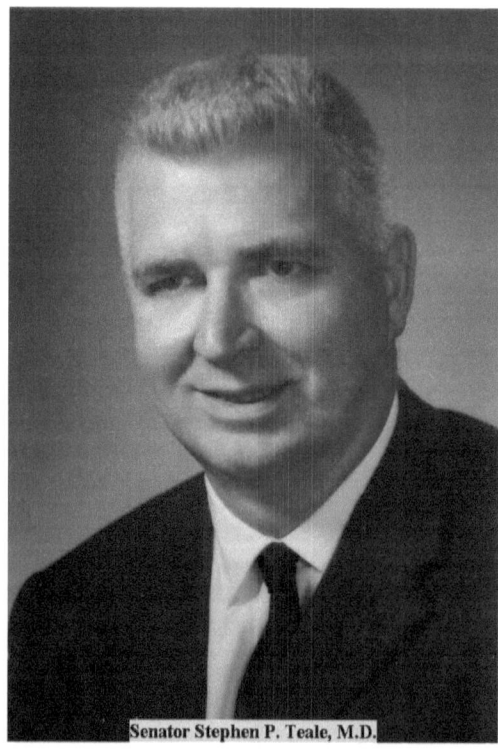
Senator Stephen P. Teale, M.D.

Figure 12. "Senator Stephen Teale, D.O."

Medical education

At the end of the 1950s California's public colleges and universities were growing rapidly. Westward migration and California's low tuition drew many students to campuses. Since the early 1950s enrollment had doubled, and an even larger influx of students was anticipated in the near future. Class sizes were often huge. Dr. Steedman and Dr. Passy attended UCLA at that time. **Dr. Steedman** recalls:

> *"During UCLA's period it was a very difficult time, at that time you had to have a very high grade-point-average, and you had very tough classes—Vic [Dr. Victor Passy] probably remembers because he went to UCLA also, only he was 2 years ahead of me—that in the undergraduate classes it was extremely difficult to pull grades.*
>
> *"This was in 1951 through 1955. At that time the undergraduate courses—as I mentioned—were very difficult, and I recall that one chemistry professor one time—we had about 600 individuals in his classroom he made a comment—'I see everybody's interested in taking this course'—there were about 100 people more than there were seats—then he says 'I thought I'd give a little announcement-he says—before I finish this presentation, there will be enough seats for everyone.' At that time, the doors opened in the back and the hundred people who didn't have a seat, they left and there were enough seats for everyone. So, it was a difficult 2 years."*

At the business level, huge class sizes meant that there was money to be made in education. Indeed, Senator Teale wrote regulations in the 1950s that increased the money set aside for medical education. Additional incentives at the local business level to build colleges and medical schools resulted in strong competition between universities. The University of California took action and by 1958 three new campuses were approved, one in San Diego, one in Orange County, and one in the Santa Cruz area.

Negotiations toward a merger between the two medical professions

A side-by-side practice of medicine of osteopathic and allopathic medicine and equal status for both professions were not the objectives of all leaders at that time. Warren Bostick, M.D. aimed instead toward the dissolution of the osteopathic profession to be brought about by a merger between the CMA and the COA.

In 1959, **Counselor Hufstedler** was assigned to effect the merger and make the situation acceptable to both CMA and COA members by writing legislation, meeting with D.Os. and M.D.s up and down the state, and representing the COA nationally to the AOA to try to effect a national AOA-AMA merger.

One approach to persuade practicing D.O.s to view a merger favorably was to raise fears about their survival, given the fierce academic and medical competition. Heightened anxiety increased many D.O.s' motivation to merge. There were perceived threats of being marginalized if socialized medicine succeeded. **Dr. Ryder** remembers Dr. Marsh's arguments about socioeconomic threats, including rising insurance costs:

> " . . . while I was interning at Long Beach Osteopathic, the California Osteopathic profession had their convention in Long Beach. **Dorothy Marsh** was president that year of the California Osteopathic Association. I can remember her talking at that meeting about the possible amalgamation of the osteopathic profession with the medical profession. I'll paraphrase what I remember her saying. 'Well boys, we are either going to get this amalgamation proceedings underway or we are going to have to forget about it altogether.' At the time everyone in the profession felt that socialized or state medicine was coming and feared the osteopathic profession would not be included in the new state scheme or would be marginalized and our practice would be limited."

In addition, an imminent rise of osteopathic medical education costs at COP&S was given as an argument in favor of the merger.

Dr. Ryder:

> "It was at the 1960 COA meeting that I remember Dorothy Marsh giving the primary reason for joining with the medical profession. To paraphrase her, "We really have to do this because we don't have the funds to support COP&S because medical education is becoming more and more expensive." I think in 1951 or '52 the California Osteopathic Association increased their dues $400.00 a year to help support the college. It seems like a small fee, but $400.00 was a lot of money in 1951 dollars."

Fears were also being raised about losing hospital staff privileges if one remained a D.O.

Dr. Frymann:

> " . . . this was really what was behind it and the CMA made it look very attractive. They were going to give them privileges, they were going to accept the specialists into their midst, all this sort of thing.
>
> "One of the stipulations they made was that you would not be able to serve on the hospital staff if you didn't get your M.D. degree. And they used T.J. Ruddy as their demonstration. T.J. Ruddy was on the staff of I believe seven different hospitals and he really adamantly refused to have anything to do with

this business and so they fired him from all those hospitals but he was in his 80s. He was retired; it didn't bother him, but they used this as a demonstration to all the other D.O.s that if you don't get your M.D. degree, you won't serve on the hospital staff. And unfortunately these young D.O.s weren't smart enough to realize that if 50% of the hospital staff had refused to get their M.D. degree, the hospital couldn't operate. And so they could have stopped it right there but they didn't and so that was one of the major devices they used."

Apparently, many D.O.s felt pressured to merge. **Dr. Ryder** recalls: *"I felt I had no choice, the M.D. was foisted on us."*

Dr. Taylor:

> *"I didn't want the merger but felt pressured to get an M.D. degree. I felt if I maintained my D.O. degree I wouldn't graduate from the residency. I needed to graduate. I discussed it with my wife and she felt it was better to go along with the majority, both economically and socially. She was working and if I could get a well-paying job, she could stop working. With the M.D. degree I was able to get into more doors; more doors opened to me."*

Dr. Grace Bell recalled the feelings of John Bell, D.O., her husband, in an interview she gave in 1977 at age 80 at UCI:

> *"I was in somewhat an awkward position. I was married to a man who was violently opposed to this thing* [the merger] *and yet he went along with it because he realized it was the only thing he could do in order to go on with his profession. In this light, the term profession meant being a physician."*

Positive anticipations also increased the D.O.s' motivation to merge, including anticipation of better opportunities to train as specialists. **Dr. Taylor** recalled, though, the difficulties in obtaining recognition as a specialist due to the merger were significant:

> *"There was a problem. Not being accepted by the D.O. Specialty Boards, after COA and CMA merged; and since I took my M.D. degree the AOA would not accept my application for certification."*

On a personal level, the hope for an end to discrimination and hurt feelings played an important role among osteopathic physicians in looking favorably at the merger. Dr. Ryder recalls that *"M.D.s never acknowledged referrals and never referred to D.O.s."* The anticipation of improved hospital privileges and communication with M.D.s increased a support of the merger among D.O.s in the community.

Some osteopathic physicians took the merger as a given.

Dr. Betsy MacCracken:

"You really didn't think about it too much. It was just sort of, well this is the way the tides are going; certainly Dad [Frank MacCracken, D.O.] *did it without any compulsion. He said this is the way the tide is going. It's not going to affect the way I practice and it's probably the political thing to do."*

Others became upset when they heard about efforts to merge.

Dr. Frymann:

"I started practice in La Jolla and centered on practicing osteopathy. The first hint that we got that something wasn't quite right was when there was a report in the L.A. Times about the convention of the California Osteopathic Association stating that negotiations were in progress to bring about an amalgamation with the CMA. That came out through the newspaper.

"At that time there was a support through dues. You had to pay with your dues a hundred dollars, I think it was a year to support the college and so I wrote to the college and I said I had no intention of paying to support the college if it was on the way to becoming an M.D. profession . . . We had the San Diego County Osteopathic Association which was suddenly very pro-medical. They didn't do manipulation, they didn't believe in doing it."

Osteopathic physicians who were practicing in communities, without involvement in their profession's political activities, might have sensed quite some secrecy about working out the details of the merger. Were there times when meetings were held in private to work things out?

Counselor Hufstedler:

"I'm not sure that you are right to say [there was] *a secrecy and under-the-table. It's true that we weren't out there announcing what we did every day. You can't conduct negotiations that way. I have negotiated all sorts of transactions. I remember I sold a dog food company once to National Can. You don't go out and tell everybody what you are doing. You may have to under FCC disclosures, if you are dealing with a stock company and that sort of thing. But the worst thing you can do is to go out and outline all the series of negotiations publicly while you are underway. The world doesn't work that way."*

Dr. Seffinger:

"Okay, that's good that you give us your insight because right now all the history books are saying that they don't know how those negotiations occurred other than they were in secrecy and all that sort of thing. I think they are missing perhaps the professionalism behind all this that you may be able to give us an insight towards, so that we understand it better."

Counselor Hufstedler:

"I must say, you know, it's been a long time ago and maybe I am misremembering, but I have no recollection at the time of anybody complaining that these were serious secret or under-the-table negotiations. I have no recollections of that."

On July 17, 1960 the AOA House of Delegates heard the **presentation by COA** and resolved that any state society entering negotiations with another profession concerning unification or merger would be subject to possible revocation of its charter by AOA.

Counselor Hufstedler:

"Fortunately, I was just a lawyer. You know you put a lawyer in with a bunch of doctors and they are not going to pay attention to a lawyer. We went back to the AOA convention at a time when it was coming to a head. That was the Kansas City Convention, I think, in 1959 [actually in 1960].

" . . . . much to the surprise to the California delegation, the chairman of the AOA, the president, I guess it was, made a speech talking about how terrible it was to have this merger and how California, if it went ahead, was going to get kicked out. They eventually had an executive session of a couple of hours or so where the matter was discussed fully by the California M.D.s as well as the California D.O.s—Dorothy Marsh primarily for the D.O.s. The net result was that the AOA didn't buy it."

"I guess in the long run it didn't matter [whether the AOA was supportive or not]. *The D.O.s in California didn't want to offend or damage the D.O.s in the rest of the country. In fact, they thought it would be helpful if the D.O.s in the rest of the country would get together with them and do the same thing which was a possibility at that point because they had the large share of the medical profession here in California and it was willing to support it. But the AOA was determined that they were not going to have it."*

Dr. Frymann:

"I was in Kansas City at the time the AOA forced the California delegation to explain what they were doing in California. They resisted, it was a very intensive battle on the floor and finally they were forced to come out and reveal that they already had a fully developed contract which they were prepared to sign with the California Medical Association. Nobody had any idea that these rumors were actual facts at that time. And the AOA gave them an ultimatum at that point, this probably was about July, July was when the House of Delegates met, that by the end of the year, the California Osteopathic Association must give a statement to the AOA that they were through with this that they had nothing more to do with this or they would lose their charter. I think it was 1960."

On November 13, 1960 the COA House of Delegates in a special session voted 66-40 to **continue talks with CMA** despite a plea by the AOA president and the earlier warning that continuation would jeopardize the COA's standing.

Dr. Frymann:

" . . . then the California Osteopathic Association called a special meeting of their House of Delegates and the way this was arranged it was, you might say, a preplanned decision before it was ever done, each divisional society had one delegate to ten members. In San Diego here, I think we had ten delegates and the delegates were either pro merger or opposed to the merger, but the voting was such that if a majority, and majority might mean one, voted for a merger then all five delegates were put in as pro merger. It was not proportionate to the vote. This was done in all the divisional societies and that's how they got a 90% vote in favor of merging."

A week later the AOA Board of Trustees in a special session **revoked the charter of COA.** Russell M. Husted, D.O. and member of the Board of Trustees of the AOA since 1956 lost his membership status. California's D.O.s were now on their own, without organizational support and status at the national level.

Dr. Ulansey:

"When the merger was just in the talking stage, our AOA, our esteemed association, became incensed by the idea that we would dare to discuss any of the problems that we had locally, which were malpractice,

the testifying of the two groups against each other; and the problems with Medicare/MediCal. These were of essential importance to us. In a dictatorial fashion, after the AOA heard of our discussions, and there were only discussions at that time between the two professions, they said, 'cease and desist.'

"Well, that was a red flag, the flag went up with the D.O.s overwhelmingly; I believe it was some 2,000, overwhelmingly rebelled. I say rebelled against the dictatorial statement and threat which the AOA did enact. They took away all of our certifications. We were Board certified, a great number of us. They took it away from us! Just absolutely took it away! The D.O.s were incensed. Now this cost the AOA eventually 2,000 members who left them with bitterness; bitterness not because of the merger itself, but it was because they were ordered to cease and desist."

Dr. Dorothy Marsh had long been playing a crucial role. Dr. Marsh was president of COA when the merger began and gave the decisive presentation at the AOA House of Delegates. While several women have been outstanding leaders and clinicians in osteopathy, Dr. Dorothy Marsh stood out among them.

Mrs. Grunigen recalls:

"She was acknowledged by the City of Los Angeles as one of the most prolific obstetricians in the City. She delivered, I don't know how many, thousands of babies. She was acknowledged for that. She practiced in Glendale most of her career. She had a lot of accolades given to her because of her long standing and her length of practice. She practiced for, I don't know, 40 or 50 years. She had a wonderful quality about her . . . . She had a lot of insight into why she wanted to be a D.O. It was very difficult for her to make the choice as to give up her D.O. degree to become an M.D., and being president of the California Osteopathic Association she did have to make a decision. So it took a lot of inner strength to make that decision. She had a hard time doing it. I know she did . . . She had to be convinced it was the right thing to do, that's for sure."

As president of the COA, Dorothy Marsh, D.O. signed the merger agreement with Paul Foster, M.D., President of the CMA, acting as "CMA Council" on March 29,1961. The agreement was approved by the CMA House of Delegates on May 3, 1961 (by a vote of 296 for vs. 63 against), and by the COA House of Delegates (100 for vs. 10 against) on May 17, 1961.

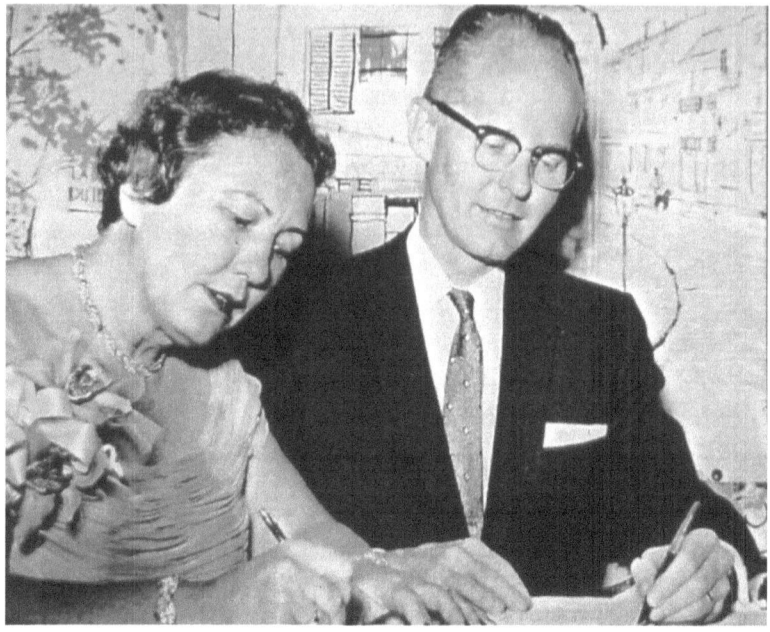

Figure 13. "Dorothy Marsh, D.O. and Warren Bostick, M.D.,
May 17, 1961, signing the merger agreement"

Dorothy Marsh, D.O. signed the merger agreement once again, this time with newly elected CMA President Warren Bostick, M.D. on May 17, 1961 after both, the CMA and the COA, House of Delegates approved the agreement.

Counselor Hufstedler:

"Dorothy Marsh . . . she was a wonderful woman. She knew about as much about that [the merger] *as anybody. You have Bostick's book, Bostick was involved from the beginning in all of those things.*

" . . . . it was really a remarkably good bunch of people. They were dealing with a very hard problem. I don't have to tell you how emotional the problem is of dealing with the potential differences and similarities of the medical profession and the osteopathic profession. The professional associations seemed to be a focus for the more difficult problems. The individuals got along a lot better than the associations did.

"But the people, both in the CMA and the COA at that point, I thought were a very high caliber people. So the best way to work this out was by approaching it from a high level point of view, not some narrow political advantage for either side. I thought the people on the CMA side were fair, and the kind of people you wanted to negotiate with. We had a lot of things to negotiate and

work out. I thought the people who primarily handled it on the CMA side were remarkably good. Dr. Cayler was kind of the grandparent for this entire plan, I think, long before I got there. Fory Grunigen had taken over, really, much of the ideological direction. Dorothy Marsh came in as president. She was a very bright and vigorous person to carry this forward. They had a very good combination of people."

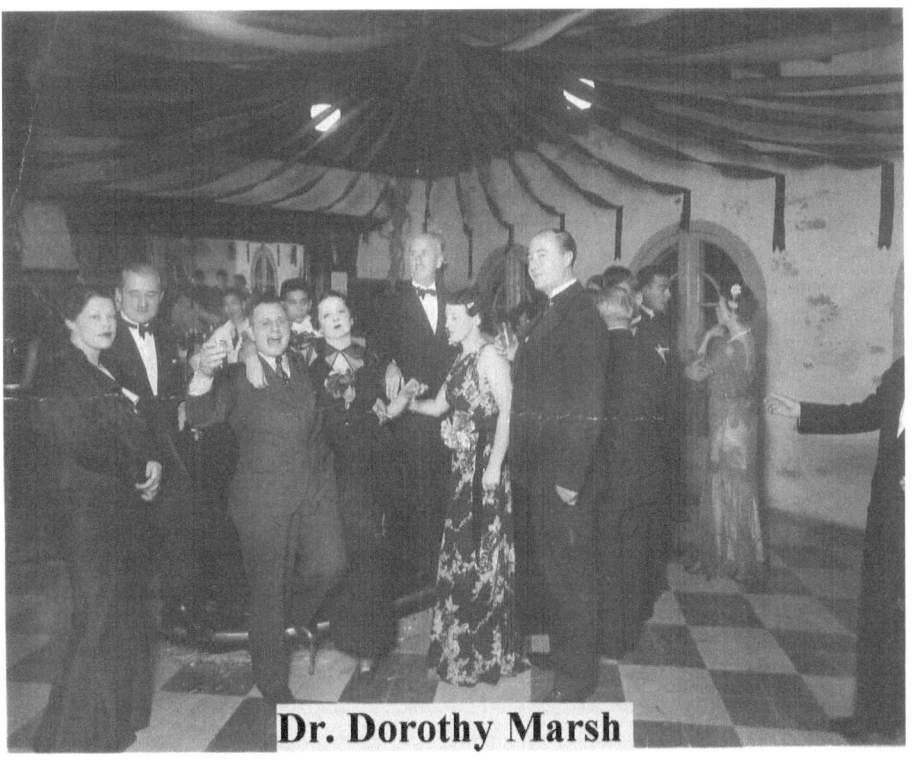

Figure 14. "Dorothy Marsh, D.O. (center) at an earlier stage of her career: COA Convention in Coronado, 1930s"

Chapter 5

Coping with the merger: 1960s to 1980s

California so far has been the only state in the U.S. where a merger agreement was signed between the professional organizations of osteopathic and allopathic medicine. Developing these agreements required close attention to the Constitutions and Bylaws of the California Medical Association, as adopted May 15, 1951. Some of the bylaws were amended during April of 1962 to facilitate the merging process. The principles of medical ethics of the American Medical Association also guided this process, as they comprise the standards by which physicians determine the propriety of their conduct not only in their relationship with patients but also with colleagues and members of allied professions.

The primary objectives of the merger agreement had to express the anticipation of improved healthcare and education for Californians, as those were the objectives of the California State government. Excerpts of the agreement are provided below in italic print:

The merger agreement

*"This Agreement is made and entered into this ___ day of **May, 1961**, by and between the California Medical Association, an unincorporated association, hereinafter sometimes called **the 'CMA'** and the California Osteopathic Association, a California corporation, hereinafter sometimes called **the 'COA',** to be effective at the time, and upon the terms and conditions as hereinafter set forth below.*

"A. General.

1. *Purposes. This agreement is made and entered into **for the primary purposes of improving the health services available to the citizens of the State of California, and expanding medical teaching facilities in the State.** The 'Governor's Committee on the Study of Medical Aid and Health' has urged immediate expansion of 'medical educational capacity in private and public institutions' and the establishment of new medical schools. These purposes are to be further accomplished by the unification, consonant with the desires of*

individual practicing physicians within the State of California, of the separate organizations which have heretofore existed in parallel structure in the State of California for the practice of medicine and surgery by persons who hold the degree of Doctor of Osteopathy and those who hold the degree of Doctor of Medicine. By accomplishing such unification, the parties hereto intend to remove any distinction among the individuals practicing medicine and surgery that is not related to skill and ability, to make available to the public at large efficient and adequate hospital facilities, and to improve the educational facilities available for those persons engaged in the practice of medicine and surgery. It is also a primary purpose of the parties hereto that upon the students at the present College of Osteopathic Physicians and Surgeons in Los Angeles or its successor becoming eligible to be licensed by the State Board of Medical Examiners, no new or additional physician and surgeon's certificates shall thereafter be issued by the State Board of Osteopathic Examiners, whether applied for under Articles 5, 6 or 11 of Chapter 5, Division 2, of the California Business and Professions Code. It is not the purpose of any party to this agreement to alter or diminish in any way the practice rights of individual physicians, or to limit their opportunity of future practice.

*"2. **Execution and effective date**. Upon approval of this agreement by the governing boards of the respective parties hereto, this agreement shall be executed by the Chairman of such board and its Secretary. Said signatures shall indicate the approval of that board only.*

"This agreement shall become binding and effective when it has been ratified by the House of Delegates of each of the parties hereto, in accordance with the appropriate rules and regulations of each respective organization.

"The parties hereto recognize and acknowledge that the consummation of this agreement will require certain amendments to be made to the constitution of the CMA, and that the constitution requires that a proposed amendment, after introduction, lay on the table for a period of one year prior to its final adoption and effectiveness. This agreement, however, shall become effective upon its initial ratification by both houses as above set forth, subject only to the conditions hereinafter set forth.

*"3. **Reference to COA**. As hereinafter provided, the COA agrees to change its name, and may in the course of the transition period change its organic structure. References to COA shall thus include such organization, although its name shall be changed, and its organic structure may be changed."*

In Schedule B, matters related to the structure of California Medical Association were spelled out, including **chartering a new component society**, and the COA agreeing to change its name to the **Forty-First Medical Society**. The dissolution of COA involved for all its members to become members of their respective county medical societies as soon as possible. *"However, such arrangement requires the consent of each of the* *respective county medical societies. When the county medical societies throughout the State of California agree to take into membership in the respective appropriate county medical society each of the members of such society, it shall be dissolved. Upon such dissolution, all of the assets then remaining of such society shall, so far as is legally possible, be transferred and conveyed to the College of Osteopathic Physicians and Surgeons, or its successor."*

Schedule C delineated the practice of medicine and use of the M.D. degree. **Schedule D** explained Statutory Amendments, including the use of the degree, the function of the Boards of Examiners, and amending the Initiative Act that had established the Board of Osteopathic Examiners.

Schedule E spelled out the requirements for the College of Osteopathic Physicians and Surgeons, including the name change, *"so that neither the word 'osteopathic' nor any similar word shall be used therein."* Accreditation involved for both parties to use their best efforts to see that the College of Osteopathic Physicians and Surgeons, or its successor, would be accredited as a medical school as soon as possible.

Schedule F described the practice rights, including the practice rights at hospitals, and *"to remove any distinction between or among persons holding a certificate as physician and surgeon in the State of California and a degree of Doctor of Medicine, where such distinction is based solely upon the ground that any such person previously held or now holds a degree of Doctor of Osteopathy."*

Schedule G specified the time schedule and conditions.

Thus, in essence, the merger stipulations resulted in three steps to be taken:

- The College of Osteopathic Physicians and Surgeons (COP&S), at that time the only osteopathic medical school in California, had to be converted into an allopathic medical school
- The Board of Osteopathic Examiners had to be repealed
- The California Osteopathic Association would cease to exist

Counselor Hufstedler represented the California Osteopathic Association, to see in their ongoing negotiations with the CMA what kind of agreement could be put together, including the terms of the agreement and how they would be carried out.

Counselor Hufstedler:

> *"There were several major headings that had to be dealt with. First of all you had all the statutory structure governing the medical profession and*

the osteopathic profession. So all of that infra-structure had to be dealt with to see if you were going to put them together—how you could combine all of those things. That's a lot of technical stuff, but it really was a lot of hard work in the long run to deal with all of the statutes and all the measures that had to be dealt with.

"You had the problem of education, the accreditation of the school, what happened to the school, who was going to own it, how was it going to be dealt with, how it was going to be supported and how it was going to get accreditation through the AMA, and the AMA related institutions that have to deal with accreditation.

"Then of course you had the practice rights, the identification of the individuals—are they going to be identified simply as M.D.s or are they going to be identified by some other kind of name or title as a result of this change. All of that had to be taken care of. And then you had the huge problem of dealing with all of the people out there who didn't agree. They wanted to prevent this from going ahead; either educationally, by accreditation, or by some other things; so you had to deal with all of those."

Converting COP&S into an allopathic medical school

The first step of turning COP&S over to allopathy required an assessment by allopathy regarding its qualifications to function as an allopathic medical school. In January 1961, representatives of the Association of American Medical Colleges (AAMC) were invited for an inspection. Dr. Glen Cayler, Secretary of the California Board of Osteopathic Examiners, invited Dr. W.N. Hubbard, Jr., Dean of the University of Michigan Medical School, and Dr. Stanley W. Olson, Dean of Baylor University College of Medicine, to visit COP&S in February 1961 to determine its qualification to be considered an allopathic medical school.

Professor Grace Bell, dean of COP&S in 1961, prepared and coordinated the visit by working with the Advisory Education Committee of the California Osteopathic Association. In February 1961 the **AAMC visit** was conducted over three days and in March Dr. Caylor received a summary from Dr. Hubbard of impressions derived at the visit and recommendations prior to a full, unqualified accreditation of COP&S as an allopathic medical school.

While the examining committee recommended provisional accreditation until the financial status seemed firm, the college would need to implement certain requirements in order to become fully accredited. On top of the list stood the pursuit of research on the effectiveness of manipulation as well as research in the basic medical sciences. They also recommended appointing faculty with an M.D. degree and deleting "osteopathy" from the name of the college.

In April 1961, **dissenting Trustees of COP&S filed law suits**, together with the Osteopathic Physicians and Surgeons of California (OPSC), contesting the legality of the merger, but the Court decided in favor of the CMA agreements on May 15, 1961.

Counselor Hufstedler recalls:

> *"With respect to the lawsuit for example, I guess there were two dissenting members of the Board of the California College of Medicine (old COP&S). I can remember Dorothy Marsh very much concerned about that lawsuit, she came down to the proceedings and promised me that, if I would win that lawsuit I would get free gynecological service for the rest of my life. So, I guess I'm entitled to it. I just was never able to use it because we did win the lawsuit."*

Negotiations continued between COA, CMA, and COP&S. On May 24, 1961, the **Board of Trustees of COP&S voted 13-11** to accede to the merger request of converting COP&S to an allopathic medical school. No action was implemented, though.

Shortly there after, COP&S received a repeat visit, this time for four days by the **Liaison Council for Medical Education** of the AMA and the AAMC. This visit resulted in action to be implemented. The Articles of Incorporation of COP&S were adapted to function as those for an allopathic college of medicine. On **November 16, 1961**, the Board of Trustees of COP&S changed the name of the college to **California College of Medicine (CCM)**. Dean Grace Bell became the Founding Dean of CCM.

In an unpublished draft from 1977, entitled "**Grace Beekhuis Bell, M.D.**", Linda Burnham at the Dean's Office at the College of Medicine at UC Irvine described Dr. Bell's view: *"The benefits of these moves, as Dr. Bell sees them, were expected to be threefold: 1) As M.D.s these doctors would have more opportunities for postgraduate education, enabling them to keep up with the current medical trends and to provide the public with better care; 2) the techniques of spinal manipulation would be fully researched, using the full resources of the medical profession, which had so long turned its back upon the subject; 3) according to Dr. Bell, the new M.D.s would receive 'a better shake under what was coming—what we see now in Medicare and MediCal insurance' ."* A few paragraphs further in the document, however, Dean Bell is quoted as having stated: *"But if you go back you will not find that Grace Bell was in favor of that change. I did what I had to do as dean of the college and I did as good a job as I could."*

Thus, the historic event occurred that COP&S which had been thriving since 1914, ceased to exist. Wayne Pollock, M.D. viewed the closing doors of COP&S not as demise but as a circular process where osteopathy returned to its wellspring. He wrote in the *World Medical Journal* in January 1962 *"Osteopathy appears to be evolving and merging back into the medical profession from which it sprang almost a century ago."*

A few months later, **Benjamin Wells, M.D.**, Assistant Chief Medical Director for Research and Education in Medicine at the Veterans Administration in Washington DC, was appointed as the first allopathic dean. Dr. Wells was a well-published researcher in the field of clinical pathology. Dean Grace Bell became Associate Dean.

Glen Cayler, D.O. who had for so long fought as the COA legislative committee chair for equal rights for D.O.s in the state of California, switched to allopathic medicine. He is listed in the CCM alumni directory with the M.D. degree. He was considered the "father" of the merger and had mentored Forest Grunigen, D.O. who worked in his office in the 1940s.

CCM received grants from the Rockefeller Foundation, the Josiah Macy Jr. Foundation, and the California Osteopathic Association to promote education and training, and to assist the College in remaining an independent, free-standing institution. When in February 1962 the Board of Trustees of CCM passed a resolution to request approval as a medical school, the accreditation was approved within two weeks.

Granting the first M.D. degree

COP&S board members struggled with their decision regarding the M.D. degree because initially COP&S had been chartered to issue either the M.D. or the D.O. certificate but only the D.O. degree had been issued. **Louis Chandler, D.O.** reflected on this issue in 1943. In a statement he made on May 17, 1943, he commented: " . . . *under present circumstances, legal considerations would make it impossible for the College of Osteopathic Physicians and Surgeons to give an M.D. degree which could be valid. For the COP&S to give an M.D. degree which could be of value in practice in the state of California, either the college must be changed to a medical college securing the approval of the Medical Board or the legal provisions governing the practice of osteopathy must be changed. Members of the State Association desiring an M.D. degree to secure for themselves greater privileges and legal recognition, should understand that the present legal status is the result of actions of the profession and not the college and that until the college brings about appropriate changes, the college cannot wisely (for the interest of the profession) alter its course"* (cited from Dr. Chandler's papers, archived at Western University of the Health Sciences).

In 1961, however, given the sociopolitical situation, about half of the Board members decided in favor of the M.D. degree.

Associate Dean Grace Bell was the first to be granted the M.D. degree on March 7, 1962 by the Board of Trustees, followed by 361 other faculty members. Dr. Bell was the first in the ceremony not only because her name was at the top of the alphabet but because she was the Dean. The graduating students followed later that spring, and 1,750 practicing D.O.s on July 14 and 15, 1962. In all, of the 2,696 D.O.s who were granted the M.D. degree, 1,953 were COP&S graduates.

Counselor Hufstedler:

"It was really a question of information, primarily on what the training was that the D.O.s had, plus the fact that when the California College of Medicine took on the job of reviewing them (you really had this body from the California College of Medicine looking at their educational requirements) to see that they had the requirements to meet the Medical Act. If they did, it was alright. So you had somebody judging it. Not everybody passed, you know. There were a

*few who asked for the M.D. degree and they were reviewed. The college said,
no, as they didn't think they measured up."*

Dr. Seffinger:

"And the $65.00 fee, what was that for?"

Counselor Hufstedler:

*"I have no recollection. Obviously there was a little cost in the processing
and that sort of thing, but I couldn't tell you about that."*

There were 400 osteopathic physicians who refused to take the M.D. degree; of these, 250 were members of OPSC. Demographically, D.O.s who did not apply for the M.D. degree were older and had more years of experience working as a D.O. than those who applied for the M.D. degree.

Repealing the licensing power of the Board of Osteopathic Examiners

The Osteopathic Initiative Act from 1922 had been of great importance to the osteopathic profession because it provided legal protection for osteopaths to be an independent, separate, self-controlling and self-disciplining profession with a separate Board of Osteopathic Examiners. The 1922 Initiative Act was also very powerful because the people of California had made that decision. A public decision, meaning a new state initiative would be needed to reverse the provisions of the 1922 Osteopathic Initiative Act.

That act had been created in 1922 *"to establish a board of osteopathic examiners, to provide for their appointment, and to prescribe their powers and duties; to regulate the examination of applicants who are graduates of osteopathic schools, for any form of certificate to treat disease, injuries, deformities or other physical or mental conditions; to regulate the practice of those so licensed, who are graduates of osteopathic schools; to impose upon said board of osteopathic examiners all duties and functions, relating to graduates of osteopathic schools, holding or applying for any form of certificate or license, heretofore exercised and performed by the Board of Medical Examiners of the State of California under the provisions of the state Medical Practice Act, approved June 2, 1913, and acts amendatory thereof"* (quoted from "Laws Relating to the Practice of Osteopathic Medicine" issued by the Osteopathic Medical Board of California, 2000).

In order for a merger to occur in California, this 1922 Osteopathic Act had to be amended by the State electorate to the effect that the Board of Osteopathic Examiners would lose its power to license new candidates. **Senator Stephen Teale**, as chair of the Senate Finance Committee, and Tom Schumaker as CCM representative, facilitated that Governor Brown introduce the required amendment to the Osteopathic Initiative Act as proposition 22 during the budget session in October 1962.

The modifications to the 1922 Osteopathic Initiative Act specified that D.O.s who elected to designate themselves as "M.D." would become subject to the Board of Medical Examiners. D.O.s who wished to remain osteopathic physicians would remain under the Osteopathic Board until there would be 40 or fewer in the state. At that point, the Osteopathic Board would be repealed and all former osteopathic physicians would be under the Medical Board.

22 Osteopaths. Initiative act amendment	Continues Board of Osteopathic Examiners with power to enforce certain provisions of the Medical Practice Act as to osteopaths. Provides that qualified osteopaths who elect to designate themselves "M.D." will be subject to the jurisdiction of the Board of Medical Examiners. Grants Legislature power to amend the Osteopathic Initiative Act of 1922 and repeal that act and transfer functions to Board of Medical Examiners when there are 40 or less licensed osteopaths.	Yes	Stats. 1962, 1st Ex. Sess. ch. 48

In 1962, this initiative was presented to the California voters as Proposition 22 and was passed by a significant margin of 2 ½ to 1 ratio. By restricting the Osteopathic Board of Examiners from issuing new licenses to D.O.s. and by permitting its existence only until there were fewer than 40 D.O.s in the state, the merger was completed in all aspects. The osteopathic profession, it appeared, would soon cease to exist.

The remaining osteopathic physicians, meaning those who did not apply for the M.D. degree, still had full privileges as allopathic physicians by law, since 1907, under the composite licensing board. Proposition 22 only denied the osteopathic right to license **new** D.O.s in the state. The proposition transferred former D.O.s who took the M.D. degree to the jurisdiction of the California Board of Medical Examiners. There were over 300 out-of-state D.O.s who were licensed by the California Board of Osteopathic Examiners. Some of them continued to pay their dues, as they were motivated to ensure solvency of the osteopathic licensing board by maintaining its licentiates above the 40 member threshold.

Dr. Allen:

> "The Board of Examiners did not cease to exist. They continued. The Board of Osteopathic Examiners continued to function through the necessary renewal of licenses, jurisdiction of misbehaving doctors, hearing patient complaints and all that for these 400 D.O.s that stayed as D.O.s. Actually, 200 were in practice and the other 200 were old enough that they were just honorary, supportive members that paid their dues, or [they lived] out of state.

"I bought the degree so that no one could say that I was not qualified. So I paid my $65 and my name is there among the graduates. But by not notifying the Board of Examiners to switch me to the Board of Medical Examiners I continued as a D.O. Each year I paid my dues to the State Board and the Board of Osteopathic Examiners continued to exist. They were stripped of their authority to examine and give new licenses. So, the state was closed as far as any new D.O.s coming in. There was no way that a new D.O. could come in and get a license. That part was taken away by a vote of the people in 1962. That was the essence of it."

Absorbing the California Osteopathic Association into the California Medical Association

August 1962, the COA was absorbed by the CMA and received its charter as the **41st Medical Society in the California Medical Association**. Dr. Joseph Cosentino, as the last COA president, became the first president of the 41st Medical Society.

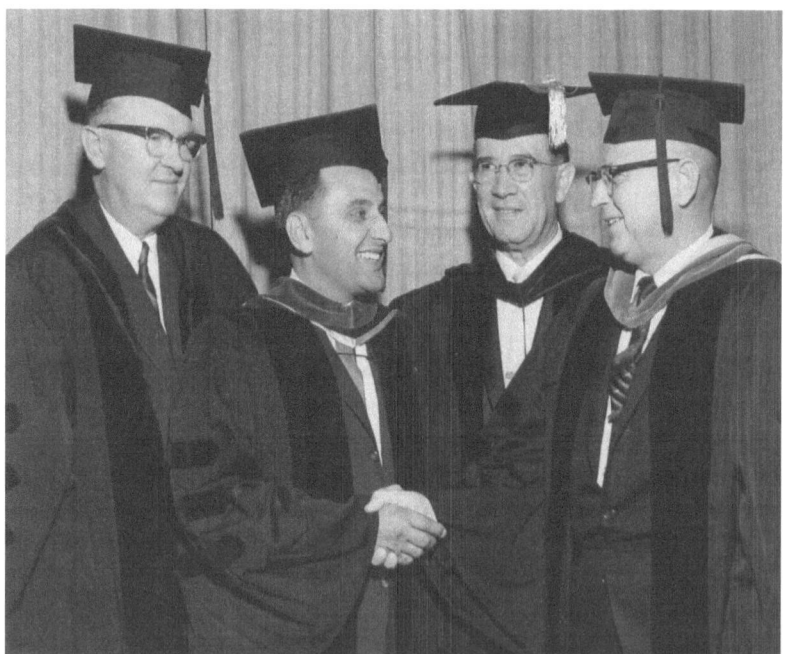

Figure 15. "Dr. Wayne E. Pollock, Dr. Joseph P. Cosentino
(COA President), Dr. Ballentine Henley, Dr. Omar Wheeler
(CMA President), June 17, 1962, Commencement"

The CMA had 40 component medical societies. The roster of the California County Medical Societies showed 40 councilor districts in California. A new component society, the 41st Medical Society was created especially for faculty and alumni of the former COP&S and new graduates of the California College of Medicine. Each former D.O. was expected to eventually become a member of his or her County Medical Society, but until such time the 41st Medical Society would be their source of continuing information and support.

Dr. Passy:

> "The doctors that were alumni that were graduating really had no affiliation with anyone, and they did not have an affiliation with the California Medical Association. At that time, they needed something to gather all of the alumni from the school and put them into one society so they could be voiced as an institution, as a unit so they could accomplish what they wanted to accomplish in terms of medicine.
>
> "There were 40 medical societies in the State. So they originated a 41st medical society to encompass all the alumni and faculty from the school. They merged into a medical society, and that is how the 41st Medical Society originated."

The CMA Constitution and Bylaws in 1960 stated that each of the 40 component societies within the CMA had the sole and final decision as to who would be members of their society. Furthermore, in order to be eligible for membership, the applicant must have received a Doctor of Medicine degree from an institution accredited by the California Board of Medical Examiners at the time of receiving the degree. Thus, in order to be in compliance with the CMA Constitution and Bylaws, COP&S had to be first converted to an M.D. school which subsequently had to become accredited by the California Board of Medical Examiners. Only then could the D.O.s be granted an M.D. degree that was acceptable to the CMA.

Each new M.D. had to apply to their local M.D. component society of the CMA and to each hospital as well. The 41st Medical Society was created to distribute this information to the newly granted M.D.s and to assist them in assimilating into the M.D. component societies of the CMA and into the hospitals as well.

To this day, a committee associated with the 41st Medical Trust (described in Chapter 6) preserved the documentation of the Forty-first Medical Society's osteopathic tradition. Archival records include about a thousand files of former osteopathic physicians and their correspondence with the COA regarding applications and licensing issues, COA membership ledgers, listing amount of dues paid per year, and correspondence dated from the years 1960 to 1964. A letter to "Dorothy J. Marsh, D.O, Chairman, Board of Certification, California Osteopathic Association", dated 1962, requested her to certify the "good moral character" of a D.O. applying to the Board of Certification, California Osteopathic Association. By 1964 topics of correspondence with the Forty-First Medical Society include letters by applicants to be released of membership.

A letter by Robert M. Garrick, Administrative Director of the Forty-First Medical Society stated that in 1967 *"the total group of supporting and sustaining members numbers nearly 1100."* Mr. Garrick's letter was in response to a request by a former D.O. to receive a list of members. The carbon copy of Mr. Garrick's letter shows that Dr. Paul D. Yates was President of the Forty First Medical Society at that time. Thirty years later, on July 31, 1997, Paul Yates, M.D. and Jordan Phillips, M.D. certified for the *"Forty First Medical Society, A California mutual benefit corporation"* that *"the corporation's known debts and liabilities have been actually paid; the corporation's known assets have been distributed to the persons entitled thereto; and the corporation is dissolved."*

While the Forty-First Medical Society came to a close in 1997, the Forty-First Medical Trust continues to pursue the objective of that unique group of physicians who were trained in the osteopathic and allopathic professions (see Figure 1 in the Preface to this book). Their work continues to this day and is described further in Chapter 6.

Adjusting to the merger

Prior to merging the COA and CMA, **Seth Hufstedler, LL.B.** (legal counsel for the COA), **Dorothy Marsh, D.O.**, and other representatives of both organizations traveled around the state to educate osteopathic and allopathic physicians about the details and ramifications of the merger and to answer their questions.

Counselor Hufstedler:

> *"I think there was a fairly strong feeling initially that it was worth a great deal of effort to try to put the two professions together, they were governed by the same medical laws, their objectives were the same (to take care of their patients), and that there didn't need to be political divisions between them that might make this more awkward. So I think they started with really a very good base among the D.O.s for the merger. I think there was more opposition among the M.D.s, and many of them thought they in some respects were superior. They really didn't think they wanted to do that. But there was also some opposition among the D.O.s, particularly the opposition that came from the American Osteopathic Association. They were in a very strong position. The major job, I guess that we all had with respect to that, was to try to get the information out to everybody.*
>
> *"We organized with what Dorothy Marsh called our 'dog and pony show.' With Dorothy, Hap Hassard, the lawyer for the CMA (or somebody else representing them), two or three doctors and I covered pretty much the state. We went to all the major state medical associations and tried to get the smaller ones together, so we could deal with them, to answer all their questions, and to tell them as much as we could."*

After the merger, Bob Garrick who represented the 41st Medical Society, arranged for **Dr. Kammerman**, a former osteopathic physician, and **Dr. Bostick** to talk to groups of physicians about the merger. They traveled to San Diego, Sacramento, San Francisco, Oakland and other cities. Together with a medical student, **Arthur Charles**, they educated the medical community about the implications of the merger. Shortly thereafter, Arthur Charles graduated as M.D. and later became chief of endocrinology at UCI.

Some former D.O.s changed their mind regarding their switch to allopathy. In 1963, the AOA developed a policy about former D.O.s who requested a reversal of their decision to convert to the M.D. degree. The AOA required the return of the new M.D. diploma. Apparently, this request was not enforced, though, and there are no data published on the number of applicants who wanted to reverse their switch to the M.D. degree.

What to do with the new M.D.s

Former osteopathic physicians with a new M.D. degree were placed under the Medical Board. Applications for licensure at the Medical Board were usually categorized according to the applicant's training. One category comprised "allied health professionals", including nurse practitioners, emergency medical technicians, physical therapists, physician assistants, podiatrists, and chiropractors. In 1962, applications by former osteopathic physicians and members of the 41st Medical Society were referred to this category of allied health professionals.

Dolores Grunigen, in her position as Assistant to the Executive Secretary in the Medical Licensing Board at the state government, was responsible for the licensing process of allied health professionals, including the newly degreed former osteopathic physicians. Mrs. Grunigen evaluated their credentials and qualifications for licensure to facilitate an expedient licensing process.

In some instances, Mrs. Grunigen represented those newly degreed physicians to different committees because they had submitted unusual application materials. Members of these committees often had little understanding of osteopathic physicians. They had heard rumors, though, of D.O.s as "cultists" and were thus inclined to place D.O.s at the same level as religious cults. Through the support of Senator Teale and Dr. Grunigen, Mrs. Grunigen was able to create awareness and increased understanding of the generally high level of medical qualification among former D.O.s. She explained to the committees that, according to the submitted documents, osteopathic training was close to allopathic medical training and comparable to many medical doctors trained outside the U.S. who obtained licensure as M.D.s in the state of California.

The California Hospital Association

As described earlier, some hospitals in California had a mixed M.D.-D.O. staff since the 1920s and were as such approved by the California Hospital Association. Most hospitals, though, accepted only M.D.s on staff. By the early 1960s, the California Hospital

Association was comprised primarily of hospitals where M.D.s practiced. There were about 450 such allopathically dominated hospitals. A parallel organization for osteopathic physicians, the California Osteopathic Hospital Association, had some 60 members staffed solely by D.O.s. While at the state level the California Hospital Association had endorsed the merger proposal, at the local level some hospital administrators and board of directors were not convinced of the value of merging the two organizations. They recognized numerous problems that would result. The change entailed a great amount of work which the administrators and boards resented.

Emery Dowell, associate executive director of the California Hospital Association, and Frank Clark, public relations director of California Hospital Association along with other staff addressed members throughout the state and through the media to make the case for consolidation. Mr. Dowell knew Senator Teale from his earlier work with the public utilities and thus had a good working relationship again with the Senator to facilitate the "consolidation between M.D.s and D.O.s", as they called the merging process.

Whereas the D.O.s became M.D.s on masse in 1962, osteopathic hospitals joined the California Hospital Association one at a time, requiring some two years for the complete integration. An osteopathic hospital administrator was added to the California Hospital Association Board of Directors to help smooth the transition. Legal medical staffs also deliberated a long time before providing privileges to their new M.D. colleagues.

The issue of recognizing specialty certification

Hospital administrators were in the position to accept the specialty certification of former D.O.s by the osteopathic Boards or to require specialty certification by the M.D. Boards. AOA Boards were under the auspices of the AOA but M.D. Boards were organized and operated separately under the approval by the AMA.

Dr. Kammerman:

"To the former D.O.s who were previously certified specialists, CMA promised as much as they could that specialists, like surgeons and orthopedists, could continue in their specialty work at most hospitals, even if those hospitals required board certification by M.D. Boards. Most hospitals continued to allow former D.O.s to maintain their acquired privileges without being boarded by the AMA approved Specialty Boards."

A difficult start for the California College of Medicine

To give CCM a jump-start several local medical societies, the 41st Medical Society, and the new Alumni Organization raised funds to help with the education expenses of the college. In spite of this support, lack of funding for CCM to continue functioning as an independent institution became a big concern. Potential donors were approached from several institutions in the Los Angeles area. Not only were these contacts unproductive, earlier governmental support to provide funds for medical education had come to an end as well, making the situation quite serious and urgent. The financial stress and rejections placed a strain on the relationship between Dean Wells and the Board of Trustees.

Dr. Wells abruptly resigned after one year of service from July 1, 1962 to June 30, 1963. A sense of uncertainty prevailed.

Dr. Passy:

> *"At that time, with the merger taking place, the college was called the California College of Medicine, which was an entity of California and not affiliated with any university at that time. There were some universities that were looking at CCM, which is what it was called, California College of Medicine, as part of a medical school. Long Beach was looking at us, Bakersfield, a school in the valley that was looking at us, and also Irvine, University of California at Irvine, that was looking at us to be part of their University system as a medical school. Finally in 1963, ' 64, '65, when we were still California College of Medicine, the University of California at Irvine elected to choose us as their medical school and we accepted."*

During the search process for a new dean, Dr. Bell was Interim Dean from July 1, 1963 till February 1, 1964 when Dr. Bostick was appointed as dean. **Dr. Bell** is quoted in a document from the dean's office at UC Irvine College of Medicine (1977) as having explained: *"In the report that was made at the time that we were approved, it was recommended that I be continued as dean until my tenure was at an end. It was my feeling that the school would go further if it had a recognized medical educator as dean. In the Association of American Medical Colleges, the dean is an important person. It needed someone who knew his way around. I didn't because I had been associated with osteopaths. As associate dean I was able to help whoever came in as dean."*

According to Dr. Bostick's recollections, the process of searching had been inefficient initially because the search committee included representatives from diverse parties who were entitled to effect the choice of a candidate most qualified in their view. When a targeted search group was selected from the committee membership, including Dr. Bostick, the process became more efficient. **Warren Bostick, M.D.**, a professor of pathology at the University of California at San Francisco (UCSF) and former president of the CMA from 1961 to 1962, was well familiar with the complexities of college politics. He had been active in gaining recognition from the state legislature for osteopathic physicians in California to receive the M.D. degree. For several years, he had been involved in the negotiations to change COP&S to an M.D. degree granting institution.

The birth of the University of California at Irvine

Grace Bell, once again Associate Dean, together with Dr. Grunigen, turned to Senator Teale who had just received the year before his M.D. degree from CCM. A plan was developed to affiliate CCM with the University of California, Irvine. The political situation was favorable for the negotiators in 1963, because the state had just decided to create three new medical schools, including one in Orange County.

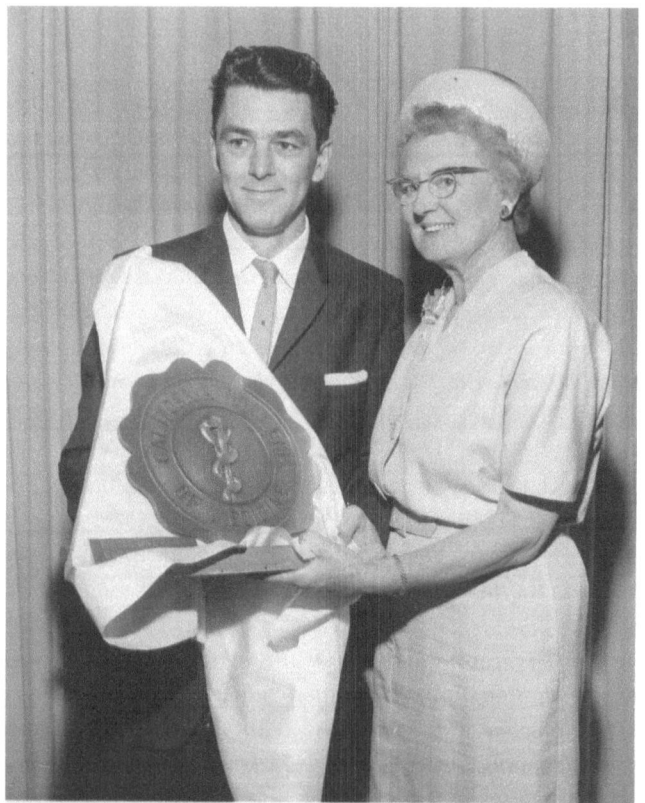

Figure 16. "Dr. Michael Moulton (left) and Dean Grace B. Bell (right) being presented with the Senior Class Gift at the Senior Breakfast, 1962"

At that time, the University of California Irvine campus began its process of birth and development. In 1957 the University of California Regents had voted to expand the institution to three new campuses in Davis, San Diego, and Orange. As a location for the campus in Orange County, the architect had decided upon the Irvine Ranch. This estate comprised "*about 156,000 acres of Orange County at that time and was owned by James Irvine who passed away before the School* [COP&S] *had been converted,*"

Dr. Kammerman recalls. "It was *mostly **Joan Irvine Burt** and the Board of Trustees of the Irvine Foundation that conceived of the campus. However, when the medical school arrived, Joan Irvine was very instrumental in developing the medical campus along with Mr. Bren."*

In 1960, the Irvine family transferred one thousand acres to the University of California. An additional 510 acres were purchased. Constructions proceeded fast, and in 1964 the UC Irvine campus was dedicated. Doors opened in 1965 and the first class graduated in 1966 under Founding Chancellor Aldrich.

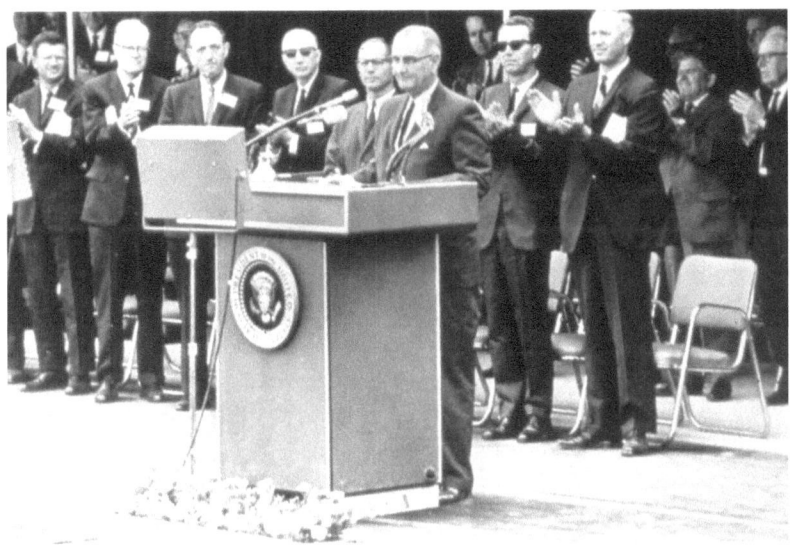

Figure 17. "Dedication of the University of California Irvine campus by
U.S. President Lyndon B. Johnson, 1964"

Transferring the California College of Medicine to UC Irvine

In order to make the California College attractive to the UC Regents, Senator Teale, former D.O. and now M.D., crafted a special bill, SB 1414, that designated the affiliation of the California College of Medicine with the University of California. In his capacity as Chair of the Senate Finance Committee, he appropriated an additional $ 500,000 to the college operational budget.

Counselor Hufstedler:

> *"We sat down with the Counselor for the Board of Regents, can't remember his name, I think it was Cunningham. He was a retired Superior Court Judge, and we worked out an agreement whereby we would now give the California College of Medicine (the old COP&S) to the University of California, lock,*

145

stock and barrel. They got the works. They invested, these numbers aren't exactly accurate by any means, but they put a hundred million dollars into a school at UCLA and were turning out just a handful of doctors. Here we had a medical school that was turning out 80 or 90 well qualified doctors every year which we were willing to give them for nothing, just there it was. And they came around on that, they liked the idea.

"We drafted the contract set it all out and then I got a call from Cunningham one day, if that was his name, I think it was. He said the Board of Regents changed its mind; we are not going to do it. That was a serious problem, obviously. And we had to make some arrangement with respect to the school. We could have continued the school as an independent non-profit and that sort of thing, so it wasn't necessarily a road block, but it certainly was inconvenient.

"Then the interesting thing was Clark Kerr was in as president, and you are well aware of the fact, and that there was a wonderful guy named Steve Teale, who was a D.O., who was the Chairman of the Ways and Means Committee of the California Senate. So the California budget came up for action, and it had to be placed first in the Ways and Means Committee in the Senate. Nothing happened. It didn't get called up. It didn't get put on the calendar, and finally after many inquiries and getting no help at all, Steve Teale comes into his office one day and there is Clark Kerr sitting there. Clark said, 'Well, Steve, how can we get our budget on the calendar and go forward?' Steve said, 'it's simple, just sign that contract and we'll get it underway.' In a couple of weeks it was back on track and we got the contract signed. As you know it's now owned by the University of California, Irvine, the California College of Medicine, a fine medical school. That's how it happened."

Thus, the Regents had responded favorably and CCM became part of the UC system in 1963. The College was to be transferred from Los Angeles to the UC campus in Irvine as soon as possible. **Dr. Kammerman** recalls: "*I do not believe it* [CCM] *was sold to the California system. It was simply acquired in an agreement with the Board of Trustees of CCM and the Board of Regents. The Board of Regents of UC had considered moving the CCM campus to another location, such as Watts or Davis or even San Diego.*"

Dr. Kammerman continued:

"I was on the alumni board at that time. Dr. Warren Bostick informed us that the Board of Regents was considering moving the medical school to Watts, San Diego, or Sacramento. Tuition had dropped for the medical students by about one half of what it was under the CCM. CCM was in the shadow of USC School of Medicine and they were planning to take over the entire county hospital system. Dr. Walter Hopps was president of the Alumni Association at that time and our board discussed the future of the school. Several of the board

members made an appointment with C. P. MacGreger who was the chairman of the Board of Trustees of CCM and informed him of the possible transition. We informed him that we would prefer that the school move to UCI if possible. In the meantime we had also met with Chancellor Aldrich at UCI and asked him if he was interested in having a medical school. He was very much in favor of the move. C.P. McGregor also met with the remaining Board of Trustees of CCM and convinced them that the move to Orange County would preserve the status of the existence of the medical school. As I understand the situation, with the advice of Dr. Bostick and the Board of Trustees of CCM, the [UC] Board of Regents, of course, made the final decision."

Dean Bostick and others considered Irvine to be the best location. Moving CCM to Irvine became quite a challenge, though. Dr. Henley, President of CCM, and Dr. Bostick differed strongly in their attitude about the move. Their differences in background led them to be motivated to move toward opposite directions. Dr. Henley favored a plan to keep the College administration under the auspices of the Regents of the University of California but maintaining the geographic location in the Los Angeles area, while Dr. Bostick felt eager to move the College to the campus of UC Irvine.

Dr. Henley was a lawyer. He had come from the Dean's cabinet at USC in 1940 and had maintained good connections to the USC administration. He was used to USC's governance but according to Dr. Bostick's perception, felt apprehensive about the UC system, especially the power and status of the academic senate. Displaying his outgoing personality and eloquent speech, Dr. Henley was used to win people over in less formal administrative negotiations than those conducted at an academic senate meeting. Dr. Bostick, however, was most comfortable in the prestigious auspices of the UC Regents. He was quite familiar with the Regents' protocols and the academic senate, while Dr. Henley shied away from having to answer to the authority of the Regents and having to participate in the unfamiliar institution of an academic senate.

Dr. Bostick was an accomplished professor of pathology who had just moved from a prestigious institution, UC San Francisco, to the less attractive downtown area of Los Angeles. He was eager to move to affluent Orange County which held the promise of a new hospital to be built that would serve an upper socioeconomic population. Dr. Henley, however, preferred to maintain his long-standing and familiar ties to hospitals in the Los Angeles area for medical training.

The promise was for a University-based hospital on the Irvine campus. Dr. Bostick lured many new allopathic faculty members to CCM with that promise. He could have used the Los Angeles County hospital as teaching and training facility but apparently did not see much promise in this option, possibly because of the presence of former osteopathic physicians. He chose his own M.D. faculty who upon their arrival provided training at the L.A. County Hospital but were being assured of a move to UC Irvine soon.

One of the new allopathic Department Chairs was **Thomas Nelson, M.D.**, Professor of Pediatrics. He came to the CCM in 1964, shortly after the College had become affiliated with the University of California. Prior to accepting Dr. Bostick's invitation to join CCM, Dr. Nelson had been Professor and Chairman of Pediatrics at the University of Kentucky College Of Medicine in Lexington and, before that, Assistant Professor of Pediatrics and Lecturer in Psychiatry at the University of California at San Francisco (UCSF).

Dr. Nelson:

"I was recruited to CCM by Warren Bostick, who was then the Dean of the College. Dr. Bostick and I had known each other for many years. I was one of his students when he was a very young Assistant Professor in Pathology at UCSF. Later I became a faculty and Academic Senate member at UCSF; and so, Dr. Bostick and I were fellow faculty members. He knew about my teaching ability at the UCSF Medical School and the research that I was doing at that time in parasitology.

"Dr. Bostick became very involved in the political process as he rose in the California Medical Association. He eventually became President of the Association. During this time, he became aware that I was involved with the State government both with the Department of Mental Hygiene as well as with the State Legislature. Thus he knew that I had experience preparing, presenting and defending large budgets to the State. In the position I held at Sonoma State Hospital, I reported directly to the Director of the State Department of Mental Hygiene and thus was only once removed from the Governor. I believe Dr. Bostick was pleased that I had had experience in administering a large institution and knew my way around state government."

This potential involvement with state politics in CCM's new administration and faculty might have caused conflict with the College's president, Dr. Henley, now called Provost, and the Board of Trustees. The state department and state legislature were probably not the places where Dr. Henley would have felt confident and in control. His "castle" was near USC and his "court" was his Trustees. He had worked for and with the Board of Trustees for over 20 years. They had their roots in Los Angeles County which was at that time the most populated and influential county in California. County representatives were determined to hold on to CCM as an economically and socially important asset.

While arguments continued about the location for the College, academic life continued at CCM by converting to an allopathic faculty.

Dr. Nelson:

"I remember that Dr. Bostick told me, 'Make this into a good department of pediatrics, one that would be nationally recognized, get a research program going that will be competitive with what's going on in other schools in the country'. I think what he also implied was to 'get the students to like you and like pediatrics

and like what they are doing and be happy with themselves as medical students in this school which is now the California College of Medicine'."

Dr. Nelson was well-prepared to turn Dr. Bostick's expectations into reality.

Dr. Nelson:

"During the first several years following my arrival, we recruited faculty from all over the country. Quite a few mid-westerners and easterners came. I recruited a pediatric hematologist who had trained at UCSF, Dr. Susie Wong Fong. Dr. David Mosier was an important recruit because he came as a full professor. He came from the University of Illinois where he was the Director of a research institute. He was a pediatric endocrinologist who was nationally and internationally known. Previous to Illinois, he had been on the faculty of UCLA, so he knew the UC system well. He was a big help to say the least. Dr. Donald Sperling came as young pediatric cardiologist out of a fellowship at USC and Los Angeles Children's Hospital. He had administrative talent and soon became the vice-chairman of the Department. Dr. Kenneth Dumars, with whom I had been a fellow faculty member at the University of Kentucky and who then had moved to the University of Colorado, came to cover the area of genetics. He also was appointed at the full professor level. Dr. Bruce Ackerman, who had just completed a fellowship in neonatology at the Geisinger Medical Center in Pennsylvania, started the Division of Neonatology and covered the newborn service and the Neonatal Intensive Care Unit in the hospital."

"At the time, there was many of the previous faculty still at the school. For instance, my predecessor as Pediatric Department Chair, Dr. Jane Hamilton, was still there, as were three others of the department's full-time faculty. So, in essence, when I came as the first chair of pediatrics in 1964, I inherited four faculty members who had previously been osteopathic pediatricians. This retention was true of other departments at the time. In fact, the previous chairmen of the Departments of Psychiatry and Physical Medicine and Rehabilitation remained in their positions for some period of time after the conversion. In that way, I became very familiar with the College and how it had been in the past (or at least in the recent past) and how it was at the beginning of the transition to a college granting the M.D. degree."

He recognized, though, a certain strain on the former osteopathic faculty having to shift to allopathy. **Dr. Nelson** recalls:

*"My predecessor, **Dr. Jane Hamilton** was someone whom I consider to be a very remarkable person. She was very positive about the changes occurring around the time of my coming. Obviously she was doing everything she could*

to make the transition easy for the students and for me. To come as the first traditional M.D. into a department with all previous D.O.s was obviously a bit of a strain for the remaining faculty, the students and for me. Dr. Hamilton did not seem to feel very much of this and she did the best she could to ease the strain felt by the other three faculty members who were there.

"Remember we had students in process; we couldn't stop the process of teaching; students were in their pediatric clerkships; teaching had to go on. We had Unit II of the Los Angeles County Hospital with its pediatric ward, with its pediatric clinics which were very busy, and with its neonatal nursery including a neonatal intensive care unit that had to be staffed. So, I was in the process of recruiting new faculty while at the same time keeping a department in operation. Dr. Hamilton was very, very helpful to me in keeping these functions going. I think that she did this with a great deal of sacrifice to herself.

"After I had been at CCM for about a year, she came in one day and said 'Tom, I think now the time has come for me to leave. I'm doing this because I want to make it easier for you. I know that you have asked me to stay on, but I just think it would be best for this transition if I moved on. I'll stay in the vicinity. I will be helpful to you and be an advisor if you need one. I'm going to stay here and take a position with Los Angeles County Government. I will be available and I will stay on the volunteer faculty.' She became the Director of Communicable Diseases in the Los Angeles County Department of Public Health, an important position to say the least."

Dr. Nelson realized *". . . . not too long after I was at CCM that there was a small close knit group of pediatricians in Southern California, primarily in Los Angeles County, who had been osteopathic pediatricians; most of them had been certified under the osteopathic board. I became interested in how they had trained, how they became pediatricians and in the history of this group. Some of them I came to know well. One of them, of course, was Dr. Jane Hamilton. Another important name in the history of pediatrics at the College was* **Evangeline Percival***. Although she was dead at the time of my arrival, it was apparent to me that Dr. Percival was a very beloved figure in the College and among recent alumni. There had been a pediatric award named after her for the outstanding student in pediatrics and I continued that award up until the time I left UCI. I hope the Evangeline Percival Award for the outstanding student in pediatrics will continue. It is a monetary award and is considered quite an honor to receive at Honors Day. I soon learned that Evangeline Percival and Jane Hamilton had been very good personal friends as well as being in a mentor/student relationship and that after Dr. Percival's death, Jane Hamilton received all of her papers. I understood them to be quite extensive having to do with events during her time as department chair, but Dr. Hamilton never offered to let me see them.*

"Another previous department chair, **Dr. Betsy MacCracken** *was also interesting because her father was an early graduate of the College* [Actually, Frank MacCracken was a graduate of the American School of Osteopathy in Kirksville, MO. He was a prominent member of the Board of Trustees of COP&S, though, and of the COA]. *She also was a graduate of COP&S and in many ways she had grown up, if you will, in COP&S with her father being a faculty member. As I became more interested in the school, I received a great deal of information about the history of the pediatric department from Betsy MacCracken. She was not at all defensive as I found some of the other people that had previously been osteopathic physicians. I think one of the reasons for this was she had gone to the University of California Berkeley some years after receiving the D.O. There she graduated with a Master's degree in Public Health and had specialized as a public health pediatrician. She was very involved with the Los Angeles County Public Health Department both in relation to the College and not in relation to it. She became the district health officer for the Public Health District of Los Angeles which surrounded the College and the County Hospital. She stayed on as an important volunteer faculty member in that aspect of pediatrics. I was very happy to have her. I found her in many ways a person who was very much like academic pediatricians that I had known in M.D. granting schools. She was an especially important person as far as I was concerned in being a very good source for the history of the College and the Department.*

"From this nucleus of previously osteopathic pediatricians, there were many others who stayed on our volunteer faculty and who were practicing in various parts of Los Angeles. Some of them were involved with Pacific Hospital and the Glendale Adventist Hospital, some of them were on the faculty and on the staff at the White Memorial Hospital, so that many of them had achieved considerable recognition within pediatrics in Los Angeles County, but they remained in this close knit group. They stayed with the College as long as we stayed in Los Angeles, but when we moved to Orange County, they did not stay on the faculty and I lost track of most of them except for Jane Hamilton with whom I maintained a considerable contact up until very recently."

The school in the initial 15 years of its existence was supported to a significant extent by the osteopathic faculty at COP&S turned CCM and especially by the alumni.

Dr. van den Noort:

"Yes, they were very helpful. The other curious thing, you see, what happened was most of the faculty of the old school were in Glendale and Pasadena and San Marino and they weren't being paid by the school. They

151

were volunteering their time to teach. When the school came down here, they weren't going to do that. Very few of them came down here. And so in a way, we got a new medical school and recruited everybody new. But we did have help from those that were down here: Vince Carroll in Laguna Beach was enormously helpful; Forest Grunigen; Richard Kammerman, and there were others, very helpful . . . . There were several people in anatomy that came down here. And there was one in biochemistry that I know came down. And there were several others. Some of the basic science faculty came down here."

While these adjustments were taking place at CCM, Dean Bostick persevered with the moving plans. The date for moving CCM to the campus of the University of California at Irvine was set for August 29, 1968.

The birth of the College of Medicine at UC Irvine and its training facilities

Dr. Bostick explained in his book that for less than a year after the move, some Trustees of CCM traveled from Los Angeles to UC Irvine to attend meetings with Dean Bostick and Chancellor Aldrich, but gradually they withdrew. Dr. Bostick recalled that they no longer attended meetings when it became apparent that they were *"no longer an element to be considered"* and *"that the Board was primarily to function as a public relations group and to be the focus for starting and generating college donations and support funds."* Dr. Kammerman recalls that *"the CCM Board* [of Trustees] *remained as co-administrative for a number of years with the Board of Regents until the assets on Griffith Avenue were sold to USC* [in 1974]. *"*

In the 1977 document from the Dean's Office at UC Irvine College of Medicine, **Grace Bell** was quoted explaining her retirement on June 30, 1969 at the age of 72: *"I retired,"* she said, *"when the whole shooting match went down to Irvine. As long as there was still work going on at the campus, I continued working, even though I had passed the necessary retirement age. Dr. Sproul who was president of the University, felt that I should be continued, but I retired by mutual consent. I wasn't about to move to Irvine."* Is [was] Dr. Bell happy with the stewardship of CCM by the University? *"I think so,"* she answered, *"particularly because of the fact that the present dean is interested in the background, not just in wanting to develop a medical school that will completely forget what the origin was."*

The move to UC Irvine occurred in two stages. For the first several years, basic sciences were still taught in Los Angeles, while clinical sciences were already taught at the University of California, Irvine. The library of CCM was moved to the Special Collection of the UC Irvine Library, as the osteopathic education literature no longer was a primary source of information. Shifting medical education from osteopathy to allopathy was quite a challenge for the medical students of the cohort that experienced this transition during their four years at the College.

Dr. Nelson:

> *"Students that I had, senior students, who had started thinking they were going to receive a D.O. degree, suddenly found they were going to get an M.D. degree. They had a lot of anxiety, a lot of questions, particularly about residencies, and how it was going to work out for them. I became quite involved in the process of helping some of these students, particularly the ones who were interested in pediatrics, in getting adjusted into the medical profession in which they now suddenly and unexpectedly found themselves. I say that was probably my main involvement with osteopathy at that time. Subsequently many of the alumni of the prior school stayed involved with CCM. I became quite active in the Alumni Association in those early years and thus I knew many of the graduates of the College going back a number of years."*

The training of physicians was conducted at the Orange County General Hospital in Orange and at the Veterans Administration Medical Center in Long Beach.

Dr. Connally:

> *"When I started the program at UCI* [the Department of Surgery], *we took in two Junior Residents from the old school* [CCM] *and they turned out to be excellent."*

Orange County General Hospital was located in the City of Orange and served the surrounding semi-rural communities of lower socio-economic status than the communities of higher income in South Orange County, including Irvine. Orange County General Hospital had a firm tradition in allopathic medicine. In contrast to Los Angeles County Hospital, Orange County Hospital had never permitted D.O.s to obtain staff privileges. Dean Bostick felt easily welcomed at Orange County General Hospital and appreciated the hospital's generosity, permitting the College to conduct its residency programs there and making available much needed office space. The County Hospital received a stipend from Orange County in recognition of the hospital's relatively large property taxes. This stipend was used to support the facility for a period of time by supplementing the costs of care for the indigent.

In spite of the good working relationship with Orange County General Hospital, Dean Bostick's objective continued to provide training at a campus-based hospital in Irvine. The first effort to build a campus hospital began in 1972 when a bond issue was passed, but these efforts were met with resistance.

Dr. van den Noort:

> *"I was the first academic neurologist at UCI* [Medical Center]. *It was then the County Hospital. Warren Bostick was the Dean. That was 1970 when*

I came here. Over the first year that I was here I became engaged a little bit in faculty politics and there was a "to-do" about the hospital on the campus. The funds had been appropriated; there was a bond issue; there was money to build a hospital here; the university hired an architect; drawings were being made of this hospital; and meanwhile doctors in Newport Beach (Fashion Island) wanted to build a hospital over here called Western World. That was a time of certificate of need, so if they built one that meant we wouldn't get one. So the faculty opposed the Western World proposal and we won. I can still remember Arnold Beckman shaking his finger at me and saying, 'You will regret this,' and I have not lived to regret this and he's dead. And I'm glad we defeated it. After that, we got Willie Brown, the Speaker of the House, who was very powerful. I got a compromise from him that we could build a hospital on the campus, but we would also run the County Hospital and develop a program in Family Medicine, which he was interested in. So we did all that. And for a long while he backed us up. Finally we got again the appropriation for the hospital through the legislature. Then Jerry Brown, just after he took office, blue penciled it and took it out. It made me furious."

In 1976, the University of California at Irvine obtained the Orange County General Hospital and renamed the facility as **University of California Irvine Medical Center.** Dr. Kammerman recalls that "*UC Irvine Medical Center was purchased from the County of Orange for $1.00 with the implied guarantee that the county would backfill the costs of care for the indigent and did until the property tax was reduced by referendum in 1982, or somewhere in that time. After that date, the county funds for property taxes were reduced to the extent that the county would not be able, or try to, pay the full fare for the indigent.*"

Transferring Manipulation Medicine to UC Irvine

The College of Osteopathic Physicians and Surgeons (COP&S) had informally organized a Department of Physical Medicine and Rehabilitation (PM&R) in the 1940s. According to the late Dr. Robert Loveland, the program was under the leadership of **William W.W. Pritchard, D.O.** who was interested in rehabilitation of patients with poliomyelitis and chronic diseases. His assistant was Dr. Robert Ruenitz. One of the first faculty members was Dr. Loveland.

On June 25, 1951, Dr. Pritchard, Executive of the Department of Osteopathic Therapeutics, sent to Dean E. L. Garrison at COP&S a copy of a paper he intended to present at the American Association of Osteopathic Colleges at their meeting in Milwaukee on July 14, 1951. In this presentation, Dr. Pritchard reported about the successful establishment at COP&S in March of 1946 of a separate Department of Osteopathic Therapeutics and called for establishing separate Departments of Osteopathic Therapeutics or Osteopathic Manipulation in each college and their associated teaching hospitals. He also suggested the formation of an American College of Osteopathic Physiatrists and an American Osteopathic Board of Physical Medicine & Rehabilitation to certify Osteopathic Physiatrists. He suggested that *"each approved Osteopathic College take steps to offer in its Clinic, after an approved internship, a residency in Osteopathic Therapeutics as part of the requirements for certification as an Osteopathic Physiatrist."*

He described that by 1951 the Department of Osteopathic Therapeutics and Rehabilitation at COP&S had expanded steadily to comprise a staff of 26 osteopathic physicians [stationery letterhead at that time included the term "and Rehabilitation" in the Department name; documents often omitted "and Rehabilitation"]. Osteopathic Therapeutics had absorbed physiotherapy from the Department of General Medicine, as it was Dr. Pritchard's goal for the Department to correspond closely with the section of Physical Medicine & Rehabilitation of the American Medical Association. In his letter to Dean Garrison, Dr. Pritchard pointed out that *"This now makes our Department of Osteopathic Therapeutics correspond very closely with the section of Physical Medicine and Rehabilitation of the AMA."*

In 1952, the Department of PM&R was formally established. Dr. Pritchard remained Chair of the Department until the merger transitions. He was succeeded by Dr. John Andrews who continued to serve as Professor and Chairman after the transition to CCM in 1962. Dr. Nancy Harding and Dr. Charles Arminski were faculty members of the Department.

When in 1968 the CCM moved from Los Angeles to the UC Irvine campus, Dr. Arminski served as the interim Chair and Chief of PM&R at the Orange County General Hospital.

In 1970 **Jerome Tobis, M.D.** was appointed Chair of the Department and Chief of Service at Orange County General Hospital. An inpatient rehabilitation service of 25 beds was established in 1971 along with the residency program. In 1973 the training program was integrated with the Long Beach Residency Program which had been organized by Dr. Michela at the Veterans Administration (VA) Hospital in 1962. The rotation of training for the residents eventually included the Long Beach Memorial Hospital, St. Jude Hospital of Fullerton, the VA Hospital and the Orange County General Hospital. There were 20 residency positions.

Education for medical students in PM&R was established by Dr. Tobis in 1971 through the approval of the Curriculum Committee for a two week obligatory rotation in the 3rd year. Musculoskeletal manipulation was included in the syllabus and was provided by Drs. Arminski and Loveland. In the residency, musculoskeletal manipulation was taught and demonstrated by Dr. Loveland.

In 1982, **Jen Yu, M.D., Ph.D.** was appointed as the Department Chair. The residency program has continued to thrive and to this day is regarded highly on a national basis. The residency involves PM&R services at the UC Irvine Medical Center in Orange, the Long Beach VA Medical Center, and the Long Beach Memorial Medical Center.

Over time, the medical student two-week PM&R clerkship in the third year was replaced by a four week required "Musculoskeletal and Rehabilitation" clerkship with

Rheumatology and Orthopedics in the 4th year in 1996. Starting in 1996, the Department also offered a one afternoon required "empathy workshop" for the first year medical students. In 2000, the required clerkship was changed to a 2 or 4 week PM&R clinical elective. The Department has always offered a 4 week clinical or research elective for medical students from UC Irvine or other schools. Musculoskeletal manipulation has no longer been included regularly in education programs.

Major clinical and associated basic science research interests in the Department have included musculoskeletal manipulation, geriatric medicine, neurorehabilitation, spinal cord injury, functional magnetic stimulation, myofascial pain, and complementary medicine. Through the 1970s, the 41st Medical Trust funded Dr. Tobis and his colleagues to carry out the first single blinded randomized clinical trial conducted in America to assess the efficacy of an osteopathic manipulation procedure for patients with low back pain.

Dr. Haldeman:

> "I got an invite from Dr. Tobis to fly with my wife [to UC Irvine]. I gave an invited talk on manipulation and what we knew about spinal lesions . . . The study [by Dr. Tobis et al.] was a combined project, using pure science, pure medicine, and a combination of the two. It was the first attempt to have a reliable outcome and to use a control observer and blinded patients. The outcome was the straight leg test, based on prior testing of various options for outcome measures.
>
> "When I came down to Irvine, I was a liaison between M.D.s, D.C.s, and D.O.s. I got to know Dr. Grunigen very well and the osteopathic physician on the study . . . . The group at UC Irvine was very dedicated. Dr. Grunigen was very committed to this. His personality was so strong.
>
> "The trial had not started before 1977 when I arrived . . . . There was no research to speak of in 1975. This was one of the few scientific islands where people started to look at science . . . When this study was published, I started the process of drawing recognition to manipulation for low back pain. It was possible to do a randomized controlled trial. Subsequently several have been done, some better than others. I started to integrate this into my lectures."

Rebuilding osteopathy in California

In 1962, OPSC had resisted most fervently proposition 22 which would amend the 1922 Initiative that had established the California osteopathic licensing board. That Initiative had meant the lifeline for the osteopathic profession for 40 years. OPSC members fought with the few resources they had, often taking their own funds to educate the public about the implications of the amendment.

The AOA could not keep its promise of monetary support, because as a tax-exempt organization AOA was not allowed to fund political campaigns. But AOA tried to help in other ways. In 1965, the AOA hired an independent marketing firm to study the effects of the merger in California by interviewing hospital administrators, M.D.s, and D.O.s about post-merger hospital practices. In February 1966, Market Facts, Inc. in Chicago, Illinois provided AOA with *"A Profile of a Merger: A Report to the American Osteopathic Association"*. Nearly 300 telephone interviews were conducted. The survey was able to obtain opinions on the effect of the merger on patient care and referrals, the use of hospital services by medical doctors and former osteopaths, overall acceptance of former osteopaths by M.D.s in hospitals, appraisal of the merger experience after 3 years, and opinions about allowing new D.O. licensing in the state of California once again.

Given that OPSC was trying to get legislation passed to allow the reinstatement of complete licensing power, this report facilitated turning to the executive branch and, after failing that effort, turning to the judicial branch, i.e., the courts. Responses given in this poll were used to mount their case, as well as opinions expressed in AOA's own mail surveys, and data obtained from American Medical Association and the California Medical Association.

Financial constraints limited OPSC to publish pamphlets through the Citizens Committee against Medical Monopoly, while supporters of the amendment advised the public by way of billboards to "Vote yes on Prop 22 for better health in California."

Dr. Frymann recalls:

> *"We had to try to devise ways in which we could combat, you might say, the juggernaut of the CMA; they got the money, and they got radio, television, and billboard advertisement for 'improved healthcare'. That was always their favorite phrase. We were reduced to things like putting announcements on peoples' cars in parking lots."*

Dr. Allen:

> *"We needed to put some kind of pressure on the legislature to try and get some legislative enactment that would help support and in time would lead to the restoration of the profession. Dr. Frymann had a patient that agreed to organize a group known as 'Californians in support of Osteopathy.' Ruth Kelley was her name. She was a dynamo of energy and an organizer; and patients of D.O.s were reached and encouraged to become members . . . When it was necessary to have some letters written to legislators supporting osteopathic bills, that was the group that could be called upon to write letters."*

Before the merger, in 1960, OPSC initiators provided a powerful example how each person with a passionate commitment can make a difference in healthcare. The AOA Board of Trustees had stated in July 1960 that it would revoke the COA's charter if the

COA continued negotiations with the CMA in exploration of merging the two professions. Some COA members considered the possibility that the COA might disobey the AOA warning and thus would lose its charter. What would happen to those D.O.s who wanted to remain in the AOA?

Dr. Frymann:

> "Dr. Eby realized there was not an organization in place for those who remained D.O.s in California. He did whatever it took to form the Osteopathic Physicians and Surgeons of California [OPSC] so that when the COA was eliminated there was an organization to accept D.O.s."

On December 8, 1960 OPSC announced officially the formation of a new state osteopathic society, OPSC, and applied to AOA for early recognition. A Board of Directors was formed, officers were elected, and committees were established, including a Legal and Legislative Committee.

OPSC began under the direction of the determined leadership of **Richard Eby, D.O**. As soon as he was chosen as the charter president, he chose his board members and set out for his first and most important task: to fly to Florida where the AOA House of Delegates was meeting, in order to make a plea for California's osteopathic profession.

On January 21, 1961 a special meeting of AOA House of Delegates at the AOA annual convention **granted a charter to the OPSC**, endorsed the actions by its Board of Trustees, and pledged support for future efforts to preserve the profession in California. The charter became important as a continued representation of the Osteopathic Association during the final merger decisions. Granting the charter to OPSC as California's osteopathic association meant that AOA was burning its bridges with the COA which had been the state's professional association for the previous six decades.

Dr. Eby:

> "Before a group which at the time had no real understanding of the situation, as only sparse rumors had reached official ears, I walked forward, never had talked to that gang, the whole AOA Board there, the Board from several states which were involved and whether they wanted to follow California or not . . . I told them what I thought: that somebody had the ingenuity to start a profession called Osteopathy, and that somebody had to have the courage to continue it, if it was valid. If they didn't continue it, then they indicated as a national group that they didn't believe in it. So I said, 'All you non-believers on the pole over there, you better think before I sit whether you want to tell the world that A.T. Still was a crap shooter that happened to get a few craps into his glove for a temporary thing, but that you're willing to throw him into the ocean and let him drown.' I forget the exact words but you get the idea. So [the

Speaker of the House] *asked, 'Are you through?' I said, 'I'm through, except telling the entire audience from all over the country, D.O.s and purported D.O.s, that either you belong to something whole-hearted or no hearted in this case; and the only thing that we will agree to in California is that osteopathy is part of the California picture in medicine.*

"That was the biggest day in my life up until then . . . when I got back that week we simply proceeded to select 12 of the D.O.s that had decided to be D.O.s come hell or high water (that's what it came to) as the board members for the first board of [what] *we would call the Osteopathic Physicians and Surgeons of California."*

Since 1961, OPSC has been representing the osteopathic profession in California. Among the osteopathic physicians who provided interviews for this project, Dr. Eby, Dr. Frymann, Dr. Allen, Dr. Dilworth, Dr. Krpan, Dr. Chesky, and Dr. Vinn have been president of OPSC.

On April 25, 1961 **OPSC filed a complaint** for injunctive relief and damages against CMA and COA, charging conspiracy to destroy the osteopathic profession in California, but on May 15, 1961 the temporary **injunction against merger was denied** on the basis that no irreparable damage would be done by allowing merger to proceed and that the merits of the case would be determined at a later trial date. No date was set, though.

On May 17, 1961, the COA House of Delegates approved the merger with the CMA. However, OPSC continued to fight to regain the power of the state osteopathic licensing board to administer new D.O. licenses. It took the fight to the state's legislative and executive branches, to no avail. Then, in 1967, the judicial branch listened to its pleas. Alexander Tobin, a lawyer familiar with civil rights issues, recognized at once that there was a breech of constitutional granted rights in the part of the Proposition 22 that removed the rights of the licensing board to grant new D.O. licenses. That part restricted the rights of D.O.s from out-of-state wishing to practice in California.

Though a small group—at times comprising only 35 politically active members, according to Dr. Dilworth—OPSC continued to fight for the reinstatement of the power of the state osteopathic licensing board to license new D.O.s in California.

Efforts to restore the osteopathic licensure

Upon the request of OPSC, hearings were conducted in December 1966 at the courts in Santa Barbara, CA on the restoration of the osteopathic licensure. The objective for these hearings was to request the re-establishment of the right to license osteopathic physicians in California. Viola Frymann, D.O., La Jolla, President of OPSC, opened the series of testimonies by briefly reviewing the history of the Board of Osteopathic Examiners. She explained that the profession as a whole had not been aware of plans for a merger until the profession's national convention in 1959. To her understanding, it was a minority of the profession that wanted the change and a minority that equally strongly felt about not changing to allopathy. A large group tended to go along where the power would fall.

A patient testified about osteopathic treatments received for sports and car accident injuries. *"Citizens in California should have access to this care, as people in other states,"* the patient stated. Dr. Frymann explained that legislature could bring back the osteopathic profession, using the mechanism of amendments to provide again the licensing ability of the Board of Osteopathic Examiners and to restore the reciprocity with other states (i.e. D.O.s from other states being able to practice in California).

William Stahl, D.O. from Pomona and a member of the Board of OPSC recalled to the legislature emotional pressure having been exerted in 1958 to leave the profession by statements like *"You are a dead or dying profession. Get the best deal you can get and get out."*

Forest Grunigen, M.D. and former D.O. testified as a member of a committee at CCM to establish a research center on manipulation. He explained that *"people in California will get better care if manipulation is taught in medical schools and researched. More people will get musculoskeletal manipulation if it is integrated rather than separate."*

Joseph Cosentino, M.D. and former D.O. and past (last) president of COA recalled that insurance companies asked him in his role as president of the COA *"Why don't D.O.s just become M.D.s?"* Dr. Cosentino felt that merger negotiations were made because of insurance companies.

Although these hearings were unsuccessful in convincing legislature to restore the Licensing Board, members of OPSC continued their efforts.

Edna M. Lay, D.O., as chair of the Legal and Legislature Committee of OPSC, repeatedly traveled to Chicago and other cities to report to the AOA Board of Trustees. Dr. Lay had been a graduate from Kirksville College of Osteopathic Medicine in 1946 and had just moved to California shortly before the merger. As soon as she received her California license, she started a practice in Ojai. She recalled being stunned by a letter in the mail, containing forms for her to sign, with the request for $65 in return for an M.D. degree. She could not believe her eyes and immediately set out to support the work of OPSC.

She "lobbied" (without any training in lobbying) in the legislature to represent the osteopathic profession; and she traveled to Sacramento countless times to support **Alexander Tobin, J.D**. She had met Alexander Tobin per chance and convinced him to take on the challenge. He remained steadfast in his commitment for the osteopathic profession, even as the case progressed and he faced the Attorney General and his large staff of lawyers.

Dr. Seffinger recently asked **Dr. Frymann** about the motivational energy that sustained this small band of osteopathic physicians in their efforts to restore the rights of their profession in California.

Dr. Seffinger: *"You in particular also had a strong desire to maintain the profession, whereas most of the D.O.s in the state didn't mind it going away."*

Dr. Frymann: *"No, it was the older people who had the experience of osteopathy for treating the whole range of human ailments that just didn't do a high velocity manipulation once in a while."*

Dr. Seffinger: *"Oh I see, the younger ones who had come out of COP&S, they thought it was just a technique add on."*

Dr. Frymann: *"Yes."*

Dr. Seffinger: *"So they didn't feel it was as much to give up, they can just do manipulation anyway, so they didn't have a sense of what osteopathy really entailed."*

Dr. Frymann: No, they didn't."*

Dr. Seffinger: *"And you saw this having grown up and being raised and taken care of by an osteopathic doctor in England, knew what the potential was, and that was worth the fight and struggle?"*

Dr. Frymann: *"Yes."*

OPSC persevered through years of frustrating legal battles to reverse the 1962 amendment and to reinstate the power of the state osteopathic licensing board.

Dr. Frymann:

"The case was filed in 1967 with representatives of

1) *Each of the osteopathic schools;*
2) *Those who were either born in California;*
3) *Raised in California;*
4) *Anyone who wanted to come back to California to practice whether they were born here or not;*
5) *Those in the armed services and could practice in Vandenberg or Camp Pendleton but couldn't step outside to treat patients.*

So, those were the represented, all of the plaintiffs in this case, because, as I said, they couldn't get a license through the M.D. board, and they couldn't get a license through the osteopathic board."

Dr. Allen:

"Members of the profession outside the state had been sending in requests to get a license in California and so it got to the Board of Osteopathic Examiners. The Board of Osteopathic Examiners answered them and said they couldn't do anything about getting them a license because of Proposition 22 in 1962. The

medical board would write them back and say 'you're a D.O. There's no way to get a license either from the medical board or the osteopathic board.'

"The court case was known as "D'Amico et al."

"It was put into the courts as a class action suit, so that when you won you covered the other arena of osteopathic doctors to be representatives of one of the schools to be representatives of the armed services to be representatives of California residents and non-California residents. So it was truly a class action suit. At this time in the history of the United States, class action suits were en vogue.

"So the court case was filed in 1968 and it proceeded in the courts up until 1974. The CMA was fighting us every step of the way . . . The AMA would also.

"An associate of Dr. Tobin was a Mr. Gasner. We went from Superior Court, we were defeated there, so we appealed the Appellate Court and we lost there and so we appealed to the Supreme Court. The Supreme Court said you got a good case but there's not enough evidence, and sent it back down to Superior Court. So, the next time we went to Superior Court we won. Then I think it went to the Appellate Court by the other side. We won again, and then it finally went to the Supreme Court for a second time for a hearing . . . .

"It was on the class action suit that a person that has a legitimate profession should have the right to be licensed in California and so this was a denial of civil rights. That was the main argument, the basic gist of it. And finally on March 19, 1974 the Supreme Court said 'action sustained', which meant we had won. I think the documents made a stack of papers about this high (36") for the 4 or 6 years that this was in the court case, about 3 feet high stack of papers with all the arguments. And the answer was on a postcard that said 'Action sustained'. So March 19, 1974 was a red letter day."

Thus, in **1974**, without further opposition and by a unanimous vote, the California State Supreme Court of seven justices reinstated the osteopathic licensing board by ruling that the restrictions imposed upon the California osteopathic licensing board in the initiative act known as proposition 22 was indeed a restriction of trade, illegal and unconstitutional. Some of the historical documents, including the arguments made to regain licensure, temporarily went to the OPSC office. They are now housed in the archives of the Harriet K. & Philip Pumerantz Library at Western University, College of Osteopathic Medicine of the Pacific, in Pomona, California.

Dr. Allen:

"One of the turnabouts that really was surprising was when we started moving through the halls of the legislature and asked to have an audience

with some of the legislatures: 'why, were you the ones that won that Supreme Court decision?', 'yes', 'well, congratulations, come in and tell us what you have to say'. It was like winning the Oscar for the movies, to win a Supreme Court decision. It just turned around a whole acceptance even though we were such a small group."

With the authority of the Board of Osteopathic Examiners returned, the newly named **Osteopathic Medical Board of California** (OMBC) has since then been empowered to regulate the osteopathic profession in California.

Dr. Allen:

"Memorial Day Holiday of 1974 the Board of Osteopathic Examiners examined about 125 new D.O.s . . . From then on, about every 3 or 4 months they had a licensing section because the applicants were coming."

Dr. Frymann:

"The first thing that we realized had to be done, almost the day after the judgment was rendered, was that we must have a Board of Examiners that provided a practical exam so that we knew that we licensed people who had hands that were of some value to them. That was how the practical exam came to be instituted."

Dr. Seffinger:

"Were other states using that as far as the licensing exam?"

Dr. Frymann:

"I think some other states were, I'm not sure what, but Mr. Tobin was thoroughly in support of this and he worked through the legislative channels in order to get this established.

"Initially the results weren't very good. About 30% of those who applied didn't pass. After about two years the governor complained. Too many people failed, and they wanted to have the requirements modified somewhat . . . And then came a time when they said that all the members of the Board should be removed and they should have a new roster of people.

"I was never an official member of the Board. I was an assistant examiner of whom they used quite a number to handle the practical exams. But I think the practical exam is extremely important because that's the only way that you can judge whether the person is competent or not. They may be able to

write the best-written exam but that doesn't tell you what they can do with their hands."

Dr. Seffinger:

"What about surgeons or people who don't treat patients as much these days that come into California, should they have to take the practical exam?"

Dr. Frymann:

"Yes, because they should be treating patients before and after surgery and there are a growing number of surgeons, certainly in the east that are doing that."

Dr. Seffinger:

"What about radiologists or pathologists?"

Dr. Frymann:

"Well radiologists have been trained in those manipulative skills and should have a rudimentary knowledge of them so that they know to use osteopathic concepts when they interpret an x-ray, which is important. They should have certain basic skills. You'll find that in most instances, the radiologists are the people who say, 'oh, yes, I treat my family, my friends'. They're not the ones who give me the most trouble. It's the people with a family practice, that don't treat their patients."

As can be gleaned from Dr. Frymann's comments on restoring osteopathic manipulative medicine as part of the licensing protocol, D.O.s in California were able to endorse again their distinctive osteopathic philosophy. Aiming for the highest professional standards in California became almost a national effort, as D.O.s from out-of-state moved to California to help rebuild the profession.

Dr. Krpan:

"We are fortunate because we had good people coming into the state. We had people coming to the state who were osteopathically oriented—D.O.s who recognized the value of their degree, including Norm Vinn and Gary Graham, of course Earl Gabriel, Gil Roth, and Stu Chesky. They all served

on the Board while I was there. Joseph Zammuto was on that early Board and they were all interested in osteopathic medicine. They had a fervor for osteopathic medicine. They did what they could to support the profession and make it grow."

Establishing new osteopathic colleges in California

Since COP&S had been converted to CCM as part of the merger and then transferred to UC Irvine to become their College of Medicine, a new osteopathic school had to be developed. In 1977 the establishment of the **College of Osteopathic Medicine of the Pacific** (COMP) in Pomona was celebrated as the profession's rise from the ashes.

Dr. Frymann:

" . . . *so they* [OPSC] *reached a point were they had no money. We only had one person in the office, and by the end of 1974 we reached a point where there wasn't even enough money in the treasury to pay the secretary's salary . . . It was at this point that Dr. Eby suddenly said, 'I make a motion that this organization should do everything possible to restore a college of osteopathy in California'. Well, everybody laughed. After all, there wasn't enough money for an office! And so that was the first words about establishing a college.*

"*It sounded utterly impossible when Dr. Eby suggested it! But Dr. Eby was a man of faith and he knew that school would be built.*

"*Shortly after that I had talked to the AOA in Chicago and with Dr. Pumerantz,* [Chairman of the Department of Education]. *He told me very bluntly that the man we got working for us as president was useless. He wasn't going to be of any help to us. So, after a while I said, 'tell me, what are the qualities we should be looking for in a president?' He listed them and I suddenly said to him, 'would you like the job?' He said, "No, no, we had basically established in Chicago; we had no desire to move' and I said 'alright'.*

"*But Dr. Allen got a call from Dr. Thompson who was president of Kirksville* [Kirksville College of Osteopathic Medicine in Kirksville MO] *at that time and he said to him 'I think if you were to ask Dr. Pumerantz again he might be interested'. So, I called Dr. Pumerantz and I asked him to come out and visit us, look over the situation. I wasn't offering him a job in my way of thinking. This was just a get acquainted meeting, but he assumed this was the real thing. However, he came out and I remember we met him in Eby's hospital up on Park Avenue."*

Dr. Pumerantz:

"We had some more discussions with Harriet, my wife, and with some of the principals here in California and went back to my office in Chicago, at the AOA office. I knew at that time a number of people also didn't know I was being considered to start the school here, but I had heard conversations in the office that went something like this, 'If they put together the ten best educators in the country and sent them to California, they couldn't start an osteopathic college.' I went home that night. I said to Harriet, 'We're going to California', which we did.

"Then I came out here to meet with those visionaries who wanted to start this school, Drs. Allen, Dilworth, Frymann, and Eby. They had identified a shopping center for us that had been defunct for a number of years. We had a little office to start in, a little rented room with some borrowed furniture, a telephone that wasn't working at the time, and a secretary who I had hired a couple of months before I arrived. The day after Labor Day 1977 I came onto this campus and we opened the door of that little rented room for the first time and that's when I date the start of the college of the university, the day after Labor Day in 1977. When I got here, I realized at that moment as I opened the door that this was an immense task I had ahead of me. This shopping center, this mall . . . it was absolutely deserted.

"There was nobody here. There was tumbleweed going down the center of the street and I turned around and I looked up at the mountains and that appeared to be a symbol—it's a metaphor for what I had to face. It's like climbing a mountain.

"I asked the secretary who joined me that morning to come with me. 'Let's go find a stationery store'. And she took me to a stationery store not far from the campus and I put into a shopping cart paper clips and papers, some pencils and all of that stuff, and we brought it back and opened the office and started. I used to tell people that we started this college from the paper clips on up, and then we started to grow."

The founding Board of Directors of the College of Osteopathic Medicine of the Pacific were Chairman Ethan Allen, D. O., Richard Eby, D.O., Donald Dilworth, D.O., Frank York Lee, M.D. (ex-D.O.), Frank Carr, Vice President of the United California Bank in Pomona, and Saul Bernat, Ph.D., Executive Director of the New Mexico Osteopathic Medical Association. Saul Bernat became the second Chairman of the Board from 1978 to 1982, when he died just as the first students were graduating.

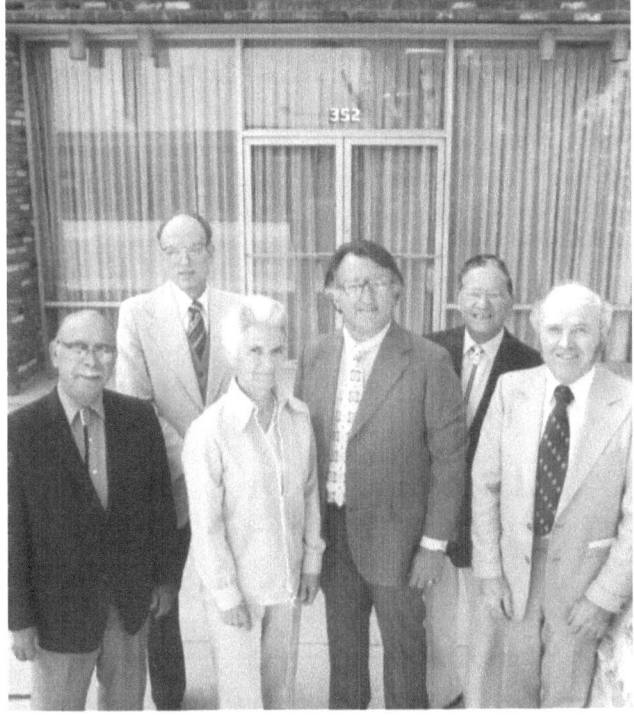

Figure 18. "Founders of the College of Osteopathic Medicine of the Pacific, 1977:
From left to right: Saul Bernat, Ph.D., Donald Dilworth, D.O., Viola Frymann, D.O.,
Philip Pumerantz, Ph.D., Richard Eby, D.O., Ethan Allen, D.O."

From the present day perspective one might wonder about Pomona as choice of location for a new osteopathic college. The previous school had relocated initially from Anaheim in the 1890s to downtown Los Angeles near the busy part of town called "Angel's flight". From there, the college relocated across the street from the Los Angeles County Hospital with its training opportunities for the students and graduates of COP&S. All these locations of the college were chosen because they were centers of a big city's activity, with many doctors and several hospitals near by. Pomona, however, was located far away from a major city and hospitals for training opportunities. **Dr. Frymann** explained:

167

> *"Yes, but one attraction was that it was a place of great need. There was a mixed population there, immigrants, and there was very little medical care. And it was felt this would be an ideal place for a clinic for service to these under-privileged people. That was one thing. Another thing was that Dr. Eby lived there and he had his hospital there. You see his hospital was still an osteopathic hospital, the only one in the state at that point I think. And because this realtor was the father of Dr. Eby's son-in-law, it was within the family and we got that Penney building for a ridiculous sum of money, ridiculous sum of money, so that was how it came to be there."*

Once Dr. Pumerantz was on board, a faculty had to be developed. Since most former faculty members had left the osteopathic profession to become M.D.s, conceiving a new osteopathic faculty became a major challenge.

Dr. Pumerantz recalls the early days of improvising medical education at COMP:

> *"The early faculty was an extraordinary group of people. I remember that several of the faculty members from the old COP&S came by in the first several months of 1977 after I arrived expressing an interest to teach here. I think we had a couple of them. One was an anatomist whose name I've forgotten, a very popular anatomist at COP&S who came to help us. Also, Cal Poly Pomona was the source of some part-time professors. In fact, four of them were loaned to me by the president of Cal Poly to teach in the basic sciences; one was in anatomy. The anatomy professor at Cal Poly helped me get the first cadavers, so we bought nine cadavers. We put them in the cold room which we had just built in our first building, which is now the research building. This was the JCPenney building at that point. Because it was important that we built an anatomy lab, as anatomy would be an important part of the curriculum, I had these cadavers before we had the faculty. I would tell people in those days that I had more cold bodies than warm bodies."*

Good faculty members they were indeed, and very generous in donating their time and effort. **Dr. Frymann** recalls:

> *"And so between the starting of school, which I think was October, until January, there was no OMM* [osteopathic manipulative medicine] *taught at all. And the president would come to me from time to time and say, 'You have to come here and teach it.' I said, 'Well, I have a practice here in La Jolla. I can't just come up here and teach it.' So, in January, he finally put the pressure on and I said, 'Alright, I will come up here and teach all day Monday, I will work Saturdays at home and so I would drive up on Saturday evening to Pomona, I would spend all day Sunday preparing my schedule for Monday's lesson, and teach on Monday.' And if we hadn't had, I think, two public holidays in*

the course of those eight weeks, I don't think I'd ever have survived, because, you see, I was it. I had no helpers, and at the end of the year they had to have final exams, practical exams. I had to do the whole thing and there were 36 students at that time."

Dr. Seffinger:

"You didn't have funds for somebody to hire to do this job?"

Dr. Frymann:

"No, there were no funds. This was a voluntary service to the college. And so the 2nd year by this time they brought in 56 students for the 2nd year, so now the AOA required two full time people. Well, now what's the definition of a full time person? [Back then]That was somebody who put in 20 hours [of teaching] a week, and so I would drive up there on Saturday, I would teach all day Monday and Tuesday morning, I'd drive back to be in the office by 2 o'clock on Tuesday, I would then drive up there on Wednesday evening after I've finished, I would teach on Thursday morning, and I'd drive back on Thursday night! And where was the 2nd full time person coming from? I couldn't get anyone. So what I did was I called upon I think it was six of the best teachers in the country, Hollis Wolf, Thomas Schooley, Harold Magoun, Herb Miller. I think there were six people. Each one would come out for one week, twice in the year. And so that blend of all these people they got the other full time person. That was accepted by the AOA. So that's how we got through the second year."

Laws and regulations to protect osteopathic education and training

With the re-establishment of osteopathic education in California, antagonism required many a legislative battle.

Matt Weyuker:

"I came on board as OPSC's Associate Executive Director on June 1, 1978, and became the "Exec" on August 1, 1978. My first three responsibilities were to move the office from South Laguna Beach to Sacramento, hire sufficient staff, and stop AB 2691. Before I was on the OPSC payroll, on May 30, 1978 I was asked to travel to the State Capitol in Sacramento to take on, and/or stop a legislative bill (AB 2691—Agnos), that was going to be heard in the Assembly Committee on Ways and Means the following day, and that already had a good head of steam up, having passed the Assembly Committee on Health with little or no opposition. If passed by the Legislature, then enacted *by the Governor, this measure would have essentially nullified the California State Supreme Court's D'Amico decision of March 1974, by permitting the state's medical board (BMQA) to license D.Os. This was a follow-up bill to SB 1044 (Garamendi).*

"On May 30ᵗʰ I literally ran around the Capitol building as if my pants were on fire. I met with at least 10 to 12 legislators of the 23 member Assembly committee. AB 2691 was passed out of the Ways and Means Committee by a vote of 14 to5 which was a far more dismal showing than the vaunted CMA had expected.

"Early in August, AB 2691 came before the 9 member Senate Committee on Business and Professions. The committee had a long agenda and didn't hear the bill until just before they broke for dinner. The Board of Osteopathic Examiners [BOE] President Dr. Billie Strumillo, BOE Executive Secretary Gareth Williams, COMP President Dr. Philip Pumerantz, OPSC Board Member Dr. Ethan Allen, and I spoke against the measure. When Committee Chairman Senator Alex Garcia called for the vote it was 3 to 3. Voting "yes" were Senators Marks, Wilson, and Presley. Voting "no" were Senators B. Green, Roberti, and Song. Immediately the bill's author Assemblyman Art Agnos (who was to become the Mayor of San Francisco in the mid 1980s) requested that the vote remain open, (technically speaking the bill was placed "on-call").

"After dinner both sides tried in vain to move the yes and no voters, and herein lies a funny story. When Jay Michael, who was the CEO and lobbyist-in-charge of the CMA's 9 member lobbyist Sacramento office, asked Senator Bill Green, who is a black man, 'Are you going to let a minority profession get away with blocking this important piece of legislation?' The Senator, who is a big man, about 6'4" and 240 pounds, with an equally large and booming voice, when I first met Bill in 1967, he was the Reading Clerk of the State Assembly—and was first elected to the Assembly in 1968, said forcefully while poking Mr. Michael in the chest with his rather large index finger, 'Jay, let me tell something about minorities!' The CMA had just inanely lost the black Senator's vote for a long, long time.

" . . . The strategy was to not allow either Assemblyman Agnos or the CMA to present the bill. Instead I had asked Senator Bill Green to make a motion for the Senate Finance Committee to send AB 2691 out for an interim study, and in the Committee passing Senator Green's motion by a vote of 7 to 4 (voting "yes" were Senators Behr, Green, Petris, Smith, Stull, Cusanovich, and Rodda; voting "no" were Senators Gregorio, Nejedly, Holmdahl, and Stiern; not voting were Senators Alquist and Carpenter), the Committee, in essence killed the measure."

OPSC supported legislation that prohibited discrimination against D.O.s in 1984 (SB 1571) and in 1988 (SB 2491). In regards to education, a bill signed by the governor in 1989 (SB 1249), provided that no medical school or clinical training program in California can deny access to elective clerkships or preceptorships. Currently, D.O. students, residents and physicians are able to train and practice in virtually any facility in the state.

Dr. Krpan:

"The Osteopathic Physicians and Surgeons of California, our state association, has a legislative bent. Our Executive Director for close to 20 years was Matt Weyuker and Matt Weyuker was probably head and shoulders above anybody we've had legislatively, [Mr. Weyuker was employed by the California Trucking Association prior to being employed by OPSC]. *He knew the legislative process; he knew legislators because he had been in the capitol for so long so when legislation would come through that looked like it was going to impact us adversely, Matt would call our legislative committee and whoever was president at that time and they would go to the legislature and get a Senator or one of the assemblymen to carry a bill for us and then we would push it to see if we could get it passed."*

Matt Weyuker:

"My daughter-in-law worked for BMQA [Board of Medical Quality Assurance] *in 1979, and she told me of an agenda item on the December 7, 1979 BMQA board meeting that was scheduled in San Diego that would be disastrous to the osteopathic profession. I alerted everyone, (OPSC board members, COMP President Pumerantz, and the BOE) about this turn of events. At that time there was a former D.O., Dr. Joseph Cosentino, from Sacramento who was the 1962 President of the California Osteopathic Association and one of the ringleaders that led to Proposition 22 in that same year, and was now serving BMQA as its Chief Medical Officer, and along with some of the 'rebels' of the now defunct COA, Dr. Taylor and others, were instrumental in the placement of this insidious item on the December agenda.*

"What that agenda item proposed was the following: that the BMQA Board adopt regulations and approve D.O. education, training, and post-graduate training institutions, for the expressed purpose of licensing D.O.s. By adopting this language, BMQA would circumvent both the essence of the CA Supreme Court's ruling in its D'Amico decision, and the CA State Legislature—as well as doing the bidding of the CA Medical Association and the 41st State Medical Association. When that day in December arrived, at least 3 of the former D.O.s

spoke in favor of the proposal, along with leaders of the CMA, representatives from the M.D. medical school community, and some CMA affiliate officials. Speaking on behalf of Osteopathic Profession were: OPSC Board member Dr. Ethan Allen, BOE President Dr. Billie Strumillio, COMP President Dr. Philip Pumerantz, and me. BMQA took all of the testimony under advisement, taking no action . . . . But the unresolved outcome gave us that were present at that December meeting a loud wake up call.

"Then the CMA did the obvious. They had State Senator John Foran, a member of the Senate Committee on Business and Professions, introduce an identical measure to 1978's AB 2691-SB 1199; Foran's Senate district contained the CMA's headquarters office located in San Francisco. Because OPSC's office was now located in Sacramento in the shadow of the State Capitol, I was in the Capitol building almost daily "schmoozing" with Legislators and staff, educating them about the Osteopathic Medical Profession, informing them that the profession was back and that they would be seeing and hearing from more of us. In as much as Senator Foran missed the bill introduction cut-off, his bill couldn't and wouldn't be able to be heard in a Senate Committee (Business and Professions) until some time in August or September, SB 1199 had become a 2-year bill. In SB 1199's situation, meaning a bill that, if enacted, couldn't take effect until January 1st of 1981).

"Suffice it to say that my lobbying efforts were so successful, that when Senator Foran took up his bill, SB 1199 in the Senate Business and Profession's Committee in August 1979, he could not get a motion to move the bill! With the election in November 1978 numerous new Senators who rode in on the property-tax-cutting-Proposition 13's back were seated. Among them were Senators John Doolittle, who is now in the U.S. Congress, and Joe Montoya, who was to become Chairman of that Committee and a good friend of the profession. The two newest members of the Business and Professions Committee and a holdover, Senator John Briggs were helpful in weakening the CMAs legislative effort. The CMA, in a face-saving move, pulled the bill off-calendar for the purpose of amending the measure. SB 1199 was not brought back to the committee again."

With osteopathic training securely assigned again solely to osteopathic medical schools in California, the College of Osteopathic Medicine of the Pacific (COMP) is thriving. By October 2007, COMP has an enrollment of 724 students in its four-year osteopathic medical program. The current first year class has 219 students enrolled with 30 designated spots for students from the Northwest region of the United States; 500 students of the 724 are Californians.

Over 2,500 osteopathic medical students have graduated from COMP and 64% of COMP alumni practice in California. They go into every specialty in medicine. The year 2007 marks the 30th anniversary of the founding of COMP, which is now one of the many professional education colleges at Western University of Health Sciences in Pomona, California. COMP started in a rented office; 30 years later, it is spreading over a significant portion of the 20 acres belonging to Western University.

At COMP, first and second year students receive over 200 hours of training in osteopathic manipulative medicine (OMM) skill development and integrative osteopathic problem solving within their clinical sciences coursework. Since 2001, third year students are required to participate in a month long clinical clerkship in osteopathic manipulative medicine (OMM).

Thus, traditional osteopathic training is alive and well in California. COMP has numerous clinical rotation sites (medical centers, hospitals, clinics, and practices) throughout the Inland Empire and Southern California that are training sites for COMP students in their third and fourth years of medical school. Sites include Arrowhead Regional Medical Center, Riverside County Medical Center, Downey Regional Medical Center and Pacific Hospital of Long Beach. COMP sponsors 20 residency programs for a total of 246 positions in California in disciplines ranging from family medicine to neurosurgery.

Northern California now also has an osteopathic college, namely **Touro University College of Osteopathic Medicine of California (TUCOM).** This college matriculated its first class of 66 students in August 1997. Originally known as the San Francisco College of Osteopathic Medicine, TUCOM opened its doors on the campus of the California College of Podiatric Medicine. The founding Dean was Bernard I. Zeliger, D.O. Soon the opportunity arose to relocate TUCOM to the former Mare Island Naval Shipyard in the city of Vallejo about one hour north of San Francisco. The College's third class matriculated here in August 1999. As the University has grown, various buildings, including some which have historical status, have been renovated for classrooms, laboratories, library, offices, student activities and dormitory space. The University now includes four colleges; in addition to osteopathic medicine.

The American Association of Colleges of Osteopathic Medicine (AACOM) recently reported that *"in the roughly 40 years since 1968, the education of osteopathic physicians has grown tremendously. In 1968, there were just five colleges of osteopathic medicine. By Fall 2007, the locations for undergraduate osteopathic medical education will have increased five-fold, with 23 colleges and three branch campuses. And, several additional colleges are in the development stage. In 1968, the five colleges enrolled 1,879 students and annually produced 426 D.O.s. In 2006, enrollment totaled 14,435 students more than a seven-fold increase, and the colleges graduated 2,713 D.O.s. By comparison, the numbers of allopathic medical students and graduates have not quite doubled in the same time frame"* (AACOM, Washington, D.C., e-letter 2-9-07).

The essence of osteopathic medicine is the continued practice of osteopathic manipulative treatment (OMT). Osteopathic physicians in California feel that their profession revitalized itself by emphasizing once again musculoskeletal manipulation for diagnosis and treatment. *"Osteopathic manipulative treatment is a series of unique manual medicine techniques applied to the patient, in both health and disease, to maintain homeostasis of the individual in health or to assist in restoring homeostasis in disease"* (AOA, 2006, The seven osteopathic medical competencies: A basis for future testing).

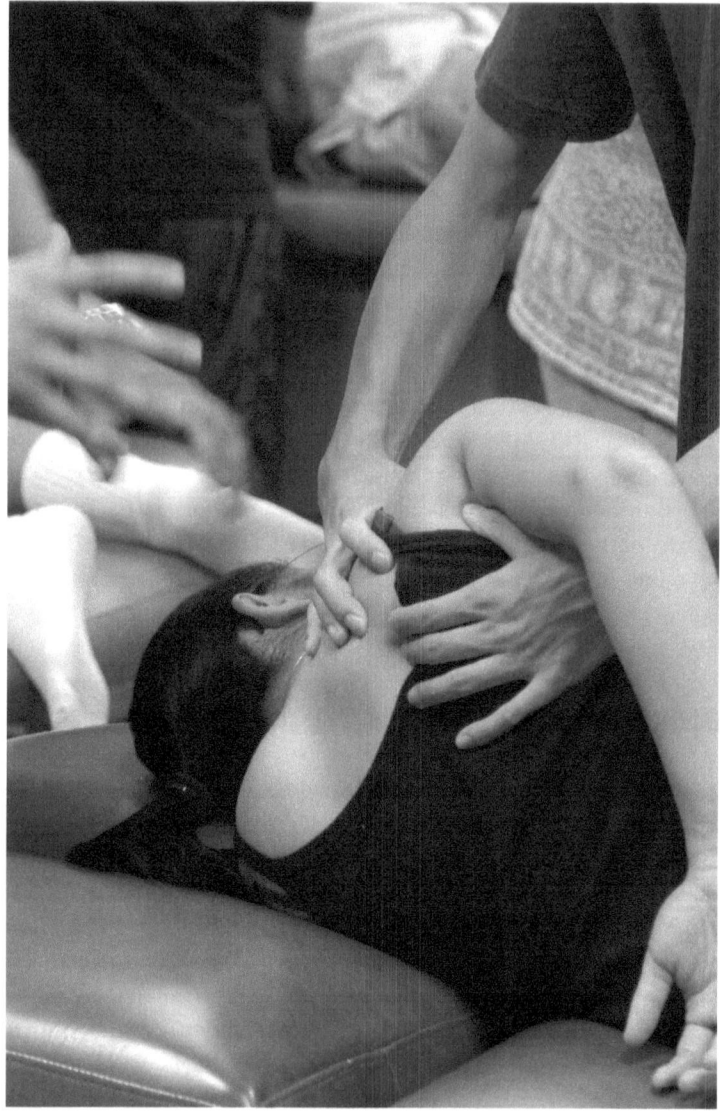

Figure 19. "Student learning the scapular myofascial release OMT procedure during osteopathic manipulative medicine class at the College of Osteopathic Medicine of the Pacific, 2008"

Seemingly then, all is well with osteopathy in California, practicing side-by-side with allopathic medicine in a mutually respectful relationship. As will be described in Chapter 6, many factors contribute to strengthen this confidence, while causes for concerns are raised as well about the survival of a minority medical profession in an allopathically oriented culture of healthcare in California and nationwide.

Dr. Van den Noort:

"At the time in 1977, I ignored it [the opening of COMP]. *I had too much on my plate to be worried about it. If they wanted to do that, that's fine with me, as the osteopathic licensing board's inability to license new D.O.s in the state was overruled by the courts. I didn't have any problem with it. I would like to see us work together that's all. I have no opposition to it."*

Chapter 6

Bridging the M.D. — D.O. divide

As described in Chapter 5, the 41ˢᵗ Medical Society served as a home base for former osteopathic physicians to transition into the M.D. world. Since former D.O.s no longer had the COA to meet their needs for social and organizational activities, the 41ˢᵗ Medical Society was established to provide such opportunities. Twenty years were anticipated for the society's existence at which time the membership would merge with the existing 40 County Medical Societies in California. As events proceeded, the 41ˢᵗ Medical Society remained in existence until 1997.

The 41ˢᵗ Medical Trust

In the years prior to the merger, when the osteopathic profession in California had become increasingly successful, their professional organization had accumulated considerable funds. These collective assets comprised about 8 million dollars, including COA cash reserves of about $717,000, medical school property valued at about $5 million, other property of about $1.5 million, and expected COA membership dues of about $450,000 (OPSC v. CMA, 224 Cal. App. 2d 378, 381, 1964).

In 1962, these assets were deposited as a trust. The trust existed separate from the 41ˢᵗ Medical Society and was run by the Board of Trustees. In 1964, the 41ˢᵗ Medical Trust was established, with the purpose to apply the trust corpus and income for furthering the unification of M.D.s and D.O.s and to support and expand the California College of Medicine, including building a hospital on UC Irvine campus and conducting research. The Trust was to exist for 20 years. Dr. Passy and Dr. Steedman explained this trust as follows:

Dr. Passy:

> *"Now there were monies that were accumulated in this society through the 41ˢᵗ Medical Society. They had a fund that was working. During these years the hospitals and the clinics that we were using for the training of the emerging physicians were sold and the money that they accumulated from that—I can't remember how much it was. Bob do you remember how much they sold that for?*

Dr. Steedman:

"Well, from selling all of the properties out there and other properties we had adjoining the College of Osteopathic Physicians and Surgeons' property, and then the money that was in the membership at that time . . . It was my impression that it was somewhere between 2 to 3 million dollars."

Dr. Passy:

"I don't know what it was at that time that the 41ˢᵗ trust was at first identified, but they needed a trust to put this money into. But I do know that as of August 1, 1983 the trust assets were approximately $486,000. Since then, it may have grown."

Dr. Allen:

" . . . there was news coming out of the college [COP&S] that the faculty and the professors were not as many or as qualified or the best [in 1961]. *So they put out a message to the membership to pay an extra hundred dollars of their dues each year of membership dues. The $100 were to be turned over to the college to improve the quality of the college. They did that quite successfully over several years and, actually, the trust fund that was in the COA at the time of the merger amounted to over $500,000 and that's the trust fund that went into the 41ˢᵗ. That money was initially requested in order to support the college and make the college have better faculty and better teaching quality and so on."*

Changes in purpose over time

After 20 years, on December 31, 1983, the 41ˢᵗ Medical Trust funds were transferred to the UC Irvine College of Medicine support foundation. Since then, the purpose of the Medical Trust has been to conduct research on musculoskeletal manipulation.

Dr. Passy's documentation:

"There was a letter from the attorney James Cordey, who was the deputy attorney general for Los Angeles. And he writes regarding the 41ˢᵗ Medical Society Trust, 'as we discussed in a telephone conversation in November of '84, I am enclosing your review and comment of the attorney generals' office documentation pertaining to the termination of the 41ˢᵗ Medical Society trust. This is a trust that only lasted twenty years, from 1964, when it first began. Since there are no private beneficiaries in the trust, it is my understanding that the trust is subject to the supervision of the attorney general's office, pursuant to California Government Code—something or another. As a background, the trust was established on

*December 31ˢᵗ of 1964, and it is required to terminate no later than December 31ˢᵗ of 1983. The trust was funded from the grant of property from the 41ˢᵗ Medical Society **for the purpose of furthering the unification of Doctors of Medicine and Doctors of Osteopathy and to support the California College of Medicine, now known as University of California at Irvine, School of Medicine.***"

Dr. Passy continued:

> *"Let me read something from the proposed Regents agenda as a member of the educational committee, that was read in 1983. 'Consent for appointment to successor trustee to the 41ˢᵗ Medical Trust to be the California College of Medicine support foundation in Irvine, California'."*

Since 1984, the unification of M.D.s and D.O.s no longer has been the objective of the 41ˢᵗ Medical Trust, but the support and expansion of the California College of Medicine has continued as a primary goal. The pursuit of research on manipulation can certainly be viewed as an effort to support the College in providing science-based education and training. Dr. Grunigen was chosen as executive director of the Board of Trustees of the Support Foundation. Dr. Passy, who was well-known and respected among former D.O.s and M.D.s, was appointed to lead a committee of the 41ˢᵗ Medical Trust to provide research funds for qualified studies on musculoskeletal manipulation.

Dolores Grunigen recalls:

> *"The 41st Medical Trust was originally created to hold the assets of the 41st Medical Society and make them available for educational and charitable purposes or, as the formal statement reads:*
> *'The parties contemplate that we would eventually determine whether or not there was an underlying reason for the favorable clinical results practitioners had experienced in using the osteopathic concepts'."*

Research on musculoskeletal manipulation

Alumni of the College who were former osteopaths fully agreed to undertake such a research program. The individual whose leadership and perseverance facilitated the establishment of the research was Forest Grunigen, M.D. He felt convinced that the integration of musculoskeletal treatments in traditional medicine would improve healthcare. To that purpose, he facilitated moving the former College of Osteopathic Physicians and Surgeons, to become the California College of Medicine, transferred to the University of California, Irvine (UCI). His hope was that UCI's strong infrastructure for conducting scientific research would provide opportunities to demonstrate scientifically the effectiveness of musculoskeletal manipulation. Based on such evidence, musculoskeletal manipulation would be practiced by allopathy as well as osteopathy. Throughout his long life he continued to search the world over for researchers who were most respected for their work in basic science and investigations into the efficacy of osteopathic manipulation.

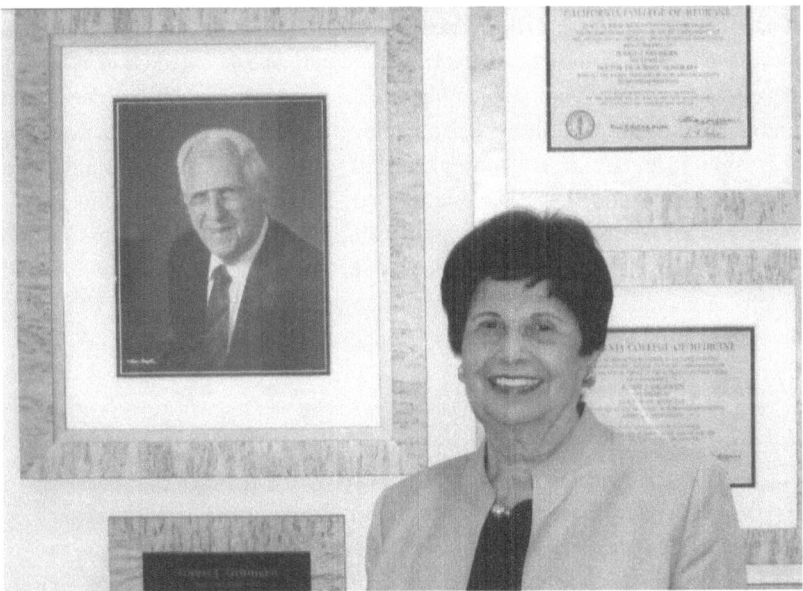

Figure 20. "Dolores Grunigen at the Forest J. Grunigen, M.D. Medical Center Library in Orange CA, 2007"

Dr. Seffinger:

"There are M.D.s now, orthopedic surgeons and physical medicine and rehabilitation doctors in Europe and Russia that do manual medicine research. All these groups developed since the merger in California."

The Fourth International Symposium on Advances in Osteopathic Research was conducted jointly with the 10th International Congress of the German Osteopathic Association in October 2007 in Germany. The scientific organizing committee includes osteopathic physicians from the United States and Professor Resch, M.D. from Germany.

Dr. Passy:

"The person who really pushed it, the person who really wanted to answer that question more than anyone was Forest Grunigen. He was the guy that made sure that this 41st trust was directed in the right way. He was on the Board. He was always making sure that I was on the right track in terms of getting this

179

together. It was his need, his feeling that if you are going to do anything, let's get this done, then we can go into medicine—then we can get to where we are going. He wanted to make sure that this object was identified".

Thus, since the merger in California, the 41st Medical Trust Fund has been a pioneer in advocating research on musculoskeletal manipulation. The 41st Medical Trust committee was among the first in the Nation to emphasize the need for mechanism research, rather than limiting investigations to the evidence about clinical effectiveness. With the support of the 41st Trust Fund and UC Irvine, musculoskeletal manipulation research and guidelines for use in clinical practice have been developed. They can be considered a product of the merger and the creation of the College of Medicine at UC Irvine from COP&S. Dr. Grunigen's advocacy, as well as the studies conducted by Dr. Tobis and others, built the foundations. It was the atmosphere and culture of the post merger era at UC Irvine that provided fertile ground for this growth in education and research.

Dr. Passy:

" . . . . they didn't want to lose it. They didn't want to lose the fact that they thought there was something in musculoskeletal treatment in the advancement of medicine. And they thought that if we all became M.D.s, that aspect of treatment would be lost, and they didn't want that. And at the time, no one really proved the fact that physical therapy, physical manipulation aided in the well being of people. They didn't have the science behind it to prove it, and that's what they wanted to do here. That's why, over the years when we had the monies delegated, we allocated about $50,000 a year to open up research—to open up the field to find out, to really pinpoint the fact, why and how did musculoskeletal treatment help in the treatment of patients with illnesses. Over the years, we've been doing this and we've not come up with anything. We've had research people come up and do various things, but it didn't really prove that point . . .

"I'm not much of a researcher. But if you're asking me a question, that I could just pick out of the air and come up with some answers, I would say, 'hey, how about coming and showing me that if I take a pill and you could tell me and show me scientifically that the pill is fixing the neuromuscular modality of that arm, so that it would be working better after I manipulated it, before and after I manipulated it'—then you could tell me that. But I'm not sure that you've got that pill. That's the pill that I want to find, or the physical manipulation that I want to discover."

Dr. van den Noort:

"I just think that manipulation medicine is good and that we need to emphasize it and make it more scientific and proceed in that direction and I

am fully supportive of, but the problem is where the money is going to come from to do it. The university has emerged into two different directions. In the old days if you did half your day in the laboratory and half your day in the clinic you could survive in a medical school. That's not true anymore. If you are going to do basic research, you've got to do it 85% of the time; at least to be competitive for grants. On the clinical side you have to make your money from seeing patients, setting up programs, and different things. You have to make your own money."

Forty years after the 41st Medical Trust recognized the importance of manipulation research, the National Institutes of Health National Center for Complementary and Alternative Medicine have made multidisciplinary research funds available. In addition, the American Osteopathic Association, the American Academy of Osteopathy, the Osteopathic Heritage Foundation, the Foundations of Osteopathic Health Systems, and other foundations have allocated research funds for osteopathic manipulation studies. Thus, the message of the 41st Trust in California has been heard and action is being taken nationwide. To this day, the 41st Medical Trust continues to be active in its role to promote research.

Dr. van den Noort:

"I would like to see manipulation taught in medical schools and I would like to see more emphasis on it. We get a lot of resistance today from orthopedists and neurosurgeons, but I think neurologists and physiatrists would welcome manipulation. The Academy of Neurology has a section on manipulation medicine and is very much involved. So I think it can be brought in, not by closing your school but by gradually working together to promote common programs, I think that's a very good idea."

Is that the main distinction between the professions?

Dr. Van den Noort:

"I think we don't have enough manipulation medicine here. To me, that's the difference. I don't know any other difference."

Projects supported by the 41st Medical Trust

In 1986, Jerome Tobis, M.D. and Fred Hoehler, Ph.D. published a monograph about musculoskeletal manipulation. This project was a result of a research program that began to develop in 1970 at the California College of Medicine at the University of California. Jerome Tobis, M.D. had just joined the faculty as Chairman of the Department of PM&R at that time, attracted by the challenge of an allopathic medical school interested in studying the efficacy of musculoskeletal manipulation as a therapeutic modality for back pain.

The investigation was the first controlled single blinded clinical trial for the study of manipulation. This was reported in the *Journal of the American Medical Association* in 1981. The study is particularly noteworthy because it was the first clinical trial of manipulation to use an appropriate placebo treatment on the control group. The experimental group received rotational manipulation of the lumbosacral spine while the control group received deep tissue massage of the same area. In order to assure the validity of this placebo treatment, patients who had previous experience with manipulative therapy were excluded from the study.

The study consisted of a large outpatient clinic pool. After x-ray screening to exclude serious musculoskeletal pathology, such as malignancy or infection, subjects with subacute low back pain were assessed by a screening examiner who did not participate as a treatment manipulator. Those patients accepted into the study received either rotational manipulation by the treating manipulator or deep tissue massage by the treating manipulator. Following a series of treatments, the patients were re-evaluated by the screening manipulator who was "blinded". A three week follow-up was conducted.

Immediately following the first treatment, there was a significant difference in various functional activities including dressing, reaching, sitting up in bed, sitting down in a chair, as well as pain relief. Three weeks after discharge from the treatment regimen the manipulated patients were significantly more likely than the controls to report that the treatment had been effective.

This clinical trial was the first to provide evidence of the validity of the controlled procedure. Three weeks after discharge, patients were asked whether they thought they had received spinal manipulation or soft tissue massage. There was no difference between the groups. Thus, the deep tissue massage controlled treatment appeared to function as an adequate course for manipulation therapy.

Dr. Tobis:

> *"I wish to emphasize that I still feel that musculoskeletal manipulation is a meaningful therapeutic intervention in selected cases, and that I feel it is part of the training of a physiatrist to be familiar with this and to use these skills in selected cases. In my own medical practice I have employed manipulation at times."*

In 1987, **Stanley van den Noort**, **M.D.** Professor and Acting Chair, Department of Neurology, and Dr. Arnold Starr, Professor, Department of Neurology, University of California, Irvine (UCI) submitted a proposal entitled *"Studies in back pain— electrophysiologic and dermatological studies of the effects of manipulation therapy"*.

The study proposed to test the scientific basis of manipulation therapy by comparing two groups of patients and controls before and after back manipulation. Three articles were published as follows:

Zhu Y, Haldeman S, Starr A, Seffinger MA, Su SH. Paraspinal muscle evoked cerebral potentials in patients with unilateral low back pain. *Spine.* 1993 Jun 15;18(8):1096-102. PMID: 8367779.

Zhu Y, Haldeman S, Hsieh CY, Wu P, Starr A. Do cerebral potentials to magnetic stimulation of paraspinal muscles reflect changes in palpable muscle spasm, low back pain, and activity scores? *J Manipulative Physiol Ther.* 2000 Sep 23(7):458-64. PMID 11004649.

Zhu Y, Starr A. Magnetic stimulation of muscles evokes cerebral potentials. *Muscle Nerve.* 1991 Aug:14(8):721-32. PMID 1890997

Dr. van den Noort:

> " . . . *I had no problem with osteopathy. I thought it was a good idea. In recent years, a lot of neurologists have gotten into osteopathy and manipulation therapy. I think it's a fine thing to do."*

Dr. Seffinger recalls about this project:

> *"When I got there* [to UC Irvine in 1989], *I was contacted by Stan Van den Noort, M.D. who was Chair of the Department of Neurology. He had called Philip Greenman, D.O. and asked if he knew anybody out on the west coast that they could collaborate with to do osteopathic manipulation and research for the 41st Trust Fund. They had money specifically designated for research in osteopathic manipulation . . . So I worked with him to write the grant, gave all the research background, and helped set-up the design and ended up working with him . . .".*

Dr. Haldeman recalls:

> *"With the 41st Trust Fund grant we went to China to do research . . . . We tested a series of patients, showing the effectiveness of muscle manipulation. Dr. Seffinger was the first to do a trial here* [in the U.S.]. *I met Dr. Seffinger through the research with Dr. Starr and Dr. Zhu. They studied cortical evoked potentials in the muscle. Dr. Zhu was the primary researcher. His study was unique because it showed you can demonstrate changes in the spine with manipulation treatment. Manipulation changed muscle tone directly. These grants made a huge impact."*

In 1992, **Dr. Yu Zhu** submitted a progress report that summarized the completed studies on paraspinal muscle evoked cerebral potentials and the H-reflex. A further research project was proposed by Dr. Zhu and Dr. Starr for an electrophysiological study of *the mechanism of the action of osteopathic manipulation therapy.* The study proceeded successfully and in 1994 **Dr. Yu Zhu** and **Dr. Arnold Starr** submitted an application for the continuation of the ongoing research project.

"Brain potentials evoked by magnetic stimulation of muscle and nerve for quantifying the efficacy of musculoskeletal manipulation of low back pain with somatic dysfunction: A collaborative study between the University of California, Irvine, the College of Osteopathic Medicine of the Pacific, and the American Osteopathic Association."

A preliminary study had dramatically demonstrated that somatic dysfunction of the lower back could be quantified using non-invasive magnetically provoked muscle contraction to evoke cerebral potentials from the scalp. This technique appeared to be able to quantify the therapeutic effect of musculoskeletal manipulation.

Dr. Seffinger:

> *" . . . . they asked me to continue working* [after graduating from the Family Medicine Residency Program at UCI], *but I moved back to Torrance . . . . So, I connected Dr. Zhu with the College of Osteopathic Medicine of the Pacific in Pomona, CA and had Dr. Zhu and the 41ˢᵗ Trust fund half of the research. I helped get the AOA to fund the other half of the research to continue the research and combine to fund the collaboration between the two institutions for the first time. They did that for a year where they did some research at Western University. Some was done here at UC Irvine as they were collaborating. Then Dr. Zhu took a job on the east coast, he left and the people at the College of Osteopathy Medicine didn't feel they could continue the research on without him and so they stopped it at that time. Since then all those people have left and moved on."*

In 1996**, Robert H. Blanks, Ph.D**. and Co-Investigators in the Department of Anatomy & Neurobiology at UC Irvine submitted a proposal entitled *"Magnetic resonance imaging of brain and spinal cord: Influence of spinal manipulation on adverse mechanical cord tension, craniosacral pump, and stress reduction-related changes in cerebral blood flow."*

The study proposed to examine three of the common factors related to the mechanisms that underlie the benefits of spinal manipulation: spinal cord tension; adequate CSF flow, sustained by respiratory movements of a flexible spine; and stress reduction. One of the objectives was to examine relaxation, as manifested by corresponding changes in cortical and brainstem flow. This study was funded in 1996 by a one year grant through the 41ˢᵗ Medical Trust.

Wadie Najm, M.D. in the Department of Family Medicine at UC Irvine Medical Center, and a multi-disciplinary team of co-investigators submitted a proposal which was funded. The study was entitled *"Reliability of spinal palpation for diagnosis in back and neck pain: A systematic review of the literature"* in 2001. Since clinicians who perform musculoskeletal manipulation rely on spinal palpatory tests to identify areas of spinal dysfunction, this study conducted a systematic review of the primary clinical research literature to determine the quality of the research and to assess the intra- and inter-examiner reliability of spinal palpatory procedures. Subsequently the systematic reviews were extended to examine the validity of spinal palpation for diagnostics as well.

Results showed that among spinal diagnostic procedures, pain provocation tests were most reliable, while soft tissue paraspinal palpatory diagnostic tests were not reliable. It was concluded, though, that the relatively poor reliability scores were due mainly to the poor quality of the studies. Once the quality of research is improved, inter-examiner and intra-examiner reliability scores may well reach levels of statistical significance.

Results on the content validity of spinal palpatory tests used to identify spinal neuro-musculoskeletal dysfunction varied greatly across the qualifying studies that were reviewed. Poor sensitivity was reported for range of motion studies regardless of the examiner's experience. Examination of cervical pain showed a slightly better sensitivity of 82%. The lack of acceptable reference standards may have contributed to the weak sensitivity findings.

The reliability and validity systematic reviews were subsequently published in several peer-reviewed journals, including *Spine,* 2004, 29(19): E413-E425*; BioMedCentral Complementary and Alternative Medicine,* 2003, 3:1 and 2003, 3:3; *J Canadian Chiropractic Association* 2003, 47(2):93-109*; J Manipulative Physiol Ther* 2003;26:374-82.

Dr. Seffinger recalls:

"I reunited with the 41ˢᵗ Trust Fund about 2001. I was again recruited as a consultant to a project to look at research and manipulation. We determined upon looking at the clinical trials that have been done in the past 15 or 20 years that what was missing were reliability studies and validity studies on palpation because most people determined where to manipulate in the body by palpating with their hands. But we weren't sure that method was reliable or valid. When I was at Michigan State, I studied with William Johnston, D.O. and Myron Beal, D.O. and these two osteopathic physicians, researchers, they devoted their careers to palpation and research in palpation, reliability and validity studies primarily, and so I was trained in how to setup those kinds of studies.

"So when I came here, the group that was assembled at the Samueli Center of Complementary and Alternative Medicine was determined to do a systematic review of literature. We had a multidisciplinary group, Ph.D., M.D., D.C., and I was the D.O. We also had a library scientist, and we decided to do a systematic review on spinal palpation as a diagnostic modality as well as a systematic review on the validity of palpation. We did two systematic reviews. We also looked into the problem of researching this literature because it was difficult to retrieve articles on the current system and we have an article on that as well. All in all we produced four or five articles that were published from that work."

Recently the 41ˢᵗ Medical Trust Fund supported the proposal to document the relationship between osteopathy and allopathic physicians. The foundation funded the preparation of this monograph and a corresponding website with the objective to promote communication between allopathic and osteopathic researchers who will examine the mechanism of musculoskeletal manipulation.

Dr. Seffinger:

> *"I began to research the history and found that there were no books about this anywhere. I went around to different book stores. I went to libraries in California. I went to the state library up in Sacramento. I went to various places in Washington, D.C. looking for the history of osteopathy in California. There are just no definitive books about it. I was very surprised and nothing that referenced where these important articles were in UC—Irvine or in Western University* [in their archives].*
>
> "So this is part of my impression of osteopathy in California, it's like it has been wiped out of the history books it seems. They didn't have it anywhere. I went to Sacramento, for instance. I went to their library that is right outside of the capitol. It is across the street and I think it was the state legislative library. There was another library there, the State Library, the Sacramento Library and I went and asked for information about osteopathy and they didn't have anything on their computer systems that led to any books. Yet, on the way to retrieving a particular article in a book the librarian passed by a whole shelf of journals called Clinical Osteopathy. That was a journal of the California Osteopathic Association that documented the practice of osteopathy in California from the 1930s to the 1950s. The librarian came back and said, "I don't know why this was not in our computer system, but it's on our shelves." You see? So, I'm seeing that the history of the profession is simply not logged or catalogued or documented. So if anybody wants to find out about osteopathy in California* [and the M.D.-D.O. relationship] *they don't know where to go."*

Osteopathic research in California today

California's osteopathic training institutions traditionally were not directly involved with research, mainly because taking care of patients was the beginning and end of their professional endeavors. Other contributing factors included lack of financial support for scientific investigations, lack of infrastructure and affiliation with academic institutions.

However, that has changed by the evolution of the College of Osteopathic Medicine of the Pacific at the Western University of Health Sciences and Western University's affiliation with Arrowhead Regional Medical Center and the creation of the Osteopathic Center for Excellence. Clinical research projects have begun. For example, the Osteopathic Postdoctoral Training Institute of the Western Educational Consortium (OWEC) has set up a research training program for residents. Since 2001, residents at affiliated hospitals have been encouraged through stipends and mentoring to engage in clinical research. Students and residents are also encouraged to present their projects at the annual Western United States Regional Research Conference in Monterey and the annual AOA Research Conference as well as at specialty society conferences related to their specialty discipline.

Western University is also developing research policies, allocating space for on-campus research, recruiting research-oriented faculty, and hiring professional grant writers, statisticians and epidemiologists. **Dr. Seffinger**, Associate Professor of Family Medicine and Osteopathic Manipulative Medicine at the College of Osteopathic Medicine of the Pacific, explains:

> *"I began to develop our own physiology laboratory, looking at the physiological effects of manipulation at our school and I became chair of a national research committee at the American Academy of Osteopathy, the Louisa Burns Osteopathic Research Committee. I was appointed Chair last year in 2005 of that committee, which is made up of osteopathic and Ph.D. researchers, and one M.D. researcher, who devote their careers basically to research in osteopathic manipulation. There are about 17 people on that committee.*
>
> *"Our latest project was to develop a standardized medical record, which has been done. My job this year is to create a stand alone electronic medical record that you can document the entire history and physical, including osteopathic palpatory findings, your structural exam findings, your manipulation approach, what you did and the response to manipulation, any side effects or complications and that document can then be summarized into a summary sheet. That summary sheet can then be sent to a national data base center and the information can be accumulated from around the country from various doctors' practices and we can then begin to answer questions as to where manipulation fits into medical practical in this day and age."*

Dr. Seffinger currently serves as chair of the Louisa Burns Osteopathic Research Committee of the American Academy of Osteopathy, Chair of the AOA Bureau of Clinical Education and Research and vice-chair of the Institutional Review Board at Western University of Health Sciences. He explained the objectives of the standardized osteopathic medical records at the National Osteopathic Database Center in Des Moines, I.A..

Dr. Seffinger:

> *"We learn a lot of things about what types of people come in to see D.O.s. What type of people need or get manipulation. What types of people benefit from manipulation. We also learn whether anybody gets harmed from manipulation. We've also learned whether people who have internal organ problems if manipulation helps them get better from that or not. You know,*

these are questions we will be able to answer and involve lots of people who typically would not be involved in research. They are just documenting what they are doing with their patients, but collectively we will be able to amass thousands of charts and patient records."

To a large extent then, research on clinical approaches and treatment effectiveness of manipulation medicine is conducted currently with osteopathic resources and separate from allopathic science infrastructures. Did the expectations of the merger for collaborative research on musculoskeletal manipulation as part of the unification not come true after all? Well, there has been research performed at UCI, and UCI sponsored a couple of national conferences on spinal manipulation in the 1970s and 1980s in which researchers from various disciplines shared their knowledge and programs in an open forum. The osteopathic profession meanwhile has established a national research center, sponsored by the AOA, AACOM, AAO, Heritage and other foundations, housed at the Health Sciences Center at the University of North Texas, College of Osteopathic Medicine. Several mechanistic and clinical research projects in osteopathic manipulation are ongoing. Dr. Seffinger is collaborating with them on several of the clinical trials; e.g., low back pain in the military; carpal tunnel syndrome; and manipulation for elderly hospitalized with pneumonia.

Dr. Seffinger:

"and there has been some success in getting people together to focus on these issues. I have a small group of M.D.s, small group of Ph.D.s, a small group of D.O.s that are moving in the same direction I am; [they are] working with me on these projects. On the other hand, there are not 10s, 20s, 100s, and 1000s of them, so the impact is small; [it is] a small group doing some work. I don't see the tremendous impact across the profession yet of these activities, but I can see that they should, and probably will, affect the future generations."

Together with Ray Hruby, D.O., chair of the Department of Osteopathic Manipulative Medicine at COMP, Dr. Seffinger published a book, entitled ***Evidence Based Manual Medicine: A Problem Oriented Approach*** (Seffinger & Hruby, 2007). Back pain, neck pain, shoulder dysfunction, temporo-mandibular joint problems, cervicogenic headache, carpal tunnel syndrome, and ankle sprain are the most common musculoskeletal ailments for which patients seek medical care. Since this type of pain or discomfort frequently resulted from trauma or overuse, manipulation is often employed as a primary modality of treatment by D.O.s. Thus, the book discusses the efficacy of manual techniques, as referenced in the scientific literature. A comprehensive literature review is provided listing the respective level of evidence for manual treatment for each problem. Several randomized clinical trials with grade A level of evidence are cited that show manipulation as beneficial for treating these painful conditions.

Dr. Seffinger:

"The book actually was generated from the American Academy of Family Physicians [AAFP] who began to accept D.Os. trained in D.O. residencies into their organization in 1992 and began having at their annual scientific assembly osteopathic manipulation workshops to teach M.D.s in their organization what it was about, kind of hands on how to do it. I joined that group of D.O.s that was teaching at the AAFP in 1995.

"And as we developed, they wanted more and more scientific evidence. So I produced that and eventually the AAFP said that, if you had evidence based medicine that was an approved source of evidence using, for example, systematic reviews of randomized clinical trials for your program, then doctors who took your workshop can get double credit: for every one hour of class, they get two hours of CME credit for the AAFP recertification requirements to stay in the organization. So the last three years my program has been certified and given that evidence based medicine approval; so, if someone takes my four hour course they get eight hours CME, because it's evidenced based."

Former D.O.s enter the M.D. culture

Interviews for this project provided insights about the M.D.-D.O. relationship as it developed over the half century that followed the merger.

Seymour Ulansey, M.D.:

"After the merger took place there was a physical contact between the two professions. They were working in similar hospitals, same hospitals. They were interchanging ideas. They were even consulting with each other. Most of the consultation went toward the allopathic end because they still had the edge on the educational facilities. When UCLA built a tremendous expansion, we were allowed to come into it. USC—University of Southern California built a big expansion. They took over the County Hospital where we were, but we were admitting to them. Socially, it became a better situation. You didn't have to explain what a D.O. was.

"I think that the merger had an unbelievable effect on the United States, on the situation for the D.O.s in the United States of America. When I went to school in the 1940s there were six osteopathic colleges. And there had been such for many years. But it was after the merger that there are now twenty-two I believe, some of which are part of state universities. They are financial subsidiaries to these state universities, medical schools. This was an unheard of thought before the merger. I think that the osteopathic profession owes California an immeasurable debt for the progress they

made. However, there is no question that they have improved their schools; they have raised the school standards; and they have earned some of this respect themselves.

"The AOA has lost some of its power, some of its dictatorial power. It has become more democratic. This also has raised the estimation of the public for the merits of the osteopathic physician. He [or she] has become a more valuable asset to the public."

Dr. Seffinger:

[Many former D.O.s] "felt that they still practiced osteopathic medicine even though they had an M.D. and to this day when I interviewed the 90 year-olds, the 80 year-olds, the people who are M.D.s that were trained as D.O.s, they still think of themselves as osteopaths. That just amazed me. I had no idea that they would still feel that way. Now that's not everybody, there are some that have no interest and no feelings about osteopathy whatsoever and are glad that they are M.D.s and they practice as M.D.s and they still feel that there should not be an osteopathic profession. I mean there are different sides of the story which to me makes it very interesting and very human."

One important side of the story was the dramatic change in the administration of healthcare in California. Several narratives describe the effects of these socioeconomic changes on the process of transitioning into M.D. healthcare.

Dr. Ryder described the socioeconomic impact on his career:

" . . . the merger took place just as the explosive change in medical technology occurred. I entered the profession at the end of one era and the beginning of another. The merger affected my practice but the revolution in medical care affected me more. By 1965, I concluded that my career was going to evolve and I needed more training especially some type of specialty status. I needed some type of board certification or eligibility."

Mr. Dowell:

"In mid-1965 it became apparent that President Lyndon Johnson was going to succeed where his predecessors, going back to President Harry Truman, had failed. Medicare was going to pass. Healthcare in America and California, professional and institutional, was about to change in ways few fully understood. Implementation of Medicare—and concurrently Medicaid (Medi-Cal in California)—in the spring of 1966 consumed the attention of every one involved with healthcare policy and practice."

Dr. Ryder recalls:

"Medicare came in 1965. So during the 1960s and 1970s, now referred to as the golden age of medicine, we treated the patients and Medicare and the insurance companies paid most of the medical bills. The explosion in costly new medical technology, coupled with the inflation of the 1970s, caused the cost of medical care to explode. In this period of time, CT scans and all kinds of special procedures in radiology became available. New surgical procedures became common place such as chest, open heart, and all types of vascular surgery. Medical procedure made the same rapid advances. There was a proliferation of new drugs and the PDR went from the size of a reader's digest to telephone book dimensions. I was thankful that I joined the American Academy of Family Physicians, because post graduate education was essential to keep your skills current. The problem was the cost of this new era of medicine was very expensive, and the insurance, government subsidy method of reimbursement couldn't pay for all the medical care we provided."

Dr. Kasovac:

"Then all of a sudden some M.D. hospitals started to lose their occupancy; not enough M.D.s; not enough patients coming in. Looking like it was going to close; they opened the doors to D.O.s. They helped to proliferate the growth and development of additional hospitals for osteopathic physicians. You know, I saw that in various states, mostly in the bigger states where we did have a lot of osteopathic hospitals, but there was a growth of D.O.s in those states, like Michigan, Pennsylvania, and Ohio. So there was room in not penalizing osteopathic hospitals. If D.O.s got on the staff of another hospital, it was okay. One of the reasons is that the osteopathic hospitals were 110 percent full. You couldn't get another patient in even though that was your primary hospital. When you had the opportunity to be on staff at a second hospital, well you knew you had a back up if you couldn't get somebody in the osteopathic hospital; you could get that patient in there. You didn't lose the patient because they were so critically ill; you just had to get them to some M.D. to get them in another place. You could still follow that patient; you could still take care of them. So some of that occurred and probably much of that was more in the '70s, but even into the '80s."

Counselor Hufstedler:

"What they were doing was incorporating osteopathy into the mainstream of medicine. And they accomplished it to a great deal, you know, look at the kinds of medicine that are practiced today. The kind of therapy and recovery

191

things that people are doing is really an outgrowth of many of the osteopathy things . . . The osteopaths that became M.D.s didn't change the way they practiced. They practiced the same kind of medicine they had practiced all the time. They just had a different two letters after their name. And they did a great deal to get it incorporated in mainstream medicine . . . . the various departments in hospitals and other clinics were incorporating many of their ideas."

Not all former D.O.s shared such positive experiences in their efforts to join the medical staff at relatively large hospitals. **Dr. Golanty** recalls:

"Now we are in practice and we wanted to be on the staffs of other hospitals as well as here, and the first hospital was St. Mary's Medical Center. We applied down there because of Dr. Unger, a cardiologist who had a relationship with us here. He backed us and we were able to get on staff. Long Beach Memorial Hospital, though, no way! You were an ex-DO, you can't do it! And the artificiality that they put up was that you had to have belonged to the Los Angeles County Medical Association in order to become a member of the staff. Well, all D.O.s, when they finished, when the amalgamation was over, were all put into this thing that you know, called the Forty-First Medical Society, okay.

"The Forty-First Medical Society, to my knowledge, was created as a political arm of the California Medical Association to allow the minority amalgamated D.O.s to have a voice in their future. So, we now had forty component medical societies and now a new one that was across the state, not geographic, and we were all put into that and none of us were in the components society in the area where we lived, and so we were not in the L.A. County Medical Association. Memorial Hospital used that as the barrier to keep us off staff.

" . . . There were at the time of the amalgamation several doctors who were in Long Beach who became part of the faculty of the now CCM program. One of them was the cardiologist at Memorial Medical Center, Mervin Ellestad, M.D., the cardiologist there, joined and also a Dr. Mann, a neurologist, and they were on staff at Long Beach Memorial Medical Center. They became my sponsors to join when we finally did break the barrier down. It took a long time. Dr. Berk finally backed us. The school, now Irvine [UC Irvine School of Medicine], *is using Memorial Medical Center as one of its teaching centers. My partner and I, after several years of fighting, finally got on staff of Long Beach* Memorial [Medical Center]. *We were the first ex-D.O.s to come on staff at that facility."*

Dr. Kasovac recalls:

"I did a lot of work in California with ex-D.O.s who were M.D.s. They identified this to me when I would call on them, or meet them at a medical staff

meeting, or an education meeting and they were very supportive of what was going on at that time in the 1990s. They were very supportive of training of our students at that time. That was very rewarding to me to see that they had to make their career decision way back in 1962 of what they thought was right, and to open the door for them to have some hospital privileges that they didn't have because they were blocked out. So I respected that. But I also respected that they never forgot their profession and that they were willing to give back to our students today."

Dr. Allen:

"A lot of the former D.O.s, even though they took the M.D. degree, still did osteopathic type practice and believed in the osteopathic profession. Some of them would go out of state to osteopathic hospitals in Arizona, New Mexico, Colorado and Washington and Oregon because we depended on the strength of those osteopathic hospitals to be teaching sites for our schools until we gradually began to get some of our own hospitals. The first hospitals to come on board were the ones that had been former osteopathic hospitals on the periphery. We never touched downtown County Hospital, but Long Beach Pacific Hospital came on board early as a teaching site. And there still was a good representation of former D.O.s on that staff. Rio Hondo Hospital came in fairly early to reinstitute their intern and resident training program."

Several former D.O.s are active in allopathic medical education. **Dr. Victor Passy, Dr. Richard Kammerman, and Dr. Robert Steedman** stand out as highly regarded teachers at the School of Medicine at the University of California, Irvine. As original members of the 41st Medical Society and currently serving on the 41st Medical Trust committee, they can provide insights to allopathic students as few could do.

Dr. Kammerman:

"I have had students in my office for a long time. I did clinic before that and I would always try to instill upon them the idea to treat the patient as a whole. This is not x, x, x with a gallbladder. This is Mrs. Jones with a gallbladder problem or this isn't a hot "appy" this is Michael Jones with a hot appendicitis. I think that's kind of rubbed off on a number of my residents, maybe not all of them, but a good share of them.

I was on staff at the County Hospital. I was attending . . . at Orange County Hospital and we would volunteer our time at Family Practice Clinic with the residents or interns in their clinics. They would see the patient; then we would kind of evaluate them. They would come to us as kind of a consultant then we would help them just like we are doing now. I was already on staff

193

here because it opened this hospital, the County Hospital to my status too, so I could become a member of the staff here."

Dr. Seffinger:

"And before that?"

Dr. Kammerman:

"Before that, no way!"

Dr. Seffinger:

"But the L.A. County Hospital had a place for the D.O.s, but not the Orange County Hospital?"

Dr. Kammerman:

"No. There was no place for osteopaths on the staff at the Orange County Hospital at that time. I don't know. Nobody had tried I guess. In fact we had referred a lot of our cases out here. Doctors here would see our indigent patients. I remember one lady that had a big old polyp come out of her cervix. She was bleeding. She was about 80 years old. She had no money. She was living on social security whatever it was then, $180.00 a month or so. Sent her out here and they took care of her and called me back and sent her back and everything."

As former D.O.s tried to continue to provide the best care, regardless of the type of medical degree, they encountered allopathic requirements that seemed to isolate them from their osteopathic heritage. **Grace Bell, M.D.** and former D.O. recalled these feelings in an interview she gave in 1977 at age 80 at UC Irvine to promote the Endowed Chair, *The Grace Beekhuis Bell Professorship of Biochemistry.*

Dr. Grace Bell:

"My husband was certified by the American Osteopathic Board of Anesthesiology. He was a fellow in the College of Anesthesiologists and he was due to become president of that outfit in a year or so. Now they were asking him to prove that he was qualified for certification under the American Society of Anesthesiologists, a medical professional society. So, with the exceptions of the contacts that he had in the hospitals where he worked, he was isolated from his former colleagues. There were many that felt the same way."

Dr. Allen:

"It was promised the D.O.s who were specialists that they would have the chance to become recognized as specialists by the AMA. Of course they were never able to deliver on that. In fact, about 15 years later, there was a supplemental suit that was brought to the front against the CMA and AMA. There were a number D.O.s that were surgeons, specialists, that sued the CMA for not fulfilling that part of the merger agreement. But they didn't recognize that the AMA can't speak for their individual specialty groups. It's not like the AOA that speaks for all of their different specialty groups. Each of the individual specialties under the AMA has its own rules and regulations. They pass their own acceptance for what they will do and won't do. So the suit didn't go anywhere. Really, the specialists were the ones that were at the worst on the whole merger deal.

"So they began to lose some practice because as the osteopathic hospitals now became M.D. hospitals, the M.D. would join the staff and they would use their own specialists. The D.O.s would continue to use the specialists that were D.O.s the way they had before, but some of them dropped out of staff and new medical doctors came on with the M.D.s siding with their own group. This is in the central metropolitan area that I had experienced this.

"What happened out in the smaller areas, like in Bakersfield and so on, some, like Dr. Art Moore up there at Bakersfield, stayed as a D.O. Dr. Moore was a strong advocate. I'm sure he was pretty much limited to an office practice. I don't know how much hospital work he did. He was a guy that did most of his manipulations. So he was happy just to do his manipulation in his office. A lot of D.O.s that stayed as D.O.s gained in their practice because all the other guys all of a sudden they were M.D.s. People that come from out of state and wanted an osteopath, they looked for a D.O. In the general practice, some of the converts didn't have as busy a practice, I don't think, for a while as they could have had."

While feeling cut-off from one's professional heritage might have promoted anger and hostility against allopathy for its discrimination, fears of isolation might have persuaded some to adopt a more positive attitude toward the allopathic world and to persevere in becoming accepted by hospital administrators, professional organizations, and educational institutions.

Dr. Ryder:

"I knew about it [the re-instatement of the osteopathic profession], *but by this time my career path had changed. By this time I had become boarded in family practice and become part of the medical community. To switch back at*

195

this time would have just disrupted my career and I had a wife and family with
children to raise and educate and a very large and busy practice. Before the
merger the osteopathic physician couldn't get admitting privileges in most non-
osteopathic hospitals . . . . My feelings were hurt and it just wasn't right.

"After the merger I was more or less courted by several institutions. A
few years before they wouldn't let me in their hospital, let alone any of my
patients; so I always felt a little uncomfortable . . . . After that, opportunity
for hospital privileges and post graduate education opened up. Several of
my classmates went on and took training in some very prestigious training
institutions.

"In the end the merger didn't destroy the Osteopathic Profession, but
made it stronger and was a factor in the integration of the two professions.
The Osteopathic Profession didn't lose its identity, but I believe led to full
recognition as a healing profession. We now have full recognition and full
privileges. And the doctors coming out of school with a D.O. degree now have
unlimited professional opportunities. They don't have the limitations that I had
to contend with. From working with D.O. residents I find them to be as well
trained as any M.D. school graduates."

Dr. Ryder's experience suggests that because of the merger many M.D.s have started
to value the expertise of osteopathic physicians and include them as equal partners in
patient care.

Dr. van den Noort:

"We've had that wonderful man from Lansing, Michigan come out and
talk at our meetings, Dr. Greenman. He is fantastic. I was involved with all
of the conferences that were at UCI over the years. I thought they were very
good and it was just presenting material on manipulation therapy and various
people coming to talk. I didn't play any major role in them, but I was very much
aware of them. I attended most of them."

The goal of bringing together various professionals who were using manual methods
as investigators or in clinical practice, was to improve interdisciplinary communication
and understanding.

Dr. van den Noort:

"The hostility to manipulation therapy has declined to nearly the vanishing
point in medicine; maybe not to the vanishing point in orthopedics. It's near
the vanishing point. I think that most internists, neurologists, physiatrists are
willing to embrace manipulation therapy as a technique. And I'm very anxious

to see the epidemic of back surgery that has gone on in the last 50 years held in check."

Dr. Haldeman, Clinical Professor of Neurology at UC Irvine, explains that the role of manipulation as a valuable diagnostic and treatment modality no longer is perceived as a threat to allopathy, since scientific methods progressed and produced substantial medical evidence.

Dr. Haldeman:

"Initially, none of us had strong knowledge. As our knowledge increased, communication improved . . . . The political process made science possible, and science broke down the barriers. The language of science is universal . . . . But science is a moving target—you have to be very active and stay up-to-date . . . joining professional organizations that advocate for, educate about, and fund or perform research on manipulation, reading peer reviewed journals that publish articles on manipulation, and attending educational meetings are ways to stay up-to-date."

Multi-professional societies on manipulation medicine

In the early 1980s, Dr. Haldeman formed the North American Spine Society as an off-shoot of the International Society for the Study of the Lumbar Spine, founded in the 1970s. The North American Spine Society has become large now and has evolved into the American Academy of Orthopedic Medicine. While **the International Society for the Study of the Lumbar Spine** is dedicated to the pursuit of pure science, providing no educational venues, the North American Spine Society has a clinical and educational focus that includes the effectiveness of manipulation.

Dr. Haldeman:

"A group of us decided to form the North American Spine Society. It's a power society now! Art [Arthur White, M.D. and former D.O.] *and I were very prominent in starting it up. We all were presidents. He always pushed for inter-professional connections. It might have been because of his background in osteopathic medicine but I don't know.*

"I became the first non-surgical president [1988-1989] *of the North American Spine Society. I pushed the interdisciplinary protocol. It's become a bit of a mantra. I started to teach with Phil Greenman, D.O."*

Additional valuable interactions occur through **the American Back Society**, founded by Aubrey Swartz, M.D. and former D.O., with the vision to build an inter-professional society. Former D.O.s continue their osteopathic training at the American Back Society by joining an open forum where D.O.s and M.D.s are teaching each other. The American Back Society is an exemplar organization where practitioners of the allopathic and osteopathic healing arts are training together. Increasingly, continuing medical education programs in osteopathic manipulation are attended by M.D.s.

Dr. Haldeman:

> *"I met Aubrey Swartz in the early 1980s. He made the American Back Society an interdisciplinary group. The American Back Society has probably the widest scope of presentations anywhere in the world."*

Dr. Ryder:

> *"As an osteopathic physician I was specifically trained for back problems. Most medical doctors have no training about the structural dysfunction of the back and the pain and disability that result. With my own back injury I was given a lot of insight. Most M.D. trained physicians called the back—the black box that produces pain and could only prescribe medication, surgery or physical therapy . . . For several years I worked in a back clinic. I worked with a chiropractor, an osteopath, a neurosurgeon and an orthopedist. At that time I joined the **American Back Society**. One of the leaders of the Society was Dr. Greenman from Michigan State University College of Osteopathic Medicine. I read his book and have studied his tapes. He was a great teacher and from my attending the Society conventions I learned a great deal more about Osteopathic Theory and treatment."*

Inter-disciplinary communication was the challenge in the 1970s which advanced to international communication in the 1990s. Upon the initiative of the World Health Organization, the "**Bone and Joint Decade 2000-2010**" was inaugurated (*www.boneandjointdecade.org*). The goal of this international initiative is "to improve the health-related quality of life for people with musculoskeletal disorders by raising awareness, empowering patients to participate in their health care, promoting cost-effective prevention and treatment, and acquiring research funding . . . International support for the Bone and Joint Decade included official recognition by the UN. This support, together with that of the WHO and the World Bank, greatly enhanced and strengthened the credibility of the Decade" (*www.iofbonehealth.org*).

Within every country there is a national action network of patients, scientists and clinicians. In the United States, the Surgeon General's 2004 Report on Bone Health and Osteoporosis recognized the importance of musculoskeletal diseases and defined strategies to improve bone health. The United States Bone & Joint Decade includes nearly 100 organizations working together towards similar goals. The goal is to promote a healthier America through improvements in education and advances in research and patient care of musculoskeletal disorders.

Dr. Haldeman:

> *"The spine has become so complicated. Manipulation is not a magical cure. I don't think it's possible to keep up with the literature [*on assessment and treatment*] without going to professional meetings and participate in education and training. Family practitioners have to become much more involved. They can treat the pain that does not interfere with daily life.*
>
> *"A group of isolated M.D.s formed interest groups to pursue non-surgical interventions. Osteopathic physicians have that capacity . . . . We asked, they refused. Osteopathic physicians are the only organization in the Bone and Joint Decade who don't participate."*

Dr. Seffinger:

> *"When D.O.s were not allowed to be on the curriculum development committee which was to work on creating guidelines for musculoskeletal system education within medical school curriculum throughout the United States, they withdrew their support."*

Dr. Haldeman:

> *"If they are criticized, they get offended. It's a highly controversial field. You got to have a thick skin. Why is it controversial? They* [M.D.s] *have an emotional negative response to manipulation. More and more of them incorporate it into their practice, though."*

Dr. van den Noort:

> *"I think osteopathy is fine. I think allopathy is fine. I think there ought to be some sort of effort at slowly integrating . . . You know the osteopaths now go into medical residencies (allopathic residencies). I think we ought to teach osteopathic manipulation in medical schools; and gradually see this come together rather then be a separate entity . . . . I was somewhat surprised in the Academy of Neurology to see the emergence of manipulation medicine as a major theme about 15 years ago. Lots of neurologists learn how to manipulate."*

Is there a need for two separate professions?

Dr. Ulansey:

(Deep sigh) " . . . that is a quandary that I find myself in, when I think on it. I do believe there is one major . . . Now heretofore, I didn't think there was. I couldn't see the differentiation between the two schools of thought. I think now there is more research being done to properly evaluate the effectiveness and value of the theory of osteopathy, whatever that is. That's opened to a lot of discussion and so forth . . . . I'm very interested recently hearing about some of the research work that's being done, real research, not lip service, true research to separate the wheat from the chaff, the real efficacy of manipulative therapy, the real value of it. I'm very enthused about hearing about some of it which you have brought to my mind."

"I must say from my contacts with the school in Pomona, that's the only one I have any contact with, that from the enrollment that I look at, and I do look at their enrollment every opportunity I have, they are so diversified as to color, ethnicity, religion, they seemed to be so open. This, in my mind, makes for a major justification for the continued existence, co-existence, of the two schools of thought."

Dr. Golanty:

"I personally still think the student body [of osteopathic medicine] *generally speaking is still made up of the same type of person [as in earlier days], older, more experienced, and mature. In large proportion, though, the allopathic medical schools are changing somewhat. I teach at UC Irvine still and have medical students with me from UC Irvine and I see some of the change in them, but they are still younger.*

"Obviously, the biggest change that has occurred in both schools is the high proportion of women. I was pointing this out to a woman, a UC Irvine student, that was with me just last week. As we went through the annuals, there were a large number of D.O. women that were in the school that I think was still disproportionate to the number of students who were M.D.s that were women. So, that is what I saw and still think I see of the osteopathic profession. In fact, my personal belief is that if there is a reason for there to still be two professions, it's that.

"I don't personally believe that the manipulation issue is what it's about anymore. I think that we all thirsted and wanted to know in school about manipulation and osteopathic medicine. We all wanted to see it practiced and used and we didn't see it then. I think you see it in some degrees even less now. And on the other hand, you see the allopathic profession beginning to embrace alternative medicine and so all these things are getting blurred to me personally . . ."

D.O.s prevail in an M.D. culture

Dr. Ryan was the first osteopathic family physician hired by Kaiser Permanente in 1974 and one of the first Navy osteopathic physicians in 1968. He recalls that

" . . . one of my challenges was proving that I was a competent physician in the presence of medical personnel who were not accustomed to working with D.O.s. [even though] I had taken and passed the American Board of Family Practice exam in 1974 and attended numerous continuing medical education meetings. I was unable to become a partner with Kaiser until 1987 as their by-laws at the time restricted partnership to M.D.s."

In support of Dr. Ryan's recollection, **Dr. Krpan** recalls:

"The profession was more or less decimated here. They were close to the critical number of D.O.s remaining with a D.O. license for renewal of licenses by the Osteopathic Examining Board. They were close to the point where that number would have been small enough that the Board would have been closed down and then people would have—everyone who practiced medicine would have been licensed by the Medical Board of the State of California. We had no hospitals, privileges were limited.

"There were hospitals where they would turn you down for privileges, namely, Kaiser. Kaiser wouldn't hire D.O.s to work in their programs in their first two or three years. I served as president of the Osteopathic Physicians and Surgeons of California two times. The dates I think are '81, '82 and '87, '88 and during my first term as president we had individuals who were trying to hire on with Kaiser. They couldn't get hired because Kaiser just didn't hire D.O.s. The Executive Director of our State Association at the time was Matt Weyuker and he and I went to the capitol. We introduced legislation that passed. Kaiser had to start hiring D.O.s.

"Then those same D.O.s who were hired by Kaiser found that because they were D.O.s they were unable to participate in the profit sharing and ownership plans that Kaiser had. So we went back to the legislature with another bill; got it introduced, got it passed; and then D.O.s started getting equal rights under the benefits of being employees of Kaiser."

Dr. Vinn:

"The OPSC Board was very involved with re-emerging efforts to discriminate against D.O.s in California. We noticed that some hospital staffs and managed care organizations such as Kaiser were not allowing D.O.s on staff. Collectively we were able to get legislation introduced, which I believe *was Senate Bill 2480 in the mid-80s. This bill mandated that hospitals and medical groups and other health care organizations consider osteopathic licensure and certification as an equivalent with that of M.D.s. This opened up numerous opportunities for our members to work within organizations and get on staffs at major hospitals and medical groups, including the Kaiser organization.*

"I can't take individual credit for that. It was a collective effort, but I was there when it happened. I also believe that both in California and nationally we did have a significant role in increasing awareness of the managed care delivery model for the AOA and its membership and helping prepare osteopathic physicians to function more effectively within these payer models."

Matt Weyuker:

"Early in 1985, I had heard from a D.O. Ob-Gyn from Ohio, who had applied for a position in the Hayward Kaiser-Permanente facility. He flew to the newly opened Northern California facility at his own expense for the in-person interview. He didn't get the position—the reason given was that Kaiser-Permanente had a policy not to employ any D.O.s. He was told to come back and see them when he had his M.D. degree!"

In 1994 Kaiser Permanente honored Dr. Ryan at an awards ceremony recognizing retiring partners from Kaiser. He was presented with a set of bookends engraved with an acknowledgement for his 20 years of service.

Dr. Ryan recalls that his *"fellow medical officers were very supportive . . . When I joined the Navy . . . , we did not have appropriate equipment to perform manipulation. Manipulative therapy was not a common procedure."* Recently Dr. Ryan has been notified by the AOA that he will be among those osteopathic physicians honored as the first 100 D.O.s to serve in the military.

Dr. Ulansey:

"I have met men [in the military service] *who deserved what they have achieved. I've seen and met several admirals of the navy. I believe there is a general in the army. I know they are active in the Coast Guard, commissioned officers which was unheard of in my day and I'm proud to see that these men have achieved the knowledge, position and status of what they now hold and deserve. That is a personal pride item for me."*

Indeed, many advances have been made in the social stature of the osteopathic physician, especially after the 1960s and into the '70s. They continue to grow, protected by legislature and facilitated by the increasingly positive attitude in allopathy.

Dr. Chesky, an osteopathic physician and surgeon in Chicago, felt attracted by the "California dream" in the late 1970s. He made arrangements to practice in the Long Beach area, performing his obstetrics at Long Beach Memorial Hospital—the first D.O. to have full privileges at that institution—and to perform surgery at Pacific Hospital, a former osteopathic hospital.

Dr. Chesky:

"When I arrived at Pacific Hospital, I had the most academic experience and training as a D.O. than any other staff member and I was made the Acting Director of Medical Education . . . . The College of Osteopathic Medicine of the Pacific had started a couple of years ago and the first class of students needed clinical experience. It was just a natural segue for those students to come to the Pacific Hospital, as clinical clerks (externs), where a D.O. was in charge of the training program. That started the resurgence of the post-doctoral training program.

"I campaigned to develop an internship program at the Pacific Hospital and presented my ideas to the Board of Directors and the powers-that-be at the hospital. I was able to convince the majority of the physicians that a reactivation of the D.O. post-doctoral training program might be in the best interest to the hospital. It certainly would give credibility to a small community hospital if it had a formal training program. The public would look at that in a very favorable way. If the hospital had a training program, it must be a good place to receive healthcare. My presentation was accepted.

"The executive committee of the medical staff assigned the responsibility to me of completing the application for the internship and to comply with all of the regulations of the American Osteopathic Association. The medical executive committee approved and budgeted for eight interns. When the application was being filled out, I instructed my secretary, to not put eight in the slot but rather 25. My thoughts were: that if we ever want to expand the program, we wouldn't have to go through the entire process of reapplying; and if we'd get approval for anything above eight, we would be comfortable for future growth.

"The American Osteopathic Assocation's committee on post-doctoral training, approved the twenty-five slots . . . Our graduates from the internship program went into practice, most of them at various locations outside of the Long Beach area. The problem in Long Beach was that the D.O.s after their internship could not get privileges at the Long Beach Memorial Medical Center. The Credentials Committee felt that a one-year post-doctoral educational program was not as adequate as the allopathic graduates who would have a three-year residency in post-doctoral family practice training.

"The idea of expanding our internship to a family practice residency program was conceived at that time! We were able to compete with the allopathic *programs and to obtain for our D.O. graduates privileges in some of the premiere medical institutions. If they had the same amount of post-doctoral training, it would be possible for them to apply for staff privileges and perhaps obtain them . . . The majority of our residents had a favorable experience. They did a good job and left a very good impression on the people at Long Beach Memorial Medical Center."*

A graduate of the College of Osteopathic Medicine of the Pacific in Pomona in 1988 and a graduate from the Pacific Hospital Osteopathic Internship Program in 1989, Cynthia Stotts, D.O. went on to train in Medicine and Pediatrics at Los Angeles County—University of Southern California (LAC-USC) Medical Center. In 1992, she served as President of the Joint Council of Interns and Residents (JCIR), the second oldest union of physicians of interns and residents in the United States.

Dr. Stotts:

"I really cared about the quality and the commitment to our residents while going through the process of advocacy. Because that's really what the position of the president and the union allowed. It was a platform, an obligation, and a possibility to advocate for patients and residents while you were a resident. That was the power in a collective voice, standing together, making a decision about what was in the best interest for them. As long as you're aligned and your missions are aligned with your administration, you can get a lot done and that was the tenor that I perceived during that period of time."

Then, in 1995, she became President of JCIR, representing the three medical centers that made up the L.A. County Hospital system, namely Martin Luther King Jr., Harbor-UCLA, and LAC-USC. Dr. Stotts represented about 1,800 residents. She was in a position to propose to the CMO (Chief Medical Officer), to the CEO (Chief Executive Officer), to the COO (Chief Operating Officer), to the CFO (Chief Financial Officer) equipment and services that would improve the care of patients and resident education. These efforts were strongly supported by the administration and significant improvements were made that could be seen year after year.

Dr. Stotts:

"You felt an ownership in being able to improve a system. If you can improve a system, you become part of the system and it allows you to own it and it allows you to push through those wedges for changes that are so necessary in order to make things happen differently. This institution has long been a resident-run, attending-supported institution that really allowed residents to play an active role in the delivery of care and their education. I was very honored and privileged

to be the president of JCIR during that period of time. There was our hospital (USC) which had about a thousand residents. Then there was a collective that included Harbor General and Martin Luther King. We had together our three hospitals which were banded together as a union. I actually became president of the interns and residents at all three of the hospitals."

From 1995 through 1997, Dr. Stotts held her position as the JCIR president of the three medical institutions. As her ability to advocate for residents and patients was recognized by the medical staff, she was asked to become Chief of Staff-elect of the organized independent medical staff of the Los Angeles County Medical Center. She proceeded to become the first female D.O. Chief of Staff in the 160 year history of the Los Angeles County / University of Southern California Medical Center.

Dr. Stotts:

*"The history is that there was a **Unit I** which is the big, beautiful general hospital that we see on the soap opera. We call her the stone mother. She is a magnificent art deco edifice with a phenomenal entryway that marvels the finest museums.*

*"Then there were separate facilities, referred to as **Unit II,** and those were D.O. run programs at hospitals. You and I are currently sitting in what is now known as Women's and Children's Hospital. It was **dedicated in 1956 as the Los Angeles County Osteopathic Hospital.** And I understand that it was the first and the only county osteopathic hospital in the nation. And it was a full fledged hospital, run by D.O.s, with a full operating room, and full obstetric delivery and internal medicine and pediatrics and all the subspecialties—all as a separate D.O. hospital, Unit II.*

"Each of the two hospitals coexisted on the medical campus here, until all the history occurred that prompted you to write this book. This history changed the way that we—meaning D.O.s—functioned within the structure at the L.A. County/USC Medical Center.

"I can honestly say that I expect people occasionally to say, 'Oh, you're a D.O.? I thought you were an M.D.', and I'll say, 'No. I'm a D.O.'And they might ask [about osteopathy]. *This may be another physician, or it may be a nurse. It may be somebody who says, ' . . . you're like really good. I thought you were a doctor. And I like to answer 'Yes. Thank you, and I am.' That happens very, very rarely, though. For the most part, I don't feel the pressures of having a distinct degree. I know it exists in other hospitals systems to this day in California."*

As Chief of Staff at the Medical Center, Dr. Stotts is responsible for about two thousand providers, about nine hundred house staff, interns and residents, and about two to four hundred medical students, nursing students, respiratory students, physical therapy students and the like. For all their care and the care that their patients receive, whether it is part of their training program or not, the organized medical staff is responsible.

Dr. Stotts:

> *"The Chief of Staff is the leader of the physicians, the attending physicians, the medical physicians in a facility, to perform certain duties. They have to credential and privilege; they have to be responsible for the delivery of care and the quality of care; they have to be responsible for producing medical records, for utilization management and review, for tissue and basic procedures. There's a number of things in the California Code of Regulations, Title 22, that the physicians of a hospital are responsible for, because the physicians are really the ones providing the care."*

In spite of the post-merger revitalization of the osteopathic profession and the re-generation of osteopathic education in California, students, interns and residents seem to show an increased interest in becoming accepted in the M.D. world, possibly at the expense of not adhering to osteopathic medical tenets. This observation causes worries about the survival of the profession.

Some osteopathic leaders believe that they have become victims of their own success, as their graduates have been eligible to train and be accepted in quite a few allopathic institutions. They are concerned that the increased contact of new D.O.s with the M.D. world seems to undermine a sense of identification and belonging with the osteopathic profession. During the late 1980s and early 90s it became apparent to these osteopathic leaders that many osteopathic medicine schools, including COMP, were reluctant to advertise joining osteopathic associations at the local, regional, state, or national level. There was a reluctance noted to become involved. They believe that attaining a balance between the wish to remain separate and the wish to feel accepted in the allopathic culture will be one of the challenges for years to come, both in California and nationally.

Dr. Seffinger:

> *"At the end of my internship I applied to get into a family medicine residency program at a more academic center because I wanted to get back into research. So my choices at that time were UC Irvine, and USC* [University of Southern California] *which were accepting D.O.s. At that time when I called up places like UCLA* [University of California, Los Angeles], *Long Beach Memorial, and Ventura County Medical Center, they each said, 'We don't accept applications from D.O.' This was **1989** and I decided then to go where I felt accepted. I was accepted to both UCI and to USC's California Hospital and chose to attend UCI."*

"I continued to practice family medicine, osteopathic family medicine in Torrance. I got a job with Bay Shores Medical Group; the medical director was a Dr. Peter Cullotta. He was a D.O., trained at the College of Osteopathic Physicians and Surgeons; then became an M.D. in 1962. He was the medical director. The president of the Group was John Johnson, M.D.; he also went to COP&S and became an M.D. in 1962. He was a gastroenterologist and they decided to hire me as the first D.O. ever into that organization. That organization began back in the 1950s and Dr. Johnson joined it in the 1960s after he became an M.D. and specialty trained in gastroenterology. The reason they took me partly was because I graduated from UC Irvine family medicine residency program which was ACGME accredited.

"I became board certified by the American Board of Family Practice, and at that time, in 1991, that medical group was not accepting D.O.s from AOA approved residencies. However, in 1992, the American Academy of Family Physicians began to accept D.O. graduates of AOA approved residencies and those board certified by the American Board of Osteopathic Family Physicians. This led to our medical group to consider applications from osteopathic physicians who had osteopathic board certification."

"Even today [2006], you'll see people [D.O.s] going into hospitals and they will give them name tags that say M.D. 'We don't have D.O. name tags for you. You have to be an M.D.' Even though you have graduated as a D.O., there are places that still don't want to show the public or 'confuse the public' that there are two different doctors."

The alleged effort of acting in the public's interest appears to dismiss the professional status and recognition that osteopathic physicians had worked so hard to attain, as Dr. Allen recalls:

Dr. Allen:

"Immediately when the Supreme Court decision was made we had access to more legislative benefits. One of the cardinal bills that was passed was an anti-discrimination bill. The preamble to that bill is as beautiful as the preamble to the Constitution of the United States. It reads that 'It is the policy of the state of California that there should be no discrimination between a physician and surgeon D.O. and physician and surgeon M.D.' In essence [it states] that all of the efforts will be supported by the state to make sure that discrimination does not happen. The D.O.s are named first in the preamble, as compared to the M.D.s.

"And we've used this legislative enactment to help in instances where there has been discrimination. Even though it was a bill in the legislature, some of the hospitals and some of the other doctors didn't know about it. I had a personal

incident happen in Whittier in which a D.O., newly on the staff there, had scheduled a patient for a tonsillectomy. When the M.D., house surgeon, came in and saw the D.O. listed to do his tonsillectomy, he said immediately that 'no D.O. is going to be doing a tonsillectomy at Whittier Hospital'. So the D.O. called me. I said, 'well, I'll call Sacramento and I'll also call the hospital and advise them that this is discrimination and that the state of California does not allow discrimination between doctors.' Within 24 hours the situation had been corrected and within 2 days the tonsillectomy was back on schedule, when we pointed out that the bill was written in the legislature and that there was to be no discrimination. Through the years, more and more armor plate has been put on the legislative strength and protection of the profession."

Dr. Seffinger:

"And you will see a lot of D.O.s that say the same thing, 'I'm tired of explaining what I am or who I am. I just want to put doctor after my name. I don't care about this D.O.' So I think that the issues that were present back in 1892 when this all started are still very present. Things really haven't changed that much, you know, when you look at the big picture. I find that very fascinating."

There comes a point, though, where disrespect hurts personally. How can one refrain from escalating the tension, when seemingly no attempts are made by allopathic professionals to learn about the art and science of their colleagues in osteopathic medicine? What interpersonal skills might promote the ability to set personal pain aside in order to arrive at mutual understanding?

Dr. Seffinger:

"A lot of it is ignorance, naiveté, hurt feelings or fear, you know, fear that comes up in people. You learn to address that and aim for a mutual understanding, sitting down to the table together and talking, interacting. One thing that I see myself as is a catalyst for conflict resolution."

As described in Chapter 5, Dr. Kammerman, together with Counselor Hufstedler and Dr. Dorothy Marsh had pursued that very approach, traveling throughout California to promote an understanding about the law among doctors. They focused on education to resolve conflict and to facilitate the merger between the COA and the CMA.

Dr. Haldeman:

"When you segregate, it ends up not being to the benefit of the patient or to anyone . . . .

"You have to have respect for everybody's opinion and you have to be able to take criticism. You can't get angry with people. When people attack, you sit back and ask 'where are they coming from?' If they come from ignorance, you try to show the medical evidence.

"You focus on research—no dogma but a willingness to accept truth, where ever it comes from. If there is no evidence, other than manipulation was the only treatment that worked, it forces the profession to do the research.

"When we got people together from different disciplines and examined a patient, we took turns to mark where we thought the lesion was. The marks were all close together! This made me realize we call it something different, using different terminology, but we are not that far apart."

Dr. Vinn:

"Reflecting how we accomplished what we did, I think it was through: (1) core knowledge of subjects and doing the home work; (2) being passionate about what needed to be done; (3) being able to establish strong, continuous long-term relationships; and (4) attempting to communicate and influence, such that there was a movement towards consensus on key goals and objectives."

Dr. Stotts:

"Sometimes, I'll see bewilderment. It's like, 'What do you mean you're a D.O.? . . . I thought you were a doctor.' But it's more bewilderment, it's not discrimination, and if it is here [at L.A.County USC], *no one shows it to me. The medical staff leadership, the department chairs, the CEO, everyone has gone out of their way to make my position as powerful and as helpful and a tool for change, as that helps the institution. I haven't seen discrimination. It may be here, I just haven't seen it."*

Dr. Seffinger:

"There is a great interest in osteopathic medicine internationally. There is a World Osteopathic Health Organization. There is also an international organization which the American Osteopathic Association is heading which is the Osteopathic International Alliance. So it ties together all institutions and organizations that are devoted to osteopathic medicine in the world. And they have formed guidelines for the World Health Organization for the training of osteopathic physicians worldwide so that the World Health Organization knows and understands the different training that people get around the world.

"In America, you get full training for unlimited scope of practice, where in other countries you get limited scope of practice, mostly manipulation and

natural methods. The Germans have a school in which, after you get an M.D. degree, you can go study osteopathy; the same thing in Russia. In England they have a school like that. They have a different school in England for people who just want to learn osteopathy without learning medicine or surgery. So there is a variety of schools around the world as well as scopes of practice.

"There are many countries that accept osteopathic training in America, so that you can go in that country and practice as a physician, as an unlimited licensed physician in some areas of Canada, New Zealand, Germany, and many other countries as well. I'm on the international committee of the American Academy of Osteopathy to keep track of these things; to help to develop these kinds of programs. I do what I can to facilitate that, especially in Japan where I'm involved with the Japanese development of Osteopathy."

The relationship between D.O.s and former D.O.s

Dr. Dilworth recalls:

"Well, the question would be 'What was the relationship with the large group of D.O.s that accepted their M.D. degree . . . ?' I can give a personal example.: In Escondido there were two out-of-state D.O.s that had come in and were practicing in California. They took their M.D. degree and stayed in Escondido of course. We were in the hospital. I was maintaining my D.O. because I didn't take the M.D. degree. Between the three of us, we were the ones that chose to exchange our calls on weekends. We were capable of working together very nicely with each other in the process, and of course it is true that we were all doing a general practice, so that a lot of our referrals would have to go to specialties in the medical field, but it was a personal example of good cooperation between those who had made the shift over, as compared to my resistance by sticking to the D.O. degree."

Thus, depending on the needs of the patient and the skills of the individual doctor, D.O.s referred to both kinds of doctors, new D.O.s who had recently come from out-of-state and former D.O.s who had become M.D.s.

Dr. Allen:

"They [former D.O.s] *were fully supportive of me. And when I asked for extra money to do things, they donated. In the early days, they contributed their $1000 to help start this new school and COMP, and they were proud of it and very interested.*

"Their practice went on. They were successful and maintained their income. None of them wanted to change beyond their hospital; so it made no difference to them what their degree was."

At the organizational and academic levels of osteopathic medicine not all former D.O.s felt respected.

Dr. Golanty:

"But understand that one of the prices I paid for [the M.D. degree] *was that I never could be anything in the osteopathic profession in the academic world. So, when you later hear the story on tape about my involvement in osteopathic training, you will hear that I could never be a Director of Medical Education for a residency program. It hurts me to know that because I have devoted the last 30 years of my life to the profession and training. I believe in my heart, no matter what anybody else believes, that I've done more than most and a lot more than a whole lot of people to advance osteopathy in this state, especially at a training level, and the osteopathic profession throws it up to me that thirty years ago I did this thing* [taking the M.D. degree] *and unless I change, which doesn't make any sense right now, I can't be involved in medical education.*

"Now, they made a mistake, the AOA, a couple years ago. This was just before I got sick with the cancer, so this would have been about 2001. Somewhere in there, it came out that a DME [Director of Medical Education] *had to be a graduate of an osteopathic school and have an osteopathic internship. It didn't say anything else, just those two things. So, with the help of Dr. Krpan, who was AOA president at the time, I approached him to talk to the AOA, Dr. Opipari, about the idea of why I can't be DME of my program. And then they said to me, 'Well, prove it, that you had these two things.' Proving it now is pretty hard because all the records are gone. Apparently the records from what I heard have been destroyed as far as the state of California is concerned. That is what I heard.*

"I petitioned the profession, saying, well, if I've got a license in California I had to have graduated from an osteopathic school and I had to have an osteopathic internship, to get a license. That was my alleged proof now that I had met those two qualifications. Nine months passed before I was even through with my cancer ordeal. And then when I started trying to approach the AOA [again], *I got nothing from them, and to this day they have never acknowledged the fact that I could be a Director of Medical Education."*

New beginnings

Many patients in California don't know they are treated by an osteopathic physician. All that is important to them is a good doctor taking care of their concerns. People used to be fully aware of their option to seek osteopathic medicine, when the Los Angeles County Osteopathic Hospital existed as well as many smaller designated osteopathic hospitals. Prior to the 1960s, people in California knew about osteopaths that did surgery and took care of them completely.

Dr. Seffinger:

"Nowadays it's mixed, people don't know all the time what a D.O. is. We have in the state of California once again county hospitals in San Bernardino and Riverside Counties. They are Arrowhead Regional Medical Center and Riverside County Hospital that have [osteopathic medicine] *residencies in neurosurgery, orthopedic surgery, obstetrics/gynecology, emergency medicine, internal medicine and family medicine. We have a residency in anesthesiology as well. We have these ongoing now; so, it is back up to par the way it was in the 1950s before the merger."*

While the public tends to be unbiased about the merits of the two medical professions, as long as their doctor meets their health needs, members of the two medical professions have come a long ways in their relationship, traversing rejection and prejudice until arriving at collaboration and communication. The relationship between the two fully licensed professions in California has been described as *separate but equal*. As these professions entered the 21st century, M.D.s and D.O.s view the other's profession with respect.

Dr. Kasovac:

"I think a lot of that [increase in respect was due to] *the newer generation of academic administrators in those schools who were of our* [younger] *vintage. They were not of the vintage of the people when all of this happened in the 1960s. They were graduates from medical schools in the late '60s and into the '70s, and now in the '90s they are associate deans, and deans of medical schools. They knew about what had happened, but they weren't involved with it. They didn't have negative attitudes or anything else and many of them trained in their residency program with D.O.s as fellow residents. They had a lot of respect for the education, the training, and the abilities of the D.O.s. They were respectful of the osteopathic manipulative skills of the individuals; particularly where it was used more in family medicine and the primary care arena. Whatever, it was an acceptable thing. So I think that was very helpful."*

Dr. Krpan:

"*It* [the M.D.-D.O. relationship] is *significantly better than it ever was. It's getting better all the time. Medicine's changed, you know, it's us as physicians against all the rest of them out there: Medicare; Medicaid; third-party payers; hospitals; and physicians are taking it upon the chin. They are paying you less and expecting you to do more. And so we are finding that as physicians, M.D. or D.O., that we have the same plights and we are supporting each other in a lot of those* [issues]. *The Patient's Bill of Rights is one of them. They were very supportive of that also. Reimbursement issues: we are working together on credentialing and privileging issues, and particularly* [on issues regarding] *third-party payers.*"

Separateness between the two professions includes the strong emphasis in osteopathic medicine on the interplay between structure and function, and a focus on primary care.

A concern is felt among D.O. educators that through the close association with M.D.s and equal status of the professions, osteopathic physicians might lose their separate identity and in fact become allopathic physicians.

Dr. Vinn:

"*Information sharing and learning is typically bilateral. D.O. and M.D. students can be mutually supportive in many ways. I do think that the allopathic students, if they are already in medical school, can learn from osteopathic post-graduate physicians in a number of ways. Healthy curiosity expands one's knowledge and abilities.*

"*Sharing information about osteopathic principles and practice furthers the issue of the Osteopathic paradox of inclusion vs. dilution. It's not in the tradition of medicine to withhold knowledge that would benefit the population as a whole. Yet, there is clearly a concern that if everybody knows what we know, then how are we different? On the other hand, one could also argue that, if what we know and do is the right way to practice, then osteopathic practices should become a universal standard. I think that the debate will continue to unfold.*"

The AOA believes that education and training in osteopathic principles and philosophy are of prime importance in preserving the osteopathic identity. Thus, in the past 25 years in California, osteopathic physicians like Ethan Allen and the late Earl Gabriel gave up their Saturdays to teach the new D.O. students at COMP the osteopathic manipulation techniques they had learned in the 1950s, especially the high velocity/low amplitude technique which no longer was emphasized in the new osteopathic curriculum in the 1980s. Since then, muscle energy, myofascial release, cranial approaches, and strain/counter strain types of OMT made their inroads into the curriculum.

Dr. Seffinger:

> *"I am mentoring students, now. I'm trying to bring forth an awareness of what it means to be an osteopathic physician in the state of California, so I think what my position is in this historical time line is a person that is trying to bring together loose ends from the past and to give some kind of direction for the students that are creating the profession for the future . . . . I've created a required osteopathic manipulation rotation for third year D.O. students at our school, so they have to go through and experience where manipulation fits into medical practice. They get to see it because for many, it was a dying art.*
>
> *"For many years we were trying to teach and bring back that aspect of osteopathic medicine by training students as well as residents in osteopathic manipulation. The first resident in osteopathic manipulation or manipulative medicine, we call it, in the state of California started this month at Downey Regional Medical Center. Her name is Rebecca Giusti, D.O. We are training her, as well as those to follow, in becoming specialists in osteopathic manipulation, which also will help the students. We now have about 40 practitioners in southern California that are preceptors for our students in osteopathic manipulation in clinical practice. They take students in to help train them. I'm trying to keep them together as a faculty; and build on that faculty.*
>
> *"We teach courses at school, you know 200 hours in osteopathic manipulation, so I'm trying to rekindle the profession and strengthen it in the state of California. Part of the reason to do this narrative history project is to reunite with UC Irvine and with the people who in the past have helped the profession; people that were D.Os. and became M.D.s; [they] supported even the growth of the College of Osteopathic Medicine of the Pacific. Many of those people we've interviewed."*

With all the devoted effort to strengthen the osteopathic profession by promoting its unique clinical practice, a nation-wide challenge remains for D.O.s to remain separate and distinct from the M.D. world. As they train and work side-by-side with M.D.s, osteopathic physicians in California feel challenged all the more because of their geographic dispersion in this big state with large rural areas. It is hard to have a sense of family when people are as much as a thousand miles apart. The osteopathic professional journal in California, the **California DO,** provides a vital link, though, through information dissemination and expression of shared thoughts and feelings about the profession's historical and current challenges. Electronic technology has made possible many new ways to promote a sense of family by sharing the heritage unique to California.

Dr. Krpan:

"And there are still some threats, but they are less noxious than they were in the old days. A lot of the prejudice has gone away. I was before the legislature one time. Matt Weyuker and I were sitting in front of this panel and this one Senator said, 'Doctor,' he said, 'Isn't it true that your students train with allopathic students in hospitals?' I said, 'Yes, Senator, that's true.' He said, 'Well, isn't it true, doctor, that when they graduate they go into residencies and internships together?' I said, 'That's true Senator.' And then he said, 'Isn't it true, when they are all done with their training they go into practice together?' I said, 'That's true.' He said, 'Tell me doctor,' he said, 'Why do we need two licensing boards in this state.' I said, 'We don't Senator. When the allopathic physician becomes competent in everything that we do, we will be happy to license them.' He said, 'That's it, pass the bill.' And they passed the bill and changed our [Practice] *Act."*

Rebuilding osteopathy in California entailed to develop a professional relationship with M.D.s who were active practitioners as well as deans and assistant deans from medical schools. In order to learn about allopathic medical education, several COMP educators joined the national Society of Teachers of Family Medicine (STFM) and the Association of Hospital Medical Educators (AHME). Attending national meetings eventually gave COMP educators and administrators the much appreciated opportunities for M.D.-D.O. interactions. As people became familiar, mutual professional respect increased which is bound to benefit patient care in California.

Summary of the M.D.-D.O. relationship over a century

The relationship between the two professions can be summarized as having evolved uniquely at each turn of a decade. The following development can be noted of the relationship over a century:

1896-1907: The two medical professions function separately, with little relation:

Some M.D.s were studying osteopathy and several dual degree faculty were running the osteopathic colleges and profession in the state.

1907-1921: As educational standards were deemed equal, attempts to discriminate ensued:

M.D.s and D.O.s both served on a composite state licensing board. By 1916 D.O.s were allowed to intern at government facilities and clinics. D.O.s and M.D.s were given the opportunity to sit for the unlimited licensing exam as both met the educational requirements. In 1919, unexpectedly and arbitrarily, D.O.s were no longer allowed to sit for the unlimited physicians and surgeons exam. This may have been related to the AMA's efforts to distinguish allopathic medicine from osteopathic medicine in light of the Flexner Report of 1910. The AMA did admonish the Los Angeles County Hospital to stop allowing D.O.s to intern there or face removal of their accreditation status. The denial of the state medical licensing board seemed an act of discrimination and it was taken to court by the COP&S Board of Trustees. The D.O.s won their right to be examined but now distrusted the allopathic profession. D.O. leaders created the Osteopathic Initiative of 1922, which gave them their own licensing board and freed them from further attempts of discrimination by a composite licensing board or legislation that seemingly favored the M.D.s.

1922-1938: Segregation in large hospitals created a major barrier for the practice of osteopathy:

D.O.s. worked their way into the Los Angeles County Hospital but remained segregated to accommodate the regulations of organized allopathic medicine. Osteopathic physicians built their own hospitals to provide patient care.

1938-1948: Efforts started to overcome segregation:

D.O.s tried to overcome segregation and discrimination by amalgamating with USC and with the CMA, but efforts were unsuccessful. Metropolitan University was created to grant an M.D. to D.O.s, in the hope they might become accepted at large hospitals and universities.

1948-1958: AOA and AMA were urged to resolve their differences:

California D.O.s tried to get the AOA and AMA to resolve their differences and to merge their organizations in order to end discrimination. The AMA evaluated the D.O. schools and met with the AOA several times, but decided not to merge, and instead to let the states decide individually about their M.D.-D.O. relations.

1958-1968: D.O.s and M.D.s merged in California:

Both professional organizations in California decided to merge. Without further training or improvement in the standard of care, D.O.s could apply to be awarded with the M.D. degree. COP&S was converted to an accredited M.D. school. The M.D. licensing board was willing to oversee the licenses of the new M.D.s and agreed to merge the new M.D.s into the CMA. Former D.O.s received unlimited hospital privileges and referred patients freely to M.D.s who now viewed their referrals as "improving the quality of care" for Californians.

As the merger was announced, a group of Osteopathic Physicians and Surgeons of California (OPSC) organized to preserve the osteopathic profession. They were successful and are representing osteopathy in California at present.

In 1966, the AMA officially removed the "cult" label from osteopathic medicine. D.O.s were allowed to become members of the AMA and admitted into their residencies by 1969. The free standing California College of Medicine became affiliated with the University of California Regents in 1964 and moved to the UC Irvine campus, becoming the UCI California College of Medicine in 1968.

1968-1977: Lawsuits successfully challenged the restriction imposed on the Osteopathic Licensing Board:

Osteopathic physicians from out-of-state, interested in moving to California, filed law suits to be able to get licensed in California. They won in 1974, and D.O.s from out of state became eligible again to be licensed in California. As the College of Osteopathic Medicine of the Pacific (COMP) received preliminary accreditation from AOA in 1977, osteopathic medicine was able to rebuild the profession in California. UC Irvine failed to establish a teaching hospital on its campus but continued to utilize the Orange County Hospital in the city of Orange as its primary training site. Research on musculoskeletal manipulation began in the Physical Medicine and Rehabilitation Department under the direction of Jerome Tobis, M.D. in 1970.

1978-1989: attempts to limit osteopathic training opportunities:

COMP graduated its first class in 1982. As tendencies continued to limit the clinical training of new D.O.s in the state, California legislature granted D.O.s access to all training facilities in **1989**. Since then, discrimination against D.O.s has been illegal in this state.

1990-1999: CMA and OPSC show mutual acceptance:

The California Medical Association (CMA) and the corresponding organization of Osteopathic Physicians and Surgeons of California (OPSC) started to work together on issues to which both can agree. **In 1999** the CMA officially recognized OPSC and agreed to work together on issues of mutual interest. They use the same persons now as their respective lobbyists. Very few issues affect the two groups in different ways, and a collegial relationship can be observed now. As always there are exceptions, some weighing heavier than others to leave an aftertaste of segregation.

Thus, many people who study healthcare in California feel confident that osteopathy is here to stay. Others argue that osteopathy might have outlived its aim to improve upon allopathy, as osteopathy might be inclined to forego its distinctive characteristics.

Dr. Tobis:

"There is an aspect of the development of medicine since World War II that deserves consideration. The explosive advances in technology, like endoscopy, robotics, joint replacements, radiological imaging and many others, has led to a vast expansion of the accoutrement of medical resources. As a result, musculoskeletal manipulation recently has made a relatively smaller contribution to the improvement of medical care. Historically, musculoskeletal manipulation treatment is very important and its story has to be told."

The interview with Counselor Hufstedler addressed the issue of taking osteopathy into traditional (or mainstream) medicine. Osteopathic physicians might have viewed their profession as having reached its goal of trying to improve medicine. Was osteopathy ready to come back into traditional medicine? Did they feel that they had accomplished what they were destined to do?

Counselor Hufstedler:

"No, I don't believe I heard anybody state that view. They were proud of us in Osteopathy. They thought it did a good job. They believed that it had some advantages over medicine that did not recognize what osteopathy did. But with regard to incorporating it into regular medicine, if you can call it that, you can see so many rehabilitation departments which had brought so much of that into regular medical practice. It's there now. But I don't think anybody said, 'gee, we are mature; we don't need to do this anymore.' I didn't hear it.

"I think the really important thing is that we're all trying to do the same thing. We all want to get as many good ideas as we can; put them together; and make them work. There is really no need or reason for there to be two divisions. I think that was the fundamental idea [of the merger]."

Ultimately, both professions are striving for excellence in healthcare. Allopathic medicine, with all its technological advances since WWII, is vulnerable to medical error and adverse outcomes, such that many patients seek a humanistic approach of inter-personal hands-on healing.

Once discrimination is legally out of the picture, equal opportunities arise. In the 21st century, the quality of patient care in California receives significant benefit from osteopathic medicine, whether practiced by an osteopathic physician or an M.D. who was initially educated as a D.O.

Chapter 7

California M.D.s and D.O.s in the 21st century

As described in Chapter 6, facing common challenges and collaborating on several issues served to improve mutual understanding and respect among the two medical professions. As a first step, allopathy and osteopathy alike had to find ways to lower the cost of their services. They joined forces to assure the delivery of high quality care in spite of cost cutting.

Secondly, both professions recognized the importance to base their respective treatments on scientific evidence. Traditionally, allopathy was able to procure better funding for research studies and facilities than osteopathy. The promise of increased research options served as motivator for the California merger of the two medical professions. While rebuilding osteopathy in California, studies on the effectiveness of manipulation have been conducted jointly between allopathy and osteopathy at the University of California Irvine, with grant support by the 41st Medical Trust. Possibly due to this trail-blazing endeavor of manipulation research, studies to identify the mechanisms involved in manipulation treatments have been advocated most recently at the National Institutes of Health.

Thirdly, both professions face the challenge to preserve the therapeutic effects of the doctor-patient relationship. Osteopathy's gold standard has been holistic medicine. At the joint osteopathy-allopathy conferences sponsored by the Josiah Macy Jr. Foundation in 1995-96, "holistic" was defined to include assessment and treatment approaches that lie outside a biomedical disease focus (O'Neil, 1996). With the increasing ethnic and cultural diversity among patients, mainstream medicine has recognized the importance of psychosocial and cultural aspects of the patient-doctor relationship.

Patients' needs in the 21st century

The two medical professions will need to join their respective skills to broaden the scientific evidence of health by examining health and healing approaches that are foreign to mainstream medicine. Expertise in the use of hi-tech medicine might be viewed as a particular strength that allopathy contributes to reduce pain and improve recovery time. Care delivery in communities and home-based settings can be viewed as osteopathy's expertise, addressing the needs of the whole person, including psychosocial and cultural needs (Gevitz, 1992; Riedell, 1998). Both professions must make sure to train physicians who are culturally competent to treat immigrant patients from Latin-America and Asia who might have health beliefs that are different from Angloeuropean medical values which historically served as the basis of mainstream medicine.

Allopathy and osteopathy both face the challenge to involve and engage patients. Non-adherence to scheduled physician visits and treatment plans have costly consequences for people's health. While reasons for non-adherence are complex, differences in health beliefs and values contribute to the barriers of serving patients' needs. One of the interviewed osteopathic physicians is treating patients in their homes, and many allopathic physicians in California are conducting home visits as well. Dr. Riedell's home visit project in Los Angeles in the 1940s might have a comeback in the 21st century (Riedell, 1998).

Preserving professional identity

For the osteopathic profession, there are potential adverse outcomes to the close collaboration between the two professions. Healthcare planners question the need to finance two types of educational institutions, two types of training, and two types of licensing agencies. They argue for "one [allopathic] medicine" serving all patients' needs. It seems that the clinical care environment of the 21st century does not promote the implementation of manipulation and holism, which led many osteopathic physicians to forego their time-consuming osteopathic manipulation skills. Such compromises seem to chip away from the osteopathic distinctiveness.

Norm Gevitz, a widely recognized scholar on osteopathy in America, pointed out these dangers already in the 1990s (Gevitz, 1996) and some of the interviewed participants for this project voiced similar concerns.

Answers to the challenging questions by healthcare planners might come from medical evidence, derived through basic science experimentation. Andrew Taylor Still's hypothesized self-healing capabilities of the human body might be supported through evidence obtained in psychoneuroimmunology (Hruby, 1996). The primary objective of the Forty-First Medical Trust is the support of such research efforts.

Suggestions for future directions by the interview contributors

Providing the best care for their patients is the primary goal for M.D.s and D.O.s alike. Both benefit from sharing their vision to reach that goal. During the interviews, some of the participants were given the opportunity to express their personal advice or thoughts on future directions for osteopathic physicians and allopathic physicians in training.

Dr. Allen:

"I feel that you need to stay in touch with your colleagues, you need to stay in touch with the leadership that you have and realize that our right to

practice is going to last only as long as the legislature sees us as having a purpose to serve and a place to serve. So you need to be supportive of your state association and the national association because they are watching how the health care dollars are being spent and to whom they are to be given and so I still think that we have a unique place in the overall management of patients and health care, and a unique philosophy of the management and approach to wellness."

Dr. Alloy:

"I think number one is to have an open mind and explore, as much as it is possible, and question that which you feel you need to question. I think it would be a good idea if both professions were able to learn more of one another, primarily allopathic medicine learning something of the benefits of manipulative therapy, and I know it does go on."

Emery Dowell:

"If I were to offer advice to a younger and newer generation of professional physicians it would be to work to make that distinction as little identifiable in the public and political environment as possible. Legislators, with very few exceptions, will neither understand nor be particularly excited to hear intensely partisan discussions about the pros and cons of being called one or another. The very necessity for them to understand the complexities of health care and hospitalization and health insurance renders the distinction between M.D.s and D.O.s something that they would rather not worry about and hope very much that the professions would take care of intramurally.

"I believe, as a layman, that the clinical distinctions between the professions began to diminish more than a generation ago. There really should not be much effort to impress them upon the public because those distinctions really make no difference in the way people are cared for by their physicians. Let's leave it at that."

Dr. Frymann:

Fostering osteopathic education and training abroad for 40 years, Dr. Frymann has promoted enthusiasm for traditional osteopathy beyond the United States:

"I think we ought to take some of the students overseas. I think they ought to see the enthusiasm that exists in Europe, in Russia, in Japan, and Australia and see how important this is to the rest of this world".

Dr. Golanty:

"[Osteopathic manipulation treatment] *OMT is still a skill. It's not a cognitive thing. It is important knowing when to use it and when to apply it, but actually performing it, that's another skill.*"

Mrs. Grunigen:

"*I think all of these people, Teale, Grunigen, Dorothy Marsh, had the quality that ran through this whole era which was, 'If they said they were going to do something, they'd do it.' They spoke truth. You knew if they said, 'This is truth', it was You never doubted it. You never questioned it because it was. These people had this quality and I suppose this is why the success was there for them because credibility is really how you accomplish anything . . . because truth was more visible then. And then you recognized when the truth wasn't there. It was so obvious. This is the difference.*

"*As for me, I could talk to a legislator and know that he would support me when I needed the vote. When I talked to him and explained to him the issues, I know that vote would be there. I wouldn't have to worry about it. It was a different way of life. It was simpler and less complicated I think. I suppose that's why I was successful because they knew my background and recognized that when I presented something it was for a good reason, and not trying to create additional problems or anything.*"

Dr. Haldeman:

" *. . . always focus on science, it's a unifying factor. If we anchor our opinions on science, we will reach similar conclusions.*

"*But it's so difficult to translate research into practice. There are a* small percent [of clinicians] *who come to scientific meetings. They may argue, but they come. But the vast majority of D.O.s, D.C.s and M.D.s never come and so they are not part of the discussion. Anybody who is not part of the discussion will suffer a severe culture shock—science will bite them hard! Because guidelines will dictate who gets paid. We have to find a way to communicate with the practitioner who is isolated in a corner and just does not communicate.*

"*Did the merger affect the inter-disciplinary discussions? Sure, it impacted how D.O.s view themselves in California. You can feel that. It changed the focus of osteopathy.*"

Counselor Hufstedler:

"Well, I don't think I have any wisdom to offer. My only reactions are personal reactions. But I thought the fundamentals of osteopathy were important and valuable. I ended up with a large share of my various doctors being ex-osteopaths—then M.D.s. For some years after that most of them died off unfortunately. I still think their ideas are valuable and should be included with allopathy."

Dr. Kamajian:

"Teenagers today use a term which is fascinating. They want to be unlimited. And the term that they use is 'aboxic'. To not recognize the box exists is the ultimate manifestation of your ability to be creative. If Dr. Still, as an artist, presented anything for future generations, [it] was the ability to suggest to us that we need to be 'aboxic', we need to be unlimited.

"I think the younger D.O.s have to have the ability to remember that Dr. Still in his life was a very religious person. The ability to recognize that there's something more than us. The ability to be honest and to be consistently honest in everything that we do, meticulously honest, especially to ourselves. The ability to say no, the ability not to enable. If we stick to that pattern, this profession is an 'aboxic' profession. If we are not honest to ourselves, or other people, if we don't have the ability to say no, if we enable people to be putzes [idiots-ed.] *and to make stupid mistakes, we run the risk of becoming a very 'boxic' profession, or an entombed profession even.*

"To my M.D. students, to my M.D. residents, I always remind them that my primary clinical skills are in patient history taking and physical examination. But I have something to offer them, and D.O.s have something to offer them in a differential diagnosis, both from the meticulous redundancy in the way that we're taught to do medical histories, and in our physical examination, including other things. And that we are a resource, that while rare, it's still not something that they should pooh-pooh or ignore. There are times when there are clinical challenges where you need resources that are extraordinary. And D.O.s bring extraordinary resources to the table if they know what they are doing, if they had been the sorcerer's apprentice."

Dr. Kammerman:

"The osteopathic students and physicians use their manipulation and do it wisely. So many of them get in the M.D. training programs and never use their

manipulation and then either lose the skill or lose the ability to think about it. They don't think about doing it when they get into private practice. Oh, I tell you, I have kept a lot of people working; got them back to work sooner; got them feeling better sooner because I do know how to manipulate them. In fact, I could still probably do it. But I think that that would be the one thing that I would suggest to the osteopathic students, especially in the osteopathic physicians, 'use manipulation'. "Don't rely on organized medicine or the regular medicines. You can do so much with your hands. It's unbelievable what you can do. You use the medicine to take the edge off the pain for a short while or get them to a comfortable point where you can do manipulation, but use the manipulation wisely.

"As far as the other doctors and every doctor: patient advocacy! You must be a patient advocate, you must think of the patient first. Treat that patient as though you would want to be treated, or treat the patient as you would one of your loved ones treated. I don't tell them to treat them like your brother or your sister because they may be having a battle with those. You've heard that term before, I'm sure. They might not like them when they are growing up but they tend to get better when they get older. Anyway, think of the patient as an individual, not as an entity. Those are some of the things I would think about."

Dr. Kasovac:

"My advice to D.O.s in programs today is to maintain your osteopathic manipulative medicine principles and practices, and demonstrate your skills in OMM. No matter what specialty you are in, there are applications. Do it in all fields of practice, and do it as part of your patient care. Remember to bring those principles forward in everything that you do every day. One of the other nice things to do is to share it with other professional colleagues; with other M.D.s at the hospitals and organizations that you are involved with, nursing staff at the hospitals, other allied health personnel, whether it is physical therapist, nurse practitioner, or physician's assistant. All of it helps our profession grow.

"I just say to all the D.O.s out there, and thank goodness we are into thousands that are out there now, 'Go D.O.s!'—keep up the good work and be professionals, ethical, honest, good patient care givers and continue to do all of the good work we have done over these years; and continue to maintain the respect and recognition that we've gained from the public as well as our colleagues in other professions.

"My advice to M.D.s in the training programs is that they have an opportunity to be exposed to osteopathic residents in their program and other osteopathic faculty members in their program. Then they will realize that we

have a skill that they didn't learn in medical school. They weren't even taught it. It wasn't even talked about, but we are willing to share. We were willing to share and we created courses for them to learn the principles and the techniques and to become proficient in those skills. I think it is a wonderful way to expand our osteopathic profession and maybe we can look at this and say, 'We are willing to accept 126 medical schools once they put our principles and practices into their curriculum and we will make them all D.O. schools nationwide'."

Dr. Krpan:

"We have our philosophy and our hands-on care to offer. I think as long as we have that, there's a reason for us to remain a separate profession and to protect the privileges that we have to practice as D.O.s."

Dr. MacCracken:

"I feel that they [osteopathic physicians in training] really should be considering the total individual and not strictly his medical needs. He needs to be an overall physician that considers their emotional and what-have-you that makes them tick . . . . taking care of the whole person."

Dr. Menkes:

"There is a musculoskeletal component to most diseases, but you have to look for it and you have to know what you are touching and feeling. That's how they train you in school and I don't understand how people can let that go by the wayside. It's the most intimate part of the physician-patient encounter. You're actually touching a patient.

"One of the things I showed my students to observe what happens when a patient is in the office and they come in for their exam. I'm looking in their eye grounds and they say, 'no one's ever done that before.' I then listen to carotid arteries, which some doctors do, some don't. But then, when I'm listening to their heart, I have my watch situated where they can't see I'm looking at it, I listen for one full minute . . . . That one minute is a bonding time. Then when you do your musculoskeletal exam, you're touching the patient, that's an intimacy that the allopathic physician doesn't share. And even though I did critical care medicine in California for 27 years, I never had a lawsuit. I contribute that to good luck, and the fact that I was honest with my patients, and we had a bond . . . .

"I think that it is a great anti-depressant. The fact that there is eye contact between the physician and patient, and then the touching. What can be more intimate? Well, obviously as long as you don't cross the line, and I'm sure that *happens, but most patients react positively to an interaction with the physician that has actually laid hands on them.*

Advice for future M.D physicians in in training? 'Treat your D.O. brethren as peers, they're your brothers, and learn from them'."

Dr. Norcross:

"I still think that medicine in general is a really exciting field. There's so much reward for helping people. That's still going to go on, the economic side of it is certainly not anywhere near what it was when I started. It was in the so called golden years and it was wonderful. I don't think there is anything to be concerned about there. I think if you want to be a physician and you want to help people, just go for it. It's a great occupation. I can't imagine really anything that I'd rather done than what I did. I of course gravitated towards surgery, I still like that idea because you can usually see results right away. My internal medicine colleagues, it usually takes them a lot longer. I think it's exciting.

"We were talking about the osteopathic profession. I hope the students do see the difference between a D.O. and a M.D. The D.O. gets everything that an M.D. gets in the way of training and they have this plus, and it's something that they should never forget. It's easy to forget it because in today's medicine you have to take care in a certain amount of time, and certainly to do some amount of manipulation on that patient takes part of that precious time. Sometimes it's very, very helpful in surgery. I have to admit very little of my practice was in manipulation but once in a while there was a spot I could use it. I hope they don't gloss it over or forget that extra that they have in training and ability . . . . The concepts of holistic medicine that seems to be growing now and in the forefront. I've seen that used and believed by the allopathic profession."

Dr. Passy:

*"'**Healing the Needy**' should be one unified goal. Combining the healing principles of the D.O. and M.D. philosophy should be blended into one philosophy of care to obtain optimal results in patient treatment.*

"Let us not forget our past but look deeply into our future together.

"Basic research and education is our common sword to open our minds to unify the goals of togetherness in our endeavor to look toward the future.

*"Working together in unity toward one goal—'**Healing the Needy**'."*

Dr. Pumerantz:

"I tell the students at the beginning of every year in all the programs, 'when you graduate from this University you are going to have the technical

and scientific competence you need to be a good healer. At the same time you are going to be offering compassion and caring to your patients because that's the type of people we've recruited in the first place'."

Dr. Ryan:

Dr. Ryan's advice for osteopathic physicians:

"Support the fact that they are osteopathic students. They should set their goals and stay with them."

Dr. Ryan's advice for allopathic physicians:

"They should follow their professional goals but they should also learn to respect the ability and judgment of the osteopathic students and physicians."

Dr. Ryder:

"After 45 years of practice I still like treating patients and taking histories and getting acquainted with people. I have had a wonderful career and wish I could relive my life again.

"I give this advice to any physician. Take time to talk with your patient. Take time to do a physical exam. The osteopathic structural exam is excellent. By performing a structural exam of your patient you can obtain a lot of information about their health concerns and problems it really helps the patient feel comfortable and it communicates to them that you care. When they say, 'I don't have time. I tell them, 'Well, make time, because you are not going to succeed if you don't'."

"I try to impress on the students that medicine is a dynamic profession and changes rapidly . . . . What is interesting is that our role as healers hasn't changed much, just the diseases have changed."

Dr. Seffinger's advice to students of osteopathic medicine:

"I would like them to be proud of their professional heritage; to know the history of their profession; and to take charge of the future of their profession. I'd like them to know the efficacy of osteopathic manipulative medicine. I would like them to know the strengths and weaknesses of all they learn in medicine; to constantly evaluate and investigate all the methods that they use and other doctors use.

"Dr. Still, when he started the college and he taught his students, he told them not to take what he had to say as dogma. He said, essentially, you need to

evaluate everything you hear and what you see; if it rings true and if it proves to be helpful for the patient, then you can use that. He wanted people to accept what was real and what worked not just because somebody said it worked, you see.

"It's very ironic that the M.D.s kept complaining about D.O.s doing dogma and teaching dogma. When Dr. Still started his whole idea he didn't want people to copy his techniques. He didn't want his students to watch and do his manual treatments. He told them they have to design their own treatments based on their knowledge of anatomy and physiology and pathology and what's good for that patient at that time; he admonished them not to just do something because he did it. Remember, he was an M.D. physician with 40 years practice by the time he started his school of osteopathy in 1892. He was not only a philosopher but [he also] *respected science and the use of valid interventions for identifiable causes of disease."*

Dr. Steedman:

"Be a bug on pre-operative and post-operative care and preparation of your patient! I received my most honored award I've ever received from the University of California at Irvine on the basis of the votes of all the students and also one class that I had taught for four years. They voted me for the Golden Apple Award for the individual that had taught them the most over the four years in general surgery. I was so proud of that and it really made me feel close to the profession."

Dr. Stotts:

"I don't know that there would be any difference between allopathic and osteopathic medical education. The only thing that allopathic students miss out is the extra training [in OMT] *which I think was so helpful to me because we are talking about a body going wrong, and there are signs and symptoms in the body when something is not working correctly.* [I would advise] *to be open to capturing all of that information with your eyes and with your hands and with your ears.*

"It's about being as close to understanding the true derangements and trying to head those off and change the natural course of an event if it's changeable, and recognizing when you can't, and being able to provide comfort and care. Unfortunately, life's ills and slings and arrows are carried in our bodies. If we don't address those, medications don't resolve all of them. [Recognizing] *the importance of the patient as a whole, the patient as a unit, the patient in society, and how all those components fit together, is really the bread and butter of the D.O. profession, and the M.D. profession is catching on."*

Dr. Taylor's advice to osteopathic physicians:

"1) Be proud to be a D.O.
2)   Go out and do the very best they can in healing people in whatever
specialty they are in.
3)   Know your limits and know yourself.
4)   Do an excellent job.
5)   Be concerned with helping people more than how much you can make.

Also: Make your patients well. Doesn't matter how you get them well.
The end justifies the means. They should have a commitment to service of
[their] *patients."*

Dr. Taylor's mentor was Glenn Gordon, M.D. and former D.O. Dr. Gordon
was an anesthesiologist at Los Angeles County Osteopathic Hospital and
became the chair of the Department of Anesthesiology at the Los Angeles
Women and Children Hospital at USC in 1965. Dr. Taylor recalls Dr.
Gordon's advice:

"Glenn Gordon, M.D. was my teacher. He said, 'you are a doctor
first, and an anesthesiologist second.' I never forgot that. I pride myself
on being able to act quickly, successfully and appropriately and create
a treatment for the problem at hand. I feel this is due to my osteopathic
education."

Dr. Tobis:

"I feel that manipulation is a valuable modality for patients with
low back pain, especially of acute and sub-acute duration. I feel it is
less effective for chronic pain lasting more than three months. I feel
that those trained in osteopathy as well as those trained in allopathy in
physical medicine and rehabilitation should gain the skills that have been
described over the years in numerous publications and be aware that it
is available."

Dr. Ulansey:

"To a D.O. student in training: live with what is going to be. Go ahead
and make the most of it. It [osteopathic medicine] *is never going to be what*
it was for me. I don't know what I could have done that would have given me
greater self-satisfaction in my years of practice. It's been good to me. It has

been good financially. It's been good socially. It's been good for my peace of mind. I've enjoyed being a physician.

"To an M.D. student in training: go to the county hospital. That's where you will get the best training. You are going to pay more for it, in your health, in your life, your work, your endeavor. But, you will be repaid many times over. You will be a better physician for it.

"They are going to be tired. We were tired. We didn't get paid. Now they get paid for it. The difference in the salary is major—that is during the training period, interns and residencies. The earning capacity of the profession whether it be M.D. or D.O. or PDQ, it is a new world. It is not going to be what everybody thinks the physician makes. There are a few handfuls that will always excel and succeed to be far and above the run of the mill. You won't be one of those, few of you will be, but it will give you satisfaction of having been a doctor and a warmth inside that I cannot begin to describe. I loved it."

Dr. van den Noort:

"I think they [students in osteopathic and allopathic medicine] *will gradually grow together as time goes along and manipulation will become more and more a part of everybody's medicine."*

Dr. Vinn:

"I would just encourage allopathic students to learn more about why we think the way we think about patients. They will have to make up their own mind if they feel that is additive to their practice, and their base of knowledge.

"[I would encourage osteopathic students to] *. . . always remember your roots, remember the importance of the osteopathic philosophy in your daily practice, no matter what specialty you are in, and in your hand, heart, and mind always be a D.O., no matter where you are; because it is a badge of pride to carry with you."*

Matt Weyuker:

" . . . . too many D.O.s, including some in present day leadership, would happily exchange their D.O. degree for an M.D. degree and not look back. As Pogo would say, 'We have met the enemy, and he is us.' . . . .

"You are an integral part of an irreplaceable and distinctively American healing arts profession; protect, safeguard, and nurture it—a lot of osteopathic physicians who brought the profession back from near-extinction here in California are depending on you."

Conclusion: Where do we go from here?

In reviewing the contents of this book, a complex story of the relationship between the two groups of physicians emerges. While on an individual basis the two kinds of physicians usually treated each other courteously and with appropriate respect, on an organizational level a multitude of political incentives and cultural beliefs created barriers to courteous collaboration.

Osteopathy of the nineteenth century offered a significant contribution to the care of impaired and disabled individuals for whom mainstream medicine had little to offer. But the long cultural history of mainstream medicine, emanating from the era of Hippocrates, through its development in the Christian era into the Italian Renaissance, with reinforcement from developments in many European countries, created a societal atmosphere that made its professional standards seem inviolable.

Certainly the Flexner report brought about an increased emphasis on science in medical education, possibly at the cost of losing traditional healing methods and folk medicine. Given the allopathic bias of the report, osteopathy had to struggle to gain recognition and overcome the strong prejudices that the medical societies imposed on any healthcare system that did not have the imprimatur of the AMA. With the new standards of the Flexner report of the early twentieth century, the gulf even widened.

The merger in California in 1962 can in part be understood as an effort to close the gulf between allopathy and osteopathy. Was that effort successful?

The first impact of the merger was the AMA's acceptance of COP&S graduates who had taken the M.D. degree in 1962 into its Association, followed by accepting D.O. graduates in 1969, and finally accepting the re-establishment of the practice rights for D.O.s in California in 1974. Former D.O.s who became M.D.s in 1962 through the California College of Medicine were commissioned as medical officers in the military in 1963. Doors opened for D.O.s to be promoted to the rank of medical officer in 1966 and conscripted as medical officers in the military in 1967. Certainly, removing the "cult" label from osteopathy in 1966 helped to close the gap as well and made reasonable and respectful communication possible.

Even though the merger did not lead to a merger by other state medical associations or to the conversion of other osteopathic to allopathic medical schools, the effects of the California merger spread nationwide, and gradually even worldwide, in other ways. For example, its effects can be found in the innovative multidisciplinary collaboration in education, research, and treatment approaches.

Education

When the AOA lost its California school and nearly a quarter of its D.O.s to the merger, it had to rebuild. Its first endeavor, sparked by California D.O.s who left the state, was to open a school in Michigan in 1967. This school, originally started in Pontiac, MI as a free standing institution, became the Michigan State University College of Osteopathic Medicine (MSU-COM) in 1969. The College was the first state-supported osteopathic medical school and the first to exist simultaneously with an allopathic college, the College of Human Medicine, on the same campus.

The founding Dean, Myron Megan, D.O. (who died on February 13, 2008) was determined to make it a research based D.O. school and hired several D.O. faculty dedicated to research in osteopathic manipulation. In 1975, Dean Megan visited M.D.s in Europe who practiced manual medicine in an attempt to open doors to international collaboration.

Also in 1975, Murray Goldstein, D.O., who was at that time affiliated with the U.S. National Institutes of Health (NIH), led an NIH sponsored research symposium on the research status of spinal manipulative therapy, to which M.D.s, D.O.s, D.C.s and Ph.D.s were invited to present papers and attend open forum discussions. It was at that meeting that John Mennell, M.D. and Philip Greenman, D.O. met and began discussions how to bridge the gap between the two professions, partly so that M.D.s could get better training opportunities in manual medicine from the D.O.s.

John Mennell, M.D. was one of the founders of the North American Academy of Manual Medicine (NAAMM), which was this continent's affiliate in the Federation of International Manual Medicine (FIMM), whose members were exclusively M.D.s who practiced manual medicine. For the first time, George W. Northup, D.O. was invited to present a lecture to NAAMM in 1973. In 1977, Paul Kimberly, D.O. from Kirksville College of Osteopathic Medicine and Robert Ward, D.O. and Philip Greenman, D.O., both from MSU-COM, attended an executive session of the Board of Directors of NAAMM, and subsequently D.O.s were allowed to become members of NAAMM and therefore of FIMM which in turn invited Drs. Greenman and Ward to their conference in Copenhagen—the first time that D.O.s were allowed to attend.

Scott Haldeman, M.D., Ph.D., D.C., who participated in the historical interview project of this book, followed Dr. Greenman as president of NAAMM in the early 1980s. NAAMM was absorbed into the American Association of Orthopedic Medicine (AAOM) in the 1990s and the American Academy of Osteopathy became the Canadian representative to FIMM while the AAOM represented the U.S. (Oral communication: Phil Greenman, D.O., May 9, 2008 to M. Seffinger, D.O.).

On the local front, in California, in 1965 two M.D. graduates of the California College of Medicine, who had started as osteopathic medicine students at COP&S in 1961, namely Arthur White, M.D. and Aubrey Swartz, M.D., organized two international musculos keletal study societies that have manual medicine as a component. Dr. Haldeman was of great help to garner the acceptance of D.O.s by M.D.s as well. His decision to teach and conduct research on manipulation together with D.O.s at UC Irvine in the 1970s was prompted by Jerome Tobis, M.D., a recognized scholar in physical medicine and rehabilitation at UC Irvine. These successful initiatives can be understood as a direct result of the merger.

International acceptance and collaboration also occurred as a result of the merger. Viola Frymann, D.O. who contributed her interview to this project, has taught manipulation regularly in France, England, Russia, Italy, and Japan to M.D.s and D.O.s since the 1970s. However, many M.D.s abroad, such as the members of FIMM, still do not acknowledge or interact with D.O.s trained in countries other than the U.S.A.

In the 21st century, several California D.O.s teach Manual Medicine to M.D.s in America and abroad. Jerel Glassman, D.O. and Harry Friedman, D.O., graduates of Michigan State University College of Osteopathic Medicine, were recruited by Arthur White, M.D. to the St. Mary's Spine Center in San Francisco in the early 1990s. They developed, along with Wolfgang Gilliar, D.O., the San Francisco International Manual Medicine Society, teaching in Germany and throughout Europe, Australia, and New Zealand, as well as in North America. Dr. Grunigen's vision for osteopathy was to become integrated in healthcare internationally. Even that lofty goal seems reachable in the 21st century.

Research

Under the leadership of Murray Goldstein, D.O., NIH sponsored another interdisciplinary and international research conference on the neurological basis of manual medicine held at MSU. In 1978, Dr. Mennell, Dr. Greenman, and several other allopathic and osteopathic physicians began teaching manual medicine post graduate courses to M.D.s and D.O.s. In 1978, Dr. Mennell argued that there were not enough physicians to provide the manual medical care required in this country and recommended to train physical therapists as well. Thus, by 1982, physical therapists were allowed to attend these interdisciplinary manual medicine courses as well.

Jerome Tobis, M.D. coordinated and co-chaired international interdisciplinary research symposia on spinal manipulation at UC Irvine in 1975 and published the proceedings with Dr. Buerger as "*Approaches to the Validation of Manipulation Therapy*" (Springfield IL, Charles C. Thomas Publisher, 1977). Contributors included scholars from Canada, England, Sweden, and New Zealand. A decade later, Dr. Tobis and Dr. Hoehler reported on the first randomized clinical trial about the efficacy of spinal manipulation in patients with low back pain and published their findings in *JAMA* in 1981 and later in "*Musculoskeletal Manipulation: Evaluation of the Scientific Evidence*" (Springfield IL, Charles C. Thomas Publisher, 1986).

Dr. Haldeman continued on a national scale to facilitate the collaborating between M.D.s and chiropractors to develop guidelines for the practice of manipulation in American health care. It was largely through his efforts that in 1994, the U.S. government recommended that its people receive spinal manipulation in the event of an incidence of simple, mechanical acute low back pain. The NIH established a fund for research in manual therapies soon thereafter. In 2008, once again, the NIH co-sponsored an interdisciplinary international research symposium on the systemic effects of manual therapies held at the national Osteopathic Research Center at the University of North Texas Health Science Center in Fort Worth, Texas.

It can be argued that these advances would have happened gradually with time, as discrimination became no longer acceptable. Perhaps so, but the effects of social awareness probably would have taken much longer to result in respect and collaboration than the dramatic impact of the California merger's original goal to improve healthcare through collaboration and research.

It is in this historical light, that the remarkable achievements can be appreciated of that small band of osteopathic leaders, with the assistance of several allopaths, who brought about the merger of the two professions. Undauntedly, though, osteopathic medicine emerged again in California, equal to allopathy legally, although not always socially. As the future progresses, how will the relationship between the two medical professions proceed? How can we nurture the camaraderie, so fondly recalled in medical education at COP&S and CCM half a century ago?

Dr. Passy:

> "How can we find an avenue to build a liaison and combine our activities in education and research? How can we work together to build one unit and aim in the direction of positive change? Both medical professions have something to offer [to improve the quality of healthcare in California]."

Dr. Nelson:

> [Regarding] " . . . the integration of the two professions as the future progresses, it has been my observation that each of the professions has something to learn from the other. The future relationship is dependent on each profession learning about and feeling comfortable with the other. I see future, improved integration occurring within the system of post-graduate education, i.e. residency programs. Can we look forward to a time when allopathic graduates will choose to attend osteopathic related residencies as they develop in this State? The postgraduate training programs may be the best place for individuals of the two professions to learn about each other and learn to work together."

Dr. Krpan:

> " I think we are seeing a trend among allopathic physicians in this country and abroad; they have become more interested in our hands-on techniques and I'd like to see more of them take advantage of that component. I think it develops a couple of things: number one, a more touchy-feely physician on their behalf, and number two, respect for what it is that we do as physicians when we have more M.D.s out there learning some of our skills. It's going to eliminate some of that bias that exists."

Dr. Seffinger: *"Should allopathic students think about practicing and working with osteopathic physicians?"*

Dr. Krpan: *"Oh, you know that situation is here. Our physicians and their physicians are working side by side everywhere right now."*

Dr. Seffinger:

"My goal is to unite various forces and people interested in the same mission, the same goal which is to improve patient care, and have everybody work together to achieve the common goal; the common goal being to improve patient care, including natural methods, especially manipulation, integrated with all other forms of medicine and surgery that work for people, to make them healthier and to educate them how to improve their health."

Dr. Kammerman:

"I am convinced that the merger in California resulted in a positive arena for acceptance of the osteopathic physician throughout the United States as well as in California."

The lives of those who experienced the California merger with its trials and tribulations are described in the Appendix. Their personal narratives, cited throughout this book, served as a second layer of evidence for this project. Their experiences documented an era, unique so far in the United States, which without their narratives might have remained an untold story, hidden in archival manuscripts.

Appendix

Individuals shaping the M.D.-D.O. relationship

"Never doubt that a group of thoughtful committed citizens can change the world. Indeed, it is the only thing that ever has." Margaret Mead

This appendix briefly describes the professional life of persons who provided interviews. While these biographies do not adequately describe their career, the descriptions hopefully provide a summary of their work in osteopathic and allopathic relations. Similar brief biographies of key historical osteopathic and allopathic physicians and surgeons are provided in the second part of this appendix.

Contributors to the historical narrative project

Ethan Allen, D.O.

Dr. Allen was born in 1923 in North Dakota and educated in Laramie, Wyoming. As a 1943 graduate of the University of Wyoming in Engineering, he was recruited for a project which turned out, unbeknown to him, to be the Manhattan project. Upon his requested transfer to a different engineering project he started to explore possibilities of combining his expertise in engineering with medicine. Osteopathy was recommended as a particularly open-minded profession that might give this idea a chance to blossom. As he was drafted into the U.S. Navy in 1945, the realization of his career plans was delayed until 1946. The following year, though, he was able to enter COP&S. He graduated in 1951. He practiced in Norwalk and performed home deliveries for 13 years.

Since he had little involvement with organized osteopathy, he did not become aware of the implementation of the merger until about 1961. Together with Dr. Dobreer, Dr. Linden and Dr. Eby, he formed a component society of osteopathic physicians loyal to the AOA called Osteopathic Physicians and Surgeons of California (OPSC) to take the place of the California Osteopathic Association (COA) which was at that time preparing to merge with the California Medical Association (CMA). OPSC filed a law suit in attempt to block one component of the merger process, namely the transition of COP&S to an allopathic medical school that granted the M.D. degree. Their case was denied and seemingly endless legal battles ensued. In 1962 Dr. Allen paid the fees required to obtain the M.D. degree from the California College of Medicine for which he was eligible, so that no one could say he was not qualified in case some person or institution would later hold it against him. He didn't turn in his D.O. degree to the AOA, nor did he ever use his M.D. degree after all, as he found that it indeed was not necessary in order to continue his practice as usual without it. He didn't lose any hospital privileges as a result of remaining a D.O.

Four times Dr. Allen served as president of OPSC. In 1968 their lawyer, Alexander Tobin, filed a class action suit that the CMA fought all the way until 1974. It essentially called for a repeal of the part of the 1962 Proposition 22 initiative which removed the licensing power of the State Board of Osteopathic Examiners. Finally on March 19, 1974 the California Supreme Court upheld their case and the licensing power of the Board of Osteopathic Examiners was re-established.

Next, Dr. Allen set out to found an osteopathic medical school in California. He and his colleagues and supporters sought to replenish the decimated profession since three fourths of the 2400 D.O.s in California exchanged their degrees and professional affiliations to the M.D./AMA in 1962. Funds had to be obtained and a feasibility study to be conducted. In 1977 these preparations resulted in the first incorporation papers for the College of Osteopathic Medicine of the Pacific (COMP) in Pomona, CA. Dr. Allen, Dr. Dilworth and Dr. Frymann recruited Dr. Pumerantz as president of COMP and the college officially opened its doors in 1978. Dr. Allen is the only founding member of the Board of Trustees still serving on the Board and continues with his contributions to OPSC and COMP, which is now part of Western University of Health Sciences. The Ethan Allen, D.O. Memorial Park was named after him on the campus of Western University of Health Sciences on December 9, 2006.

Dr. Seffinger interviewed Dr. Allen on April 6, 2002 at COMP in Pomona, CA

Paul Alloy, M.D.

Paul Alloy was born in 1924 and raised in the city of Philadelphia. In 1943, he matriculated at the Philadelphia College of Osteopathy and graduated in 1946. While waiting to start his internship at the Los Angeles County General Hospital, he worked for about five months in a small hospital in Audubon, New Jersey. The facility had no house staff and Dr. Alloy had an opportunity to fulfill that task. He felt that he learned a lot in that period of time, the years during and immediately after the Second World War.

His internship and residency at the County Hospital in Los Angeles, having started in February of 1947, were compressed because of the war. The twelve months of internship were condensed to nine months, and four years of residency were compressed into three. Having trained in several departments, including urology, he got onto the service of general surgery. He gave up urology and continued in general surgery until he left the County Hospital in 1949.

Having worked for several years in a family practice group, he opened his own office for general practice and provided anesthesia work in concurrence. When in 1952 one of the hospitals at which he was on staff was approved by the AOA for internships, he was appointed the Assistant Director of Interns. His interest in surgery continued, though, and he was able to obtain a preceptorship / residency program in surgery at Park View Hospital primarily involving Dr. Robbins. He worked also with several other surgeons at the hospital until he was well-prepared to practice on his own.

He was accepted as a candidate with the American Osteopathic College of Surgeons for membership and Board Certification. In 1957 he passed the Boards and received his certification from the American Board of Osteopathic Surgery. He was accepted on the staff of the County Hospital which included teaching and training interns and residents. He provided his services in the outpatient department and in surgery, working with the residents. He was also made a clinical instructor of surgery and was asked to provide lectures at COP&S.

Dr. Alloy served on the Professional Adjudication Committee of the COA from 1960, continuing under the auspices of the 41st Medical Society until December 1964. He conducted insurance reviews relative to doctor complaints or complaints from insurance companies regarding physician charges. He also served on the Committee on Certification, the Board of Certification of the COA from 1961 and later the Committee on Medical Specialties through the 41st Medical Society until 1965. He was the president of the southeast district of the 41st Medical Society from 1962 to 1963.

At that time, there was talk of a merger between the two professions, which involved review of specialty certification. While he was not actively involved with the merger, he was not against it, primarily because of potential advantages to the many individuals that were looking for extended training, unavailable to them at that time. Subsequent to the merger in 1962, he was appointed to the committee on insurance review for the Los Angeles County Medical Association where he served until 1981. He was appointed by the Department of Education, State of California, to an ad hoc committee of the Office of Private Postsecondary Education to evaluate the application of the College of Osteopathic Medicine of the Pacific in 1978.

Dr. Alloy was a Fellow of the American Society of Abdominal Surgeons (FASAS) and a Senior Fellow of the American College of Gastroenterology (FACG). Upon his retirement from clinical services in 1982, he became active with the Alumni Association at the California College of Medicine and later at the University of California at Irvine. Dr. Alloy served on the Board of Associated Alumni, CCM from 1981 to 1994 and was the president from 1984 to 1985. At UC Irvine, Dr. Alloy was appointed to the Committee on Admissions to the medical school. He was instrumental in achieving the presentation of a diploma from the University of California Irvine College of Medicine to all its graduates. The cooperation provided by Dr. Forest Grunigen and Dr. Stanley van den Noort, who was Dean of the College of Medicine at that time, was invaluable in obtaining faculty senate approval for the diplomas.

At the University of California Irvine College of Medicine, Dr. Alloy functioned on several committees, including a committee, established by the Dean, to promote a liaison between the Alumni and the College of Medicine. He also served as chair of the annual scientific sessions for the annual Alumni meeting as part of a homecoming reunion at the University. He initiated to include individuals of the reunion classes as speakers for the scientific sessions in order to attract their former classmates and to provide visibility to the graduates' accomplishments.

Dr Seffinger interviewed Dr. Alloy in Palm Springs, California, on August 27, 2005.

Stuart Chesky, D.O., J.D.

Born in 1943 and raised in Chicago, IL, Dr. Chesky knew already in elementary school that he wanted to become a physician. Toward the end of his pre-med education he chose the Chicago College of Osteopathy for his medical education. Upon graduation in 1968 he completed a one-year internship and a four-year Ob/Gyn surgery residency at the Chicago College. In 1973 he joined the faculty of the College and the staff of the Chicago Osteopathic Hospital.

Hoping to migrate to California he obtained his California license in 1974 by the newly re-instated California Osteopathic Licensing Board. In 1978 the opportunity arose to take over a practice associated with the Pacific Hospital of Long Beach (PHLB), in Long Beach, CA. In short time he became the first osteopathic physician to obtain full staff privileges at the Long Beach Memorial Medical Center, a much larger facility with an obstetrics department.

Given his academic background, Dr. Chesky soon became Director of Medical Education at PHLB for the foreign student program at this institution. Dr. Chesky recognized the opportunity to provide internship experience for the first cohort of graduates from the College of Osteopathic Medicine of the Pacific (COMP). As these new D.O.s applied for privileges at the Long Beach Memorial Medical Center, they were confronted with the stipulation of an equivalent to the 3-year allopathic post-doctoral training.

Thus, Dr. Chesky set out to develop the first osteopathic family practice residency in California since 1962 at Pacific Hospital of Long Beach, with Stanley Golanty, MD (former D.O.), as director. Osteopathic physicians, like Drs. Thomas, Vinn, and Adams taught, as well as the allopathic surgeon, Dr. Horowitz who was instrumental to convince other M.D.s of the value of this family practice residency.

For about 15 years, Dr. Chesky was a professor at COMP while also actively involved in the political structure of OPSC, serving even as its president. In 1993 he relocated to Ohio and built his practice there. After a few years a medical disability forced him to change careers. He became an attorney, actively practicing in Vermillion, Ohio, at the time of the interview.

Dr. Seffinger interviewed Dr. Chesky on October 9, 2005 at Dr. Chesky's home in Vermillion, Ohio.

Donald Dilworth, D.O.

Born in 1919 and raised in Chicago, California, Dr. Dilworth received his osteopathic medical education at the College of Osteopathic Physicians and Surgeons in California, graduating in 1944. In 1945 he went to Long Beach and interned at the Magnolia Hospital.

After extensive mission training, he and his family were accepted into the mission field in Ecuador where they were appointed to provide medical service to the Quichua Indians who are the famous heirs of the Incas who number some five million in the country of Ecuador and even more in Peru. Dr. Dilworth stayed in Ecuador for approximately eighteen years and was successful in establishing three clinics and lastly a small hospital. He was able to build a radio station in connection with the hospital by which he could send fixed tuned receivers with the patients at their daily return from the fields. Thus, he was able to establish contact with them every evening. He was able to introduce some components of modern medicine, like recognizing parasitic problems, in order to improve children's health and public health practices. His clinics focused on preventing parasitic infections through the hookworm, amoebas, and various combinations of Trichomonas and Ascaris.

Upon his return to California Dr. Dilworth worked with a general practice in Escondido. In the process of setting up his practice, he had the opportunity to work with the American Osteopathic Association, as he was interested in establishing a Christian Osteopathic Fellowship to work in various mission fields. In connection with this Christian Osteopathic group he was able to join the National Medical organization, now known as the Association of Medical and Dental Doctors. It was at this time that he began to think about re-establishing an osteopathic college in California and joined the Board of Directors to build the College of Osteopathic Medicine of the Pacific.

He was president of OPSC when only shortly afterward, approximately in 1984, the Governor appointed Dr. Dilworth to the Board of Osteopathic Examiners. Sensing a potential conflict of interest, Dr. Dilworth resigned from the Board of Directors for the new college. The Board of Osteopathic Examiners had established a rather strict criterion by which to recognize D.O.s from out-of-state. The Board insisted on a strong emphasis in the applicants' abilities to perform the osteopathic side of manipulative therapy and conducted hands-on examinations in order to maintain the quality of the profession.

During all these years of service to rebuild the osteopathic profession in California, Dr. Dilworth maintained his practice in Escondido until he sold it recently to an osteopathic colleague.

Dr. Seffinger interviewed Dr. Dilworth on August 22, 2005 at Dr. Dilworth's home in Escondido, CA.

Emery (Soap) Dowell

Mr. Dowell was associate director of the California Hospital Association in the Spring of 1962. The concept of an association between M.D.s and D.O.s which had been percolating for years was now in full professional and political bloom. The CMA and COA were in agreement. Both were ready to present the necessary legal changes to the California legislature and to the public for ratification.

The California Hospital Association was then comprised of hospitals where M.D.s practiced. These were about 450 in California. A parallel organization for osteopathy with some 60 members also existed. The California Hospital Association was in favor of the merger, and Mr. Dowell's job was to help promote the idea to the hospitals, legislature and public. An amendment to the State constitution had to be approved in the November 1962 election.

Mr. Dowell was not a policy maker. His strength was to function as a cheer leader. The California Hospital Association endorsed the proposal, but at the local level some hospital administrators and board of directors were not convinced of the value and furthermore recognized numerous problems that would result. The changeover entailed a lot of work which the administrators and boards resented.

The California Hospital Association was obliged to accept into its membership the 60 osteopathy hospitals many of whose boards and administrators were also dubious. Dowell and Frank Clark, public relations director of California Hospital Association along with other staff covered the state and the media to make the case for consolidation.

The leader for the consolidation was Senator Steve Teale, D.O. who practiced in Calveras County in the Sierra foothills, and was a leader in the State Senate. By coincidence, a CMA leader who also advanced the case was Ralph Teall, MD.

Whereas the D.O.s became M.D.s on masse in 1962, osteopathic hospitals joined the California Hospital Association one at a time, requiring some two years for the complete integration. An osteopathic hospital administrator was added to the California Hospital Association board of directors to help smooth the transition. Legal medical staffs also deliberated a long time before providing privileges to their new M.D. colleagues.

Mr. Dowell submitted his written narrative on October 8, 2006 from his office in Sacramento, CA.

Richard E. Eby, D.O.

Richard Eagle Eby was born in 1912 in Pittsfield, Massachusetts. He attended Wheaton College from 1931 to 1933 and graduated from the College of Osteopathic Physicians and Surgeons (COP&S) in 1937. He completed his internship and residency in obstetrics and gynecology at the Los Angeles County Osteopathic Hospital in 1939.

He co-founded the Park Avenue Hospital in Pomona, where he practiced from 1942 to 1962. He served as clinical professor at COP&S from 1948 to 1958. He became chairman of the Board of Directors at Park Avenue Hospital in Pomona in 1958 and Chief of Staff and Director of Medical Education in 1973. He also served as professor and chairman of the Department of Obstetrics and Gynecology at COP&S from 1958 to 1962. He became a Fellow and was president of the American College of Osteopathic Obstetricians and Gynecologists from 1957 to 1958.

In 1961, being not in favor of the merger between the California Osteopathic Association (COA) and the California Medical Association (CMA), he became the founding president of the Osteopathic Physicians and Surgeons of California (OPSC) and subsequently was appointed to the American Osteopathic Association (AOA) Board of Trustees, replacing Russell Husted, D.O. who lost his seat due to allegations of his pro-merger stance. In this role, Dr. Eby became the representative from California's newly chartered osteopathic medical society, OPSC. From 1962 to1963, Dr. Eby served as assistant executive director of the AOA.

He then served a short term as president of the Kansas City College of Osteopathic Medicine from 1963 to1965. Following that, he became professor and chairman of the Department of Obstetrics and Gynecology at the Kirksville College of Osteopathy and Surgery from 1965 to 1967.

He returned to California, practicing once again at Park Avenue Hospital in Pomona. He became president of OPSC for a second term in 1973 to1974 and helped OPSC battle to regain the right for the California state osteopathic licensing board to license osteopathic physicians. This effort finally culminated in a unanimous California state Supreme Court decision to restore that right in 1974. Dr. Eby then co-founded the College of Osteopathic Medicine of the Pacific in 1976 to 1977, along with fellow osteopathic physicians Dr. Frymann, Dr. Dilworth, and Dr. Allen.

Dr. Eby's life was changed dramatically by an accidental fall off a balcony in 1972 after which he had no pulse and was declared dead. He survived, though, and had a vision during that period of suspended life. He decided to devote the rest of his life to telling the world about that experience, wrote several books, and traveled the world as an evangelist through the 1980s and 1990s. He died at age 90 on December 26, 2002.

Dr. Seffinger interviewed Dr. Eby in 2001 at his home in Victorville, CA. It was Dr. Eby's recollection of events throughout his life that motivated Dr. Seffinger to dig deeper into the archives to unearth the details of the history of osteopathic medicine in the state of California, the merger between the COA and CMA, the founding of OPSC, UC Irvine School of Medicine and the College of Osteopathic Medicine of the Pacific at Western University of Health Sciences.

Viola Frymann, D.O., F.A.A.O., F.C.A.

Dr. Frymann grew up in Nottingham, England where she was exposed to osteopathic care when she was four years old. When the osteopathic college in London closed during WWII, she matriculated at the University of London and then the Royal Colleges, earning the British equivalent to the M.D. degree in 1945. However, she had the aspiration to find opportunities to resume her study of osteopathy, as she strongly believed in the effectiveness of osteopathic manipulation. After World War II she was able to finance her move to Los Angeles to study at the College of Osteopathic Physicians and Surgeons (COP&S).

Because of her British allopathic education, she received advanced placement at COP&S which had the unintended disadvantage of skipping training in osteopathic manipulation, offered at COP&S during the first two years. Thus, it was her impression that in the late 1940s no one was teaching or practicing osteopathic manipulation at COP&S.

She felt fortunate when she had the opportunity to train individually with an advanced student who had learned OMT from an osteopathic physician in Hawaii. She graduated with the D.O. degree in 1949 but continued to further her understanding of osteopathic manipulation. She submitted her work to the Academy of Applied Osteopathy and won two essay contests, in 1950 and 1952, for applying osteopathic principles and practice to heart and kidney diseases.

For many years, she conducted an osteopathic family practice with special emphasis on the problems of children in La Jolla. Then in 1982 she founded the Osteopathic Center for Children (OCC) which became a clinical teaching affiliate of the College of Osteopathic Medicine of the Pacific. The OCC, now located in central San Diego, is concerned with the treatment of all children including those for whom the primary consideration is prevention of sub optimal health, as well as those with deep and complex problems who seek to reach the optimum of their potential. The new Center now provides continuing education courses for M.D., D.O., and D.D.S. practitioners who recognize the significance of osteopathic medical practice relative to their various areas of special interest.

In addition to her clinical work, Dr. Frymann devoted much of her time to rescuing the osteopathic profession after the merger. She was President of OPSC three times, Secretary of the Board of Trustees, and founding Chair of the Department of Osteopathic Manipulative Medicine at COMP. She has been teaching osteopathy at many of the colleges of osteopathic medicine in the U.S. as well as colleges, universities and institutes throughout the world.

She is the author of many published journal articles. She has published research on newborn babies, the cranial rhythmic impulse, learning disabilities of children and the effect of osteopathic manipulative treatment of children with neurologic developmental problems and articles on other aspects of the profession, its philosophy, concepts, and practice. The American Academy of Osteopathy (AAO) published her collected works in a book in 1998.

She has served as President of the Cranial Academy and Osteopathic Physicians & Surgeons of California. She served on the Board of Governors of the American Academy of Osteopathy.

She has received many awards and is considered a living legend of osteopathic medical leadership by her peers. Awards have included: Andrew Taylor Still Medallion of Honor, the highest honor of the American Academy of Osteopathy; the William G. Sutherland Award of the Cranial Academy; Honorary Doctorate of Science in Osteopathic Medicine from the College of Osteopathic Medicine of the Pacific; Osteopathic Physician of the Year from the Osteopathic Physicians and Surgeons of California; the Philip Pumerantz Medal for "Distinguished Service and Extraordinary Commitment to the College of Osteopathic Medicine of the Pacific and the Osteopathic Medical Profession" and life membership in OPSC for "the sacrifices and labor of love in bringing the osteopathic profession back from extinction."

Dr. Seffinger interviewed Dr. Frymann at the Osteopathic Center for Children in San Diego, CA on June 29, 2002.

Stanley Golanty, M.D.

Dr. Golanty was born in 1933 in Ohio. In 1949, at age 16, he moved with his family to Los Angeles, California where his father set up a Kosher butcher business with home deliveries. One of the customers was an osteopathic physician who had a brother studying at the College of Osteopathic Physicians and Surgeons (COP&S) in Los Angeles. These acquaintances raised Dr. Golanty's interest in osteopathic medicine, an interest that became intensified by meeting Munish Fineberg, D.O. as a speaker for pre-med students at UCLA. At an open house orientation program for COP&S he met Dr. Papageorges whose enthusiasm inspired Dr. Golanty. Even though his friends chose allopathic medical schools, Dr. Golanty chose COP&S and graduated in 1959 with the D.O. degree.

He hoped for an internship at the Los Angeles County Osteopathic Hospital but those opportunities were reserved for veterans of WWII or the Korean War. Fortunately opportunities for interning arose through a newly built osteopathic hospital in Long Beach, with two months training at Magnolia Hospital and ten months at Pacific Hospital.

Obtaining a residency in obstetrics, his initial choice, presented with even bigger hurdles. Dr. Golanty, through the support of his mentors, took a residency in internal medicine at the newly built, larger L.A. County Osteopathic Hospital which had just opened its doors.

In the middle of this residency the amalgamation between COA and CMA occurred in 1962. Together with most of his classmates Dr. Golanty, fearing for the legitimacy of his osteopathic residency, took the M.D. degree from the California College of Medicine and finished his residency in 1964.

He has been teaching and training osteopathic and allopathic medical students throughout his career. For the past twenty five years of his life he has devoted himself to the advancement of postgraduate osteopathic education at PHLB.

Dr. Seffinger interviewed Dr. Golanty at the Pacific Hospital of Long Beach, CA on July 1, 2005.

Dolores Grunigen, B.S., B.A.

Mrs. Grunigen was born in 1933 and raised in Modesto, California. At the University of Redlands she obtained a B.S. degree in business administration and additional administrative training. She was the Assistant Executive Officer and Consultant for the State Board of Medical Quality Assurance. Her responsibilities included to oversee the licensing of allied health professionals and to promote legislation for these professions. In 1962 she became responsible for evaluating the credentials and to determine the qualifications for licensure by the State Board of Medical Examiners of the newly M.D.-degreed former D.O.s.

Dolores met Dr. Forest Grunigen through her work at that office. They married in 1976 and lived happily in Newport Beach for 23 years in a home filled with art work that they collected during their world-wide travels. Dr. Grunigen passed away in 1999.

Since her retirement, Dolores Grunigen continues to contribute to excellence in medical education and training by supporting learning endeavors in mainstream and osteopathic medicine. She has been serving on the committee of the 41st Medical Trust for many years.

245

The Dean of the Medical Center at that time, Dr. Cesario, proposed to establish the **Forest J. Grunigen, M.D. Medical Center Library** at the University of California, Irvine, Medical Center in 1999. Since then, Mrs Grunigen has supported the library.

Mrs. Grunigen published an attractive book about her late husband, *"A strength born of giants: The life and times of Dr. Forest Grunigen"* (Raven River Press, Van Nuys CA, 2002). In her spare time she enjoys writing short stories.

Dr. Seffinger interviewed Mrs. Grunigen at her home in Newport Beach, CA on June 13, 2006.

Scott Haldeman, M.D., Ph.D., D.C.

Dr. Haldeman is known as an international leader in promoting manual medicine. With his extensive experience in chiropractic, neurophysiology, and neurology, he has obtained a broad multidisciplinary perspective on manipulation research, healthcare policy, and the pursuit of innovative directions. Even within osteopathic medicine, few clinicians have become such influential advocates of manipulation medicine.

In 1975, he helped to organize a conference at UC Irvine and published two chapters, discussing causes of back pain and the relevance of manipulation, in the conference proceedings entitled *"Approaches to the Validation of Manipulative Therapy"*, edited by Dr. Buerger, Dr. Tobis, and Dr. Hoehler (1976). When in the 1970s the 41st Trust Fund started to support the study of musculoskeletal manipulation to facilitate its integration into allopathy, Dr. Haldeman was invited to join the research team at UC Irvine in 1978. He became the most influential researcher and clinician trained in manipulation medicine and neurology at the UC Irvine College of Medicine. His early mentors included Dr. Tobis in Physical Medicine & Rehabilitation and Dr. van den Noort in Neurology. Presently Dr. Haldemann mentors himself countless students, as clinical professor of neurology at UC Irvine.

While still a medical student, but empowered by a doctorate in chiropractic and a Ph.D. in the basic sciences, Dr. Haldeman participated in a workshop at the National Institute of Neurological Disorders and Stroke to identify the research status of spinal manipulative medicine (DHEW Publication No. (NIH) 76-998, 1975). When Murray Goldstein, D.O. published the proceedings, it became undeniably evident that such research was inconclusive (NINCDS Monograph No.15). Since then, Dr. Haldeman devoted his efforts to examine the efficacy of manipulation.

When he joined the International Society for the Study of the Lumbar Spine in 1979, he brought attention nationally and internationally to the science of manipulation mechanisms and treatment effectiveness. He also became a member of the American Back Society (and its president), the North American Spine Society (and its president in 1988-89), and the North American Academy of Manipulation Medicine (and its president in 1983).

In 1994, Dr. Haldeman served as a panel member for the Agency for Healthcare Policy and Research to establish clinical practice guidelines on acute low back pain.

When the World Health Organization initiated the *Bone and Joint Decade 2000-2010*, Dr. Haldeman was elected Chair of a task force on spinal manipulation research. He became Ambassador for the Bone and Joint Decade in 2003.

Dr. Haldeman helped to bridge the gaps between chiropractic, allopathy, and osteopathy by giving presentations to the U.S. Government and to worker's compensation plans. He lectured internationally as well at numerous occasions. Thus, with the initial support of the 41st Trust Fund and the mentoring he received at UC Irvine, Dr. Haldeman became a leader worldwide, integrating musculoskeletal manipulation with allopathic treatment approaches.

It was the atmosphere and culture of the post merger era at UC Irvine that provided fertile ground for the growth and education of a leader in pursuit of multidisciplinary research in manual medicine. Dr. Haldeman continues to put UC Irvine and the 41st Trust Fund on the map world-wide, and his name is synonymous with research in musculoskeletal manipulation, originated by the 41st Trust Fund at UC Irvine. For these reasons Dr. Haldeman became an important bridge between the M.D.s, former D.O.s and current D.O.s. Also many chiropractic researchers are now consulting with the osteopathic profession to build an integrated infrastructure and research network for the study of manipulation and its mechanisms.

Dr. Seffinger interviewed Dr. Haldeman in his office in Tustin, CA, on May 9, 2007.

Seth Hufstedler, LL.B.

Counselor Hufstedler was born in Oklahoma in 1922, apparently under an osteopathic star, because 1922 was an important year for the osteopathic profession. In 1922, the Osteopathic Initiative Act was passed, establishing a separate licensing board for the profession and placing osteopathic medicine firmly into California's healthcare arena. As the attorney for the California Osteopathic Association, Seth Hufstedler played an important role for organized osteopathic medicine.

After completing four years of education at USC he entered the Naval Reserve and obtained an ensign's commission at the same time he graduated from USC. He spent three years in the Navy in WWII. Upon his return, he studied for three years at Stanford University and graduated in 1949. He has practiced law in Los Angeles ever since and is recognized as a distinguished attorney.

In the 1950s he represented San Gabriel Valley Hospital, an osteopathic hospital at that time. Several years later, about 1958, members of the San Gabriel Valley Hospital and members of the California Osteopathic Association, asked him to represent them in their negotiations with the California Medical Association.

Counselor Hufstedler wrote and co-wrote eight bills and two California constitutional amendments, the merger agreement, the documents for COP&S to become the California College of Medicine and subsequently the College of Medicine at the University of California, Irvine. He successfully defended these acts of legislation and merger in lawsuits twice, fending off two members of the COP&S Board of Trustees.

Dr. Seffinger interviewed Counselor Hufstedler at the law offices of Morrison & Foerster in Los Angeles, CA on December 14, 2005.

Steven Kamajian, D.O.

One of Dr. Kamajian's distinctions is his contribution to establishing the clinical courses in osteopathic medicine at COMP which at that time was the first osteopathic college to have opened in California after the merger. Starting in 1981, he served as clinical instructor to the third year students. He also provided care as osteopathic physician to students, staff, and faculty at COMP.

Another of his distinctions is his perseverance in overcoming barriers for osteopathic physicians to obtain staff privileges at hospitals. When in 1981 he was denied a position at Glendale Adventist Hospital because of his non-mainstream medical training and his ethnic background, he prevailed in the application negotiations and succeeded, over the years, to rise to the top. In 2002, he was elected by the hospital's 700 physicians to serve as chief of staff.

He also dedicates much of his service to the profession's social and political goals. He is the former editor of the *California D.O. Journal*, the professional journal of California's D.O. organization, OPSC (Osteopathic Physicians and Surgeons of California). He has a long history to organize volunteer medical services to the homeless and patients without financial resources for medical care. For years, he has directed three health clinics at churches in Glendale, Westlake Village, and Thousand Oaks where the homeless and uninsured receive free medical care.

Dr. Kamajian was born in Waco, Texas in 1952. He entered the Philadelphia College of Osteopathic Medicine in 1974 and graduated in 1978. After completing a family practice residency and an additional year in geriatrics, he moved to California in 1981. Since he was without a license at that point, he pursued pre-exam refresher course work at COMP, succeeded in obtaining his license, and conquered the next challenge to find a position as hospital staff.

To this day, he loves to be a clinician and employs osteopathic manipulation not only for treatment but for diagnostic purposes as well.

Dr. Seffinger interviewed Dr. Kamajian in February 2007 in Palm Springs, CA.

Richard Kammerman, M.D., F.A.A.F.P.

Richard Kammerman has the most interesting history since he achieved political leadership roles in both the Osteopathic Medical Society and the Allopathic Medical Society.

Born in 1930 in Glendale, CA, Dr. Kammerman attended COP& S from 1951 to 1956. He found that the school created a culture of compassionate medicine. Throughout his career he has been interested in osteopathic manipulation and used such modality until his retirement as a physician. After his graduation from COP&S in 1956 he sought specialty training, but the few positions that existed in California for osteopathic specialists were filled. Further, he was unsuccessful to obtain privileges in allopathic hospitals. One exception was the Santa Ana Hospital which had a dual staff of both M.D.s and D.O.s.

Early in his career he would seek surgical consultation for his patients from Los Angeles osteopathic physicians. With the passage of time, he developed a professional relationship with allopathic specialists, including a urologist and an orthopedist. At the Santa Ana Hospital, allopaths and osteopaths often worked together, a professional relationship which was relatively rare throughout the country at that time.

Dr. Kammerman was not directly involved in the political maneuverings that were under way concerning the merger of the two medical professions. He first began to hear information about such a merger in 1960. Dr. Kammerman spoke to Vincent Carroll, D.O., concerning this matter and was told that the merger was inevitable. Further, that the AOA was not supportive of the COA or of osteopathic physicians in California. On the other hand, about this time he was advised by Dr. Eby that he was collecting money to fight the merger.

Although the merger did not change his practice referrals, Dr. Kammerman was able to obtain privileges at Children's Hospital and St. Joseph's Hospital in Orange County. The fact that he now was associated with such prestigious hospitals made several of his patients feel that his professional resources were more attractive to them. Because of his extensive experience in doing minor procedures, such as dilatation and curettage, tonsillectomy and adenoidectomy, and conization of the cervix, he was permitted to carry out those procedures at the new hospital affiliations. However, few general practitioners were permitted such surgical procedures as more specialists appeared in Orange County.

Dr. Kammerman's association with the UCI College of Medicine began early. He was on the Alumni Board of COP&S when it became the California College of Medicine, still located in Los Angeles. As a member of that Board, he and other members of the Associated Alumni met the first Chancellor of UCI, Dan Aldrich. They recommended to the Board that CCM move to the UCI campus. With the merger he was appointed to the staff of the Orange County Medical Center. He attended a weekly clinic in Santa Ana and thereby became involved with the school. He began to teach UCI medical students and has continued to do so to the present time.

Early in his career in Orange County he became the Chairman of the Orange County branch of the California Osteopathic Association and served as President of the Orange County Osteopathic Society from 1960 to 1962 when it became dissolved. Following the merger he became a delegate to the California Medical Association and from 1991 to 1992 became President of the Orange County Medical Association. Thus, he has served as President of both local medical professions. His activities with the Orange County Medical Association involved him in developing the CAL Optima program in Orange County, an important contribution to the healthcare program for the indigent of Orange County.

Throughout his career, Dr. Kammerman has maintained a holistic approach that he acquired as a medical student at COP&S and in turn has attempted to instill in his teaching sessions as Clinical Professor in the Department of Family Medicine at UC Irvine School of Medicine to the present. At the Orange County Medical Center, he served as President of the Voluntary Faculty Association.

Dr. Seffinger interviewed Dr. Kammerman at the University of California, Irvine, at the Forest J. Grunigen, M.D. Medical Center Library in Orange, CA on May 2, 2006.

Mitchell Kasovac, D.O.

Born in 1937 in Michigan, Dr. Kasovac attended Wayne State University from 1955 to 1959 for his pre-med education. Through a premed fraternity at Wayne State University he learned about the Osteopathic School in Des Moines and the Chicago College of Osteopathy. He decided to matriculate at the Chicago College of Osteopathic Medicine in 1959, graduated in 1963, and proceeded to obtain his internship at Phoenix General Hospital.

He had just married and started a practice in family medicine in Phoenix, when he heard about the merger and decided to contribute to a legal fund, starting in 1964, until the osteopathic licensing board was re-established in 1974.

Together with a colleague he made a commitment, at the request of the D.O.s in California, to become licensed in California. From 1975 until his retirement a few years ago, Dr. Kasovac maintained his active California license.

Fifteen years of family practice in Phoenix were followed by nine years as director of medical education at his hospital until its closure. In 1989, Dr. Kasovac welcomed the opportunity to become Assistant Dean of Clinical Affairs to Dean Krpan at the College of Osteopathic Medicine of the Pacific (COMP). The hospital in Phoenix had been one of the major osteopathic teaching hospitals through the 1980s when COMP was developing clinical training opportunities. Thus, Dr. Kasovac was well prepared to develop third and fourth year clerkships with individual physicians at various hospitals, as well as internships and residencies. He worked with hospitals throughout California, and with hospitals in Arizona, Nevada, New Mexico, Utah, Oregon, and Washington.

The last five years at COMP, when Dr. Krpan became Provost, Dr. Kasovac became Dean of COMP. He facilitated teaching relationships with M.D.s who were former D.O.s

For 16 years, Dr. Kasovac was on the AOA Board of Trustees, from 1977 to 1993. Then, just when he had started at COMP in California, Dr. Kasovac was elected as AOA president from 1990 to 1991.

Dr. Seffinger interviewed Dr. Kasovac in Chicago, Illinois, on July 14, 2006.

Allen Korneff, M.S.

Mr. Korneff was born in Los Angeles in 1941 and grew up in Boyle Heights and City Terrace in East Los Angeles. His family later moved to Downey where Allen attended high school. Mr. Korneff graduated with a degree in industrial engineering from Northern Arizona University and obtained a master's degree in economics from USC. .

Upon graduation he worked as an applied economist for Stanford Research Institute and for many of the large corporations that were conducting economic feasibility studies for various investments and ventures. He worked with several health care facilities and was chief financial officer for Presbyterian Hollywood Hospital. Subsequently, he worked with Gateways Hospital which was a sister facility for Cedars-Sinai. He also worked closely with the Jewish Federation Consulate. At around age 30, he became executive vice president and then CEO of Downey Regional Medical Center.

Influenced by his exposure to cultural diversity in his youth—Los Angeles in the 1940s already was the goal for many immigrants from different ethnic populations—Mr. Korneff later in life obtained a degree in cultural anthropology at Northern Arizona University. He worked there at the museum where he often found opportunities to interact with Hopi Indians. He found them not much different than most other people that he had been with in life. He felt very comfortable in accepting their value systems and religions.

His experience in communicating with people from other cultures helped him to respect and appreciate values and beliefs that differed from his own. He felt convinced that this respect enabled him to deal with ambiguities in work settings and to survive in his position as CEO at Downey Regional Medical Center for almost 30 year—possibly the longest tenured CEO of one institution in California.

Dr. Seffinger interviewed Mr. Korneff at his office in Downey Regional Medical Center on May 8, 2007.

Donald J. Krpan, D.O.

Donald John Krpan, D.O. was born in 1936 in Rocks Springs, Wyoming. His family were immigrants from Croatia who worked as coal miners in Sweetwater County in Wyoming. When his uncle became a victim of coal mining, Donald Krpan's family started to build a new life in Long Beach, California. In his early teens at that time, Dr. Krpan suffered from migraine headaches and encountered for the first time the benefits of osteopathic medicine.

In 1963, he graduated from the College of Osteopathic Medicine in Kansas City, did a rotating internship at Phoenix General Hospital and then went into practice. He practiced his first year in Houston, Texas and then returned to Phoenix where he practiced from 1969 to 1976. He obtained his license to practice in California in 1975 and established a practice there in Yorba Linda from 1976 to 1987 at which time the Dean at the College of Osteopathic Medicine of the Pacific (COMP), Dr. Jerry Bayles, recruited him to come to COMP and help him with post-doctoral programs. Dr. Krpan was at COMP for 16 years, from 1987 until 2003. He served for six years as the Dean and the remainder of the time as Provost and Chief Academic Officer. He successfully took on the challenge to improve the quality of clinical training for students and post-doctoral training for graduates.

As Dean, Dr. Krpan brought in full-time faculty into the Osteopathic Medicine & Manipulation Department, with John Jones, D.O. as Chair. He set about developing post-doctoral training programs at county hospitals in California and Arizona that provided care to the underserved patient population. He established relationships and affiliations and then post-doctoral programs in those hospitals. He started an internal medicine program at San Joaquin General in Stockton, an internal medicine program in Maricopa County in Phoenix, an internship family medicine program at Highland General in Oakland, and multiple post-doctoral programs at San Bernardino County and Riverside County Hospitals. The family medicine program had 54 residents. It was the second largest family medicine program in the country, with all slots fully accredited by the American Osteopathic Association and the Accreditation Council on Graduate Medical Education. Subsequently Dr. Krpan started an OB-GYN program, with about 12 residents, an orthopedic program, and a neurosurgical program.

He served as president of the Osteopathic Physicians and Surgeons of California two times, 1981 and '82, and 1987 and '88. He also served as president of the AOA in 2001-2002.

Dr. Seffinger interviewed Dr. Krpan in Palm Springs, CA on February 17, 2006.

Betsy MacCracken, M.D., MPH

Betsy MacCracken was born in Nebraska in 1914 as the daughter of two osteopathic physicians, graduates of the American School at Kirksville. Upon moving to Fresno, California she pursued her education in combination with her enthusiasm for sports, especially baseball. One of her pre-medical classmates was Stephen Teale, who later entered COP&S as well. Her father, Frank MacCracken was a member of the Board of Trustees of COP&S during the 1930s and was involved with the California Osteopathic Association. Once she decided to become a physician, education and training in osteopathy at COP&S seemed the indisputable choice. She graduated from COP&S in 1940. Since shortly after her graduation WWII broke out, she joined the Navy in an administrative position at the Bureau of Medicine and Surgery. At that time, D.O.s were not commissioned as medical officers in the military due to protestations by the allopathic medical profession.

After the War, Dr. MacCracken joined the faculty of the Department of Pediatrics at COP&S and the Pediatrics staff of Unit II at the L.A. County Hospital in the late 1940s. Soon she was appointed as Assistant Executive of the Department of Pediatrics and in 1958 as Executive. She had close professional relationships with Grace Bell, D.O., Forest Grunigen, D.O., and Dorothy Marsh, D.O. who got her start in Obstetrics as a resident on the City Maternity Service.

Simultaneously, Dr. MacCracken had been active with the City Health Department Child Health Conference since 1948. In 1960 she decided to devote her professional career to public health entirely and obtained the Master of Public Health degree at UC Berkeley in 1961. Upon returning to Los Angeles, she became the Northeast District Health Officer, holding responsibility for the qualifications of nurses, social workers, health educators and other health professionals.

In 1962, Dr. MacCracken took the M.D. degree from the California College of Medicine and served on the volunteer faculty of the California College of Medicine at Los Angeles and, upon its move, at the University of California at Irvine. She became Board certified by the American Board of Preventive Medicine in Public Health. When

252

in the late 1960s the County Hospital System had to be merged with the Public Health Department System, Dr. MacCracken was responsible for maintaining and improving the strengths of the Public Health system. She retired in 1976.

Dr. Seffinger interviewed Dr. MacCracken in her home in Fresno, CA on September 8, 2005.

Alan Menkes, D.O.

Dr. Menkes was born in 1943 in Brooklyn, New York, where he was raised. He became involved with the osteopathic profession because of the care the family received from an osteopathic physician, without realizing he was a D.O.

He applied to the Philadelphia College of Osteopathic Medicine in 1963. As a senior medical student, he attended grand rounds at the University of Pennsylvania and cardiology lectures by Dr. Leonard Dreifus at Hahnemann Medical School. Dr. Dreifus invited him to go on rounds with him at Lankenau Hospital. Alan gladly noted that he never felt discrimination or condescension at these occasions.

Dr. Menkes finished his internship in 1968 and was encouraged to go into a residency. He felt torn, though, between going on to residency in internal medicine or family practice or whether to start immediately as a general practitioner. A residency in internal medicine required three years, a major commitment for a young physician with three boys to raise at that time. He chose to do a residency in internal medicine and became a highly trained intensivist.

After finishing his residency, and practicing in Florida for a short time, Dr. Menkes came to California in March1976 to take the state licensing exam. He was examined by Dr. Frymann, Dr. Allen, and Dr. Dilworth. He was asked to demonstrate his manipulation skills and he did well enough to be encouraged to come to southern California. He gladly seized the opportunity.

Eventually Dr. Menkes became one of the commissioned examiners on the licensing board himself, a function he served for more than twenty years. He always emphasized that the manipulative portion of the licensing exam was essential to differentiate a physician as an osteopathic physician and surgeon.

In 1976, Dr. Repel and Dr. Menkes came together to southern California and worked with others to obtain a charter for a new school in osteopathic medicine, the College of Osteopathic Medicine of the Pacific (COMP). In 1977, Dr. Repel became the first Dean of the College of COMP.

Though Dr. Menkes was not intimately involved in the planning stages of the college or the associated political process, he was appointed as the first professor and chairman of the Department of Osteopathic Medicine. His goals were to bring to California more osteopathic family practitioners, to help with the teaching load at COMP, and to make apparent the equality of osteopathic and allopathic physicians. Because of his advanced skills and training, he was given staff privileges at local hospitals. There, M.D.s were at first skeptical of the education and training of osteopathic physicians, but soon this changed. Thus, Dr. Menkes

253

opened doors to hospitals in southern California to provide clinical training opportunities for students of the newly formed College of Osteopathic Medicine of the Pacific.

Dr. Seffinger interviewed Dr. Menkes in Palm Springs at the OPSC convention in February 2007.

Jay Michael, M.S.

Jay Michael was one of Sacramento's leading lobbyists. Born in Kansas in 1932 and raised in California, he was educated at the University of California, Berkeley and obtained a graduate degree at the University of California, Los Angeles. He studied public administration to be a city manager of the city of Claremont.

Mr. Michael met Senator Teale in 1957 when he worked as a lobbyist for the League of Cities, an organization of legislators. He was Vice President of the University of California during the student revolts in the 1960s and 1970s. He convinced the state legislature to defeat constitutional amendments that would have decreased the autonomy of the University of California (UC). In 1976 he left the UC system and represented the physicians and healthcare interests for 24 years. He retired in 2002.

Dr. Seffinger interviewed Mr. Michael at the Hilton Hotel in Sacramento, CA on June 30, 2006.

Thomas L. Nelson, M.D., F.A.A.P., F.A.A.A.A.I.

Dr. Nelson is the Founding Chair of the Department of Pediatrics at the University of California, Irvine where he currently is Professor of Pediatrics, Emeritus. He was born in Barranquilla, Colombia, South America where his parents were missionaries and lived there until he was two years of age. He was raised in California, graduated from Bakersfield High School, attended the University of California, Berkeley, and obtained his medical degree at the University of California, San Francisco. He became Board certified in Pediatrics as well as in Allergy and Clinical Immunology. He is a Fellow of the American Academy of Pediatrics and a Fellow of the American Academy of Asthma, Allergy, and Immunology.

Dr. Nelson became Assistant Professor of Pediatrics and Lecturer in Psychiatry at the University of California at San Francisco (UCSF). At the same time, he was Superintendent and Medical Director of the then Sonoma State Hospital (SSH), which was affiliated with UCSF for residency training in several specialties. His laboratory and clinical research during this time was being conducted at SSH. This was a very large hospital with about 3500 beds for developmentally disabled persons of which about half were children.

In the position he held at SSH, he prepared, presented and defended large budgets to the State government, both with the Department of Mental Hygiene as well as with the State Legislature. He reported directly to the Director of the State Department of Mental Hygiene and thus was only once removed from the Governor.

He then was recruited as Professor and Chairman of Pediatrics at the University of Kentucky, College of Medicine in Lexington.

Dr. Nelson first became involved with the osteopathic profession when he was recruited by the dean of the California College of Medicine, Warren Bostick, M.D. to become the Chair of the Department of Pediatrics at the California College of Medicine (CCM) in Los Angeles. This was in 1964 and shortly after the College had become affiliated with the University of California.

He became interested in a small close knit group of pediatricians in Southern California, primarily in Los Angeles County, who had been osteopathic pediatricians. Most of them had been certified under the osteopathic board. He became interested in how they had trained, how they became pediatricians, and in the history of this group. He has collected a great deal of information and data about osteopathic pediatrics within the College of Osteopathic Physicians and Surgeons in Los Angeles.

He traced the history of osteopathic pediatrics in California back to a woman who went to Europe around 1910 to receive the training she could not obtain in the U.S. at the time. She was at the Children's Hospital on Great Ormond Street in London which was probably the greatest pediatric institution of that time. Following London, she went to the Vienna Polyclinic where she studied with one of the great pediatricians of that day. On her return to Los Angeles, she limited her practice to infants and children and most importantly established a Division of Infants and Children within the Department of Medicine at CCM and an infant feeding clinic. There were other early graduates and faculty members who, wanting post-graduate training in Pediatrics, had gone to Europe. Some had even received an M.D. degree there.

While Dr. Nelson has not yet published these historical materials, he did take the time to produce an exhibit of the history of the College of Osteopathic Physicians and Surgeons in Los Angeles. The exhibit can be viewed at the Forest J. Grunigen, M.D. Library and Medical Education Center at the University of California, Irvine, Medical Center in Orange, CA.

Dr. Seffinger interviewed Dr. Nelson at his home on May 24, 2005, in Davis, California.

Robert Norcross, M.D.

Dr. Norcross is a native Californian who grew up in the Hollywood area. He went to the University of California, Los Angeles and the University of Southern California for his pre-medical education and graduated from the University of Southern California as a Bachelor of Science in Zoology in 1947. He received his training as an osteopathic physician and surgeon at the College of Osteopathic Physicians and Surgeons and graduated in 1951, followed by a one-year internship and a three-year residency in orthopedic surgery at Doctor's Hospital. He continued working at the clinic and assisted his uncle Howard Norcross, D.O. in surgery until 1957. Dr. Howard Norcross had been a graduate of the College of Osteopathic Physicians and Surgeons in 1935. Dr. Robert Norcross became Board Certified in General Surgery and went into practice at Bay Harbor Hospital in Lomita, California, which initially was an osteopathic hospital until 1962. In 1962 he obtained the

M.D. degree from the California College of Medicine. Although his practice and referrals from former D.O. general practitioners remained relatively unchanged throughout the 1960s, by the mid-1970s he became more accepted within the local allopathic community. He obtained staff privileges, received referrals and performed surgeries in previously 'M.D. only' hospitals such as Little Company of Mary in Torrance.

Dr. Seffinger interviewed Dr. Norcross at his home in Rolling Hills, CA in 2003.

Victor Passy, M.D., F.A.C.S.

Dr. Passy was born in 1930 in Brooklyn, NY. After having served in the U.S. Army with a High Company Award, he graduated with a B.S. degree from the University of California, Los Angeles, in 1953. He matriculated at the College of Osteopathic Physicians and Surgeons, Los Angeles, in 1955 and graduated in 1959 with the D.O. degree as a member of the Honor Society. He completed a rotating internship at the Los Angeles County Osteopathic Hospital and seven years of residency at the same institution in Ear, Nose, and Throat, and General Surgery.

It was during this residency that the merger occurred between the California Osteopathic Association and the California Medical Association. In 1962 Dr. Passy obtained the M.D. degree from the California College of Medicine. In order to ensure his specialty certification would be recognized, he repeated another residency under M.D. trainers in ENT at the Los Angeles County Hospital after the merger. In May 1970 he became certified by the American Board of Otolaryngology. Dr. Passy is a Fellow of the American Academy of Surgery.

For nearly 40 years Dr. Passy has been a full-time Professor in the Department of Otolaryngology at the University of California, Irvine, College of Medicine (UCI-COM). He has served on numerous committees at UCI-COM. He published his extensive research in professional journals and books. His forte has been teaching at all levels of medical education.

In his endeavors to facilitate the relationship between allopathic and osteopathic physicians he has been a member of the 41st Medical Trust Committee since 1981. He is presently the Chair of the 41st Medical Trust Committee at the University of California, Irvine. He is Past President of the California College of Medicine Alumni Association.

Dr. Passy continues to serve on the active staff at UC Irvine Medical Center in Otolaryngology, Head and Neck Department. For many years he was acting Head of the Otolaryngology Division.

Dr. Seffinger interviewed Dr. Passy at the University of California, Irvine, Forest J. Grunigen, M.D. Medical Library in Orange, CA in March, 2003.

Philip Pumerantz, Ph.D.

Philip Pumerantz, Ph.D., founding president of Western University of Health Sciences may very well hold the unique distinction of being the longest-serving founding university president in the nation.

Now celebrating its 30th Anniversary, Western University of Health Sciences is comprised of five colleges; the College of Osteopathic Medicine of the Pacific (the flagship college); the College of Pharmacy; the College of Allied Health Professions; the College of Graduate Nursing; and the College of Veterinary Medicine. To date, more than 2,200 students are enrolled, and the May 2007 commencement increased the number of alumni to approximately 6,200 caring and compassionate health care professionals who practice across the country and around the world. The Strategic Plan calls for opening three additional colleges in 2009, Dentistry, Podiatry, and Optometry.

Dr. Pumerantz has been the recipient of numerous awards including the 1995 Distinguished Alumni Award from the University of Connecticut and the 1995 Dale Dodson Award from the American Association of Colleges of Osteopathic Medicine for national leadership.

Prior to coming to California in 1977 with his wife, Harriet, and his family, Dr. Pumerantz was a professor of education at the University of Bridgeport in Connecticut, the co-founder of the University of Bridgeport's College of Continuing Education and, the director of education for the American Osteopathic Association.

Dr. Pumerantz co-authored four college textbooks in education. In addition, he has numerous articles published in professional journals. He is listed in Who's Who in the East, Who's Who in the West, Who's Who in California, Who's Who in America, as well as in the Directory of International Biography, and Outstanding Educators.

Dr. Seffinger interviewed Dr. Pumerantz at Western University of Health Sciences on June 30, 2006.

William J. Ryan, D.O.

Several members of Dr. Ryan's family were osteopathic physicians including his father, John Ryan, and two of his great uncles. He attended what was then referred to as the Kansas City College of Osteopathic Medicine and Surgery. He graduated in the class of 1962. He feels especially proud of his daughter, Susan Mackintosh, who is also a D.O., graduate of Western University.

Dr. Ryan was born in 1933. He came to California in July of 1967 as one of the very first military physicians where he was stationed in San Diego as a Navy physician. He was the very first D.O. hired by Kaiser Permanente in November of 1974, with the support of an M.D. colleague with whom he worked when stationed in Hawaii. He was certified by both the American Board of Family Practice and the American Board of Osteopathic Family Practice and attended numerous continuing medical education meetings. He had been unable, though, to become a partner with Kaiser because their by-laws at the time restricted partnership to M.D.s. In 1987, Dr. Ryan became the first D.O. partner at Kaiser.

He did not practice manipulation after graduating from osteopathic medical school. Manipulative therapy was not as common a procedure performed by D.O.s in the 1970s.

He retired with more than 20 years of service from Kaiser and also retired from the U.S. Navy, including both active and reserve time. In his Navy career he served during the Viet Nam conflict as well as being recalled to Desert Shield/Desert Storm.

Dr. Ryan answered Dr. Seffinger's interview questions in writing in March 2007.

Richard Ryder, M.D.

Dr. Ryder was born in 1931 at Monte Sano Sanitarium and Hospital, one of the few, if not the only osteopathic hospital in Los Angeles, aside from the Los Angeles County Hospital Unit II, at that time. His family had been under the care of osteopathic physicians, connected with the L.A. Clinical Group, an early group practice. He attended UCLA for undergraduate studies from 1949 to 1953 when he was drafted into the army. Two years later he was able to resume his studies and graduated from UCLA with a B.S. degree in 1956. He intended to proceed with medical school at UCLA, not realizing that there was an additional way to be a doctor, namely to become an osteopathic physician.

Chance led to a decisive conversation with Professor Grace Bell, D.O., and within a few months he matriculated at the College of Osteopathic Physicians and Surgeons. Upon his graduation in 1960 he interned at the Long Beach Osteopathic Hospital where he met Willis Tunnell, D.O. who soon became his medical office partner in a spacious, beautiful building in Lakewood for many years.

In 1962 Dr. Ryder obtained the M.D. degree from the California College of Medicine. His practice as a family physician did not change with the allopathic degree, as he continued to provide a wide range of service, including obstetrics and assistance with surgery. When in 1968 the American Board of Family Practice (ABFP) was organized as a medical specialty, he realized the importance of becoming Board certified. In 1973 he met this goal and a few months later became president at the local chapter of the American Academy of Family Physicians (AAFP). He was the first former D.O. to become board certified by the ABFP and officer in AAFP.

When in 1973 Pacific Hospital of Long Beach closed its obstetrics units, Dr. Ryder moved his obstetric patients—and eventually all his patients—to St. Mary's Hospital in Long Beach. He joined the medical staff of several hospitals, including Long Beach Memorial, Doctors Hospital of Lakewood, Woodruff Community Hospital, and Los Alamitos General Hospital.

In the early 1980s, legislative changes pertaining to medical practice in California shifted the practice of medicine away from private physicians. Dr. Ryder who had felt these changes in his solo practice, joined a group practice at the Harriman-Jones medical clinic in Long Beach. He primarily provided urgent care and for several years practiced in the Back Clinic, together with a chiropractor, an osteopathic physician, a neurosurgeon, and an orthopedist, until the clinic was closed. In 1974 he joined the American Back Society where he continues to refresh his osteopathic skills.

Even though Dr. Ryder retired fully in 2002, he teaches and mentors students in the Family Practice Clinic at the Pacific Hospital in Long Beach once per week, as part of the medical education program for osteopathic students and residents from the College of Osteopathic Medicine of the Pacific and from other osteopathic colleges across the country.

Dr. Seffinger interviewed Dr. Ryder on October 11, 2005 at his home in Long Beach, CA.

Michael Seffinger, D.O., F.A.A.F.P.

Dr. Seffinger is a native Californian, born in 1954 and raised in Los Angeles. He is a graduate of Michigan State University College of Osteopathic Medicine in 1988. He interned at the Pacific Hospital in Long Beach under the tutelage of Stanley Golanty, M.D., a graduate of the College of Osteopathic Physicians and Surgeons. Dr Seffinger completed a family medicine residency at the University of California, Irvine in 1991 while conducting research funded by the 41st Medical Trust, in the Department of Neurology, chaired by Dr. Stanley van den Noort.

In 1991, he joined a large multi-specialty group practice, Bay Shores Medical Group in Torrance, CA, which was directed at the time by Peter Culotta, M.D. and John Johnson, M.D., both graduates from the California College of Medicine. He practiced family medicine in Gardena and Torrance with HealthCare Partners Medical Group until 1999. At that time he was recruited to teach at the College of Osteopathic Medicine of the Pacific (COMP) at Western University where he is now a tenured Associate Professor of Family Medicine and Osteopathic Manipulative Medicine.

When he started to teach he realized that there is no definitive, referenced text on the history of osteopathy in California and the relationship between the two medical professions. He thus set out to conduct this project, interviewing those that made significant contributions to California's medical history, from both medical professions. His goal is to have these sources available for teaching and research worldwide.

Robert Steedman, M.D., DABTS, DABS

Dr. Steedman was born in 1933. After a demanding undergraduate education at UCLA, Dr. Steedman entered the College of Osteopathic Physicians and Surgeons in 1955. Upon graduation in 1959 he interned for one year and trained for three years as a surgeon at the Los Angeles County Osteopathic Hospital, followed by two additional years of extended training in thoracic, pancreatic and bowel surgery. He obtained the M.D. degree in 1962 from the California College of Medicine.

He taught at Rancho Los Amigos and supervised Residents. Then he became a thoracic and cardiovascular resident at Long Beach Veterans Hospital, while functioning at the same time as chief of the residents staff. He was so well-liked among students that they voted for him to receive the University of California Golden Apple Teaching Award. He was the first resident to receive this award.

After one more year of training at the Orange County Medical Center he became a Diplomat of the American College of Surgeons and a Diplomat of the American Board of Thoracic Surgery. He became a successful and well-respected cardiovascular surgeon at Western Medical Center in Santa Ana, CA.

He had just started his practice when he was contacted by the Associated Alumni of the California College of Medicine to become a member of the Board of Directors of the Alumni Association of the California College of Medicine, University of California, Irvine. He also served as its president. Since 2005 he has been a member of the 41st Medical Trust Committee.

Dr. Seffinger interviewed Dr. Steedman together with Dr. Passy in March 2003 at the University of California, Irvine, Forest J. Grunigen, M.D. Medical Library in Orange, CA.

Cynthia Stotts, D. O.

Dr. Stotts was born in 1953 in Fort Leonard Wood, Missouri, into a military family who often was required to move. For young Cynthia, the frequent changes required adaptation to five different elementary schools, two junior high and two high schools. After graduating from high school and taking time to see parts of the United States and Central America she decided to embark on a profession in the medical field.

She started her college education at Santa Monica College and proceeded to study at the University of California Los Angeles (UCLA). She graduated from UCLA with a Bachelors degree in Psychobiology.

In college, she tried to learn about service in the healing arts. She had long been a vegetarian and was very interested in leading a healthy life and advocating for health. She obtained a master's degree in nutrition but soon realized that as a dietician, she could only make recommendations to patients, while depending on a physician to write the order. She became aware of her desire to become a physician rather than working as a dietician.

Her first experience with medicine was the care she received as a child from an osteopathic physician. It had been her mother's choice to seek out D.O.s in Iowa and Missouri and wherever the family went. Thus, when in 1984 she had the option of matriculating into an osteopathic or allopathic medical school, she felt in her heart that she would be a better D.O. than an M.D., because being a D.O. would offer her the opportunity to provide osteopathic manipulative treatments and touch. With those skills, she felt she would practice as a complete doctor.

Even though she was aware of prejudices against D.O.s, she chose the College of Osteopathic Medicine of the Pacific (COMP) over an M.D. program because training at COMP fit her model of the type of physician she wanted to become, i.e. practicing as a solo, general practitioner in the wilds of Idaho Snake River Valley. Indeed, as a D.O. intern at Pacific Hospital of Long Beach in California she was given opportunities to provide as many procedures as she felt prepared, including delivering babies. She developed a great fondness for her mentors and the osteopathic training she received from Dr. Golanty, Chief of Medicine, and Dr. Horowitz, chief surgeon at the time, and Dr. Chan, then Head of Obstetrics at Pacific Hospital.

She finished her internship at Pacific Hospital, Long Beach, in 1989. She continued her training at the Los Angeles County-University of Southern California (LAC-USC) Medical Center in the Medicine-Pediatrics dual residency. Soon, she was representing the Pediatrics Department to the Joint Council of Interns and Residents (JCIR), the second oldest union of physicians of interns and residents in the United States. Proceeding through the leadership, she was elected President of JCIR at LAC-USC and had the opportunity to advocate for better patient care and better resident education. As the JCIR President, she represented about 1,800 residents. She was in a position to propose to the CMO (Chief Medical Officer), to the CEO (Chief Executive Officer), to the COO (Chief Operating Officer), to the CFO (Chief Financial Officer) equipment and services that would improve the care of patients and resident education. These efforts were strongly supported by the administration and significant improvements were made that could be seen year after year.

She held her position as the president of JCIR at LAC-USC Medical Center for three years and from 1995 through 1997 served as the JCIR president of three institutions that made up the L.A. County Hospital system, namely Martin Luther King Jr. Medical Center, Harbor UCLA Medical Center, and L.A. County-USC Medical Center. As her ability to advocate for residents and patients was recognized by the medical staff, she was asked to become Chief of Staff-elect of the organized independent medical staff of the Los Angeles County Medical Center. In 2002, she proceeded to become the first female D.O. Chief of Staff in the 160 year history of the Los Angeles County / University of Southern California Medical Center.

As Chief of Staff at the Medical Center, Dr. Stotts is responsible for about two thousand providers, about nine hundred house staff, interns and residents, and about two to four hundred medical students, nursing students, respiratory students, physical therapy students and the like. For all their care and the care that their patients receive, whether it is part of their training program or not, the organized medical staff is responsible.

Dr. Stotts' plans for the future include the challenges of ordering a new custom hospital, moving to the new facility, and making sure that care is delivered in the proper fashion while learning new ways in doing things. Dr. Stotts anticipates spending much of her time with administrative duties, in-patient hospitalization duties, and resident education. She is looking forward to becoming involved in more formal academic pursuits to align patient care and resident education. She would like to advance her education with a Master's degree of Health Administration or a Master's of Medical Education in academics.

Dr. Seffinger interviewed Dr. Cynthia Stotts at the L.A. County—USC Medical Center in Los Angeles, California on March 29, 2007.

James Taylor, M.D.

Dr. Taylor was born in 1925 in Texas, obtained his pre-medical education in Torrance CA, and attended the College of Osteopathic Physicians and Surgeons in Los Angeles from 1954 to 1958. As a student he helped to promote the Los Angeles population to vote for funds to build a new osteopathic hospital, the Los Angeles County Osteopathic Hospital.

Dr. Taylor interned at the Los Angeles County Osteopathic Hospital, followed by a three-year residency in Anesthesiology at the same institution. He became Assistant Professor of Anesthesiology at the University of Southern California in 1961, while working at night and on weekends at Daniel Freeman Hospital in Los Angeles.

Hoping for a better future, economically and professionally, Dr. Taylor obtained the MD degree from the California College of Medicine and then practiced for 30 years at Bay Harbor Hospital near Los Angeles. He opened a pain clinic at this facility, providing neurolinguistic programming, hypnosis, thyamine, osteopathic manipulative treatment, and epidural injections. At age 72 he retired, enjoying his hobbies of wood carving and painting with watercolors.

Dr. Seffinger interviewed Dr. Taylor at his home in Fresno, CA on August 24, 2002.

In June 2007, Dr. Taylor passed away. His obituary states:

"Taylor, Dr. James"
1925-2007

Jim Taylor passed away on Tuesday, June 5, 2007 from multiple health related issues. Jim was born in Perryton, Texas. He was raised in Aztec, New Mexico with three brothers and one sister, all of whom preceded him in death. He came to California after high school. He worked as an iron worker to put himself through medical school. He was married to his first wife, Fay Louise, an organist and music teacher, for 43 years before her death in 1988, and they had three children. After medical school he taught anesthesia and did research at the University of Southern California. He loved his Trojan football team. He was Chief of anesthesia at Bay Harbor Hospital in Torrance and had a private pain therapy practice for over 30 years. He moved to Fresno and practiced anesthesia with community hospitals from 1992-1995. Following his retirement he took up a career as a watercolor artist specializing in humming birds and as a sculptor. He married his second wife, Maryna "Sam" Myers in 1989. Sam was a teacher at Robinson Elementary School in Fresno United School District until her retirement in 2004. Jim is survived by his wife, Sam; sons, Kenneth of Torrance, and Don and his wife Maria Elena of Lodi; daughter, Cathy of Rancho Bernado; and step son Marshall and his wife, Lora of Fresno. He had nine grandchildren, four great-grandchildren and numerous nieces and nephews.

Jerome S. Tobis, M.D.

Dr. Tobis was born in 1915 in Syracuse, NY. He obtained his M.D. degree in Chicago in 1943. He was a professor at the Albert Einstein School of Medicine in New York and Chief of the Rehabilitation Medicine Service at Montefiore Hospital in New York. He was recruited in 1970 to chair the Department of Physical Medicine & Rehabilitation at the University of California, Irvine. The historical roots of this medical school in osteopathic medicine were of interest to Dr. Tobis in forming his decision to accept the position.

Dr. Tobis was Chair of the Department of Physical Medicine & Rehabilitation at UC Irvine from 1970 to 1982. He established a 2-week training program in the field of physical medicine and rehabilitation for UC Irvine medical students, and he expanded the VA residency to include training at the Orange County General Hospital. He conducted research on the efficacy of osteopathic manipulation, an area for scientific study that had high priority in the conversion of the College of Osteopathic Physicians and Surgeons into a mainstream medicine educational institution.

Dr. Tobis was the first physician to conduct a randomized blinded clinical trial on the treatment efficacy of osteopathic manipulation in America. He was the first medical researcher at UC Irvine to obtain funds for research from the 41st Medical Trust. His additional special research interests and publications were related to cardiac rehabilitation, exercise physiology, aphasia, stroke and cerebral palsy.

Dr. Seffinger interviewed Dr. Tobis at his home in Corona Del Mar in California on April 26, 2006.

Seymour Ulansey, M.D.

Dr. Ulansey was born and raised in Philadelphia, Pennsylvania. His father was an osteopathic physician and young Seymour was determined to follow in his father's footsteps, as his older brother had done by graduating at the Philadelphia College of Osteopathy (PCO). Seymour completed three years at PCO. Having heard of the greater opportunities afforded to students and graduates of the College of Osteopathic Physicians and Surgeons (COP&S) in Los Angeles, California, he decided to graduate from there. Upon his graduation from COP&S in 1945, he served a clerkship or externship at the County General Hospital and was most impressed by that experience. He continued to obtain his residency there in anesthesiology and subsequently a fellowship.

He then became a junior attending physician and remained on the teaching staff at the County Hospital and at COP&S, teaching students, interns, and new residents. He served in that role for about 25 years. He also was on staff of a small osteopathic hospital with about 35 beds, the Hollywood Leland Hospital, performing anesthesia for D.O. as well as M.D. surgeons. When he was offered to buy the hospital he formed a group of 16 osteopathic and allopathic physicians to conduct the purchase. The hospital thrived and expanded to 125 beds in a six story structure.

The advent of Medicare and MediCal, the financial structure changed to the point where after several years it was converted into a nonprofit structure. In the 1980s, the group had to sell it to a private corporation. The hospital still exists in the heart of Hollywood, one block off Sunset and Vine.

In 1962, Dr. Ulansey received the M.D. degree, with his diploma showing that he was a graduate of the California College of Medicine. Sensing his dual loyalty to the College of Osteopathic Medicine of the Pacific as well as to the College of Medicine at UC Irvine, he started to support both colleges at the same time.

He also showed his dual loyalty as a teacher, first serving on the teaching staff as Assistant Professor of Anesthesia at the College the Osteopathic Physicians and Surgeons, and after the merger on the staff of the California College of Medicine. He held the same teaching status after the college affiliated with the University of California and moved to Irvine. Eventually, traveling daily between the Beverly Hills area and Irvine became too arduous and he resigned but retained his emeritus status.

Dr. Ulansey is a member of numerous national and international professional associations, including the American Medical Association, the International Association of Anesthesiologists, and the World Medical Association. He has been certified by the California Board of Certification in Anesthesia, by the Review Committee of the California Medical Association, and the American Osteopathic Board of Anesthesiology. He is a Fellow of American Geriatrics Society and the International College of Surgeons.

Dr. Seffinger interviewed Dr. Ulansey at his home in Malibu, California, on August 2, 2006.

Stanley van den Noort, M.D.

Dr. van den Noort was born in 1930 in Lynn, Massachusetts. He graduated from Harvard Medical School with the M.D. degree cum laude in 1954. He became a Diplomat of the Board of Neurology in 1963. His university appointments included Associate Professor of Neurology at Case Western Reserve University; Professor of Neurology, California College of Medicine, University of California, Irvine; Dean of the California College of Medicine, University of California, Irvine for 12 years; and Chair of the Department of Neurology, University of California, Irvine. He has held numerous hospital appointments and memberships in professional organizations.

In his endeavors to facilitate the relationship between allopathic and osteopathic physicians he has promoted research in the area of manipulation. He worked closely with Dr. Grunigen for 30 years on administrative and leadership tasks. Establishing a hospital on campus of UC Irvine had been Dr. van den Noort's fervent goal. When instead the county hospital in Orange was obtained, he supported its development and expansion no less strongly. Although he officially retired from his tenured university position in 1996, he continues to speak at professional meetings at the national and international level.

Dr. Seffinger interviewed Dr. van den Noort in his office at the University of California, Irvine on April 26, 2006.

Norman Vinn, D.O.

Dr. Vinn was born in 1949 at Houston Osteopathic Hospital. His father was an osteopathic general practitioner in Houston (class of 1941, Philadelphia College of Osteopathic Medicine). His father originally came to Texas from the east coast and completed his internship at Sparks Hospital in Dallas. He settled in a small town, Velasco, a suburb of Freeport, Texas, with a large strategic chemical plant known as Dow Chemical. He practiced there and hospitalized patients in the front room of his house because he couldn't get privileges at the local allopathic hospital.

Norman Vinn went to college at Tulane University in New Orleans and eventually chose to go to Philadelphia College of Osteopathic Medicine; graduated in 1977 and did an internship at Botsford Hospital in Farmington Hills, Michigan before he came to California to set-up practice in Long Beach, California, in 1978. Impressed by the example of his father and people during his training who provided care with a holistic approach, he realized that osteopathic medicine was a primary care-oriented profession. He chose to follow that path.

Dr. Vinn became involved with osteopathic organizational activities in the state of California because he was practicing out of a hospital named Pacific Hospital of Long Beach which at that time was re-emerging as an osteopathic hospital. Several times he represented the hospital at the osteopathic licensing sessions in Sacramento and became acquainted with Matt Weyuker, who at that time was the Executive Director of the Osteopathic Physicians and Surgeons of California (OPSC).

After serving for several years on the legislative committee of OPSC, he was asked to serve on the Board from 1982 to 1986, and again in 1988. He became president of OPSC in 1989-90 and attended the House of Delegates for the AOA for the first time in the summer of 1988 at the Fontainebleau Hotel in Miami. Subsequently he remained on the Board for a number of years and is now an Emeritus Board member.

Together with Dr. Howard Levine, then Chair of the Bureau of Research of the American Osteopathic Association (AOA), and later President of the AOA (1997), he developed the first Managed Care Task Force in 1993. That managed care task force eventually became a standing committee called the Committee on Health Care Delivery Systems, of which Dr. Vinn was Vice-Chair and ultimately Chair. The committee became permanent and was later renamed the Committee on Socio-economic Affairs.

Dr. Vinn was elected to the Board of Trustees of the AOA in 2003, serving two terms; one term as Second Vice-President and two terms as First Vice-president. He is currently serving a 3 year term on the Board of Trustees.

In addition to his legislative and administrative activities Dr. Vinn developed his own unique model of care in Orange County, California. He developed a house-call program where he visits frail home-bound elderly and end-of-life patients. It is a flexible model of care that produces a high degree of personal satisfaction. He believes that his home visits embrace a set of best practices and core competencies that are, in effect, a specialty practice. He calls his model of care "Residentialist Medicine."

Dr. Seffinger interviewed Dr. Vinn at the AOA House of Delegates Meeting in Chicago, Illinois, on July 15, 2006.

Matt Weyuker, OPSC Executive Director Emeritus

Matt Weyuker was born in 1933 in Brooklyn, NY and received his early education in Queens, NY. He joined the Navy in San Diego and earned 2 years of college credit while doing so. He proceeded to conduct insurance business for over 13 years and served on two school boards in Orange County, California, for 4 and 8 years respectively.

He served as legislative consultant to the California state legislature in Sacramento, CA from 1967-1977, building a strong network of associates through his work. In 1978 he was hired as the lobbyist for the College of Osteopathic Medicine of the Pacific and as Executive Director of OPSC. In this capacity, he introduced 49 bills; 40 of these bills he had authored; 39 passed the legislation process, and 36 were signed into law by three different governors. He drafted every anti-D.O.-discrimination bill.

He was the Executive Director of the Osteopathic Physicians and Surgeons of California (OPSC) for 19.5 years until retiring in 1997. At an OPSC convention in Las Vegas in 1998 he received unanimous vote to have bestowed the status of "Executive Director Emeritus" (a status which OPSC apparently failed to put into print).

From December 1997 until July 2000 he was the full-time Director of Government Relations for Western University Health Sciences. In 1999 he was elected mayor of Desert Hot Springs and served three 2-year terms.

Mr Weyuker has been the osteopathic profession's faithful and undaunted legislative advocate. He was instrumental in rebuilding the osteopathic profession by tenaciously aiming to protect the profession legally against discrimination.

Mr. Weyuker emailed his answers to Dr. Seffinger's interview questions on July 30, 2006, due to a neurologic disorder making it difficult for him to speak.

John E. Wykle, M.D.

Dr. Wykle was born in 1918 in Illinois. He lived in various states of the U.S. during his youth, as his father was a Presbytarian minister. While living in Ohio, John Wykle's sister was run over by a car. With medical help not forth coming, his father sought care by an osteopathic physician who inspired John to become an osteopathic physician.

A graduate of the College of Osteopathic Physicians and Surgeons (COP&S) in Los Angeles in 1941, Dr. Wykle did his internship at the clinic associated with COP&S while taking care of emergencies at night at a doctor's office south of Los Angeles. In 1942, Dr. Wykle moved to Shasta County to set up practice in a small lumber town and from there, a few years later, to San Andreas where a bond measure had just passed for a new hospital being built with dual (M.D. and D.O.) medical staff. Senator Teale, D.O. had written into the bond measure that there would be no discrimination against osteopathic physicians admitting and caring for their patients at this facility.

Until this hospital's completion in 1950, the only hospital available to osteopathic physicians was in Stockton. For a while, Dr. Wykle had a practice with Senator Stephen Teale and his wife, Barbara Teale, D.O., until Dr. Wykle took his patients to San Andreas. He continued, though at Mark Twain Hospital, providing anesthesiology for the county physicians.

In 1962, Dr. Wykle obtained the M.D. degree from the California College of Medicine, motivated mainly by the opportunity to be able to partake in the CME program through the University of California. Dr. Wykle was a member of the San Joaquin Medical Society, the CMA and AMA, and the California Society of Anesthesiologists. Dr. Wykle worked from his practice, providing obstetrics, house calls, and anesthesia until in 1988 he shifted to working under contract at Mark Twain Hospital. He retired in 1998 at age 83.

Dr. Seffinger interviewed Dr. Wykle by phone on August 1, 2006.

Biographies of historical persons

Andrew Taylor Still, M.D., D.O.
1828-1917

As the founder of osteopathic medicine, Dr. Still proposed concepts of health and treatment of disease that were revolutionary in America in his time. While medical discoveries of great importance were made in Europe, America had not yet been exposed to these advancements. Benjamin Rush, M.D., an influential teacher in Dr. Still's time, advocated blood letting as treatment for many symptoms.

Instead of focusing on the treatment of symptoms, for which one usually had no explanations, Dr. Still advocated seeking the health of patients. In his view, symptoms were just temporarily disrupting the human organism's continuous striving toward health. It was this natural tendency for self-repair that Dr. Still aimed to facilitate. He viewed the human organism as a dynamic, self-regulating unit of function. Anatomy and physiology were interrelated, a hypothesis that gave the musculoskeletal system a pivotal role for diagnosis and treatment.

In 1874 Dr. Still published these principal thoughts in his book *"Philosophy of Osteopathy"*. News about Dr. Still's abilities spread quickly and he became a highly sought after physician. Patients came in bus loads and a hotel had to be established in Kirksville to provide them with accommodations. As Dr. Still needed colleagues to help meet the patients' needs, he founded a medical school, the American School of Osteopathy, in 1892. Several students were M.D.s who wanted to learn his approach to diagnosis and treatment. Dr. Still accepted all qualified applicants, regardless of race and sex, and pursued a policy of non-discrimination in the training of physicians that was not the standard in allopathy at that time.

His school was based on the scientific discipline of anatomy and the physical laws of mechanics. His school was chartered to improve healthcare delivery by advancing the fields of medicine, surgery and midwifery (later called obstetrics). The curricula included microbiology, chemistry and physiology, but not materia medica. Contrary to common belief, Dr. Still, and his students, were not completely drugless practitioners. He taught his students to use medicinal anecdotes to poisons, plasters applied to the skin and anesthetics in surgery.

After the turn of the 20th century, physiological research, particularly in the neurosciences and cellular biology, including immunology, made inroads into osteopathic curricula, along with pharmacology. Even while Still was President, his school began advocating immunizations against small pox, and before his death, in 1914 the California College of Osteopathic Physicians and Surgeons added pharmacology to its curriculum and its graduates used medications. The remaining five American Osteopathic colleges added pharmacology to their curricula by mandate from the American Osteopathic Association by 1930.

The primary complaint of allopathic medicine against osteopathy was that it maintained a set of concepts and principles that the D.O.s claimed were unchanging truths, first enunciated by its founder, A.T. Still, M.D. As proponents of a system of ever changing theories of etiologies of diseases and their treatments, based on new scientifically derived research studies, and not paying homage to a "Founder of Medicine", the American Medical Association labeled osteopathy a "cult" and considered any interaction with osteopaths to be unethical and grounds for expulsion from their society.

A secondary complaint was that the education and training of D.O.s was inferior to that of M.D.s, giving them legal justification to limit interactions on a professional and economic level by barring D.O.s from their hospitals and practices. These two long held divisive attitudes were challenged often in the first 100 years of existence of the osteopathic profession, both in the courts and legislatures of each state across the country, coming to a head in the 1960s-1980s in California. They are still pervasive, however, in smaller communities around the country and internationally as well. D.O.s currently have full, unlimited scopes of practice in all 50 United States and are no longer barred from hospitals or institutions on the basis of their degree, education, training, osteopathic concepts or principles.

Dain Tasker, D.O.
1872-1964

Dain Tasker was born in Wisconsin and received his initial education in Chicago. He pursued a classical education in Greek, Latin and the sciences in order to be admitted to Rush Medical School. For financial reasons he abandoned that plan and took a job as proofreader of abstracts while attending ward walks at night with his medical school friends. Apparently he still hoped to become an M.D. some day.

Soon his health showed the strain of his busy life, and a move to California was thought to facilitate his recovery. His uncle had homesteaded 150 acres of land near Riverside and Dain took the opportunity of a Santa Fe Railroad special to buy a ticket to go to California. In 1893 he got off the train at a station that is now called March Field and found his uncle's home that consisted only of a tent. His health must have soon improved because he bicycled from Riverside to San Diego along railroad tracks to learn about a disease that afflicted California's citrus growth at that time.

His scientific mind soon returned to medicine when the wife of a Riverside banker became ill. She was successfully treated by a physician at a new school of medicine in Anaheim, called the Pacific Sanitarium and School of Osteopathy, which had just opened in 1896.

As he had learned about osteopathy already earlier through his mother, a registered nurse, he enrolled at the Pacific Sanitarium where he soon was recognized as an outstanding student. Even before his graduation in 1898 as a member of the first class, he had been made an assistant to the professor of anatomy. On graduation he became the head of the Anatomy department.

He taught the principles of osteopathy for years and published these in 1903. His book, "*Principles of Osteopathy*" was soon recognized as an essential textbook in the training of the profession, not only in California but also at Dr. Still's American School in Kirksville. Beautiful drawings by his physician friend Dr. Comstock as well as photographs by Dr. Hunt, another physician friend, contributed to the book's popularity.

Dr. Tasker pursued photography as his great hobby which might even have contributed to choosing roentgenology as his professional specialty. He became a renowned roentgenologist in Los Angeles. He managed to turn roentgenology into his hobby too by developing the new art of X-raying flowers to show their internal structure. His flower X-ray pictures were on display world-wide. He was so scientific about his work that he was never burned by X-rays, like many other doctors at that time.

Once the school (PSO) was established in Los Angeles, he started to fight for gaining practice rights for D.O.s in California. The first step was to form the COA in 1900. As the Association's first president he biked all through Sacramento to win over legislators for the cause of osteopathy.

In March 1901 the profession gained its right to practice. In 1907, a composite licensing board was organized, including allopathic, osteopathic and homeopathic physicians. In 1910 it was Dr. Tasker's turn to be the president of that board. In that role he signed over 200 diplomas, giving MDs their practice rights. When he continued as a member of the Board, hundreds of MDs had to pass the anatomy exams administered by Dr. Tasker.

He worked untiringly for the profession to gain recognition and practice rights in California. Yet, several years into his retirement, he joined the majority of osteopathic physicians and took the M.D. degree in 1962 from the California College of Medicine. Dr. Tasker was the designated historian of the California Osteopathic Association from 1950-1960. His 80-chapter, typed, double spaced manuscript, titled the *History of Osteopathy in California,* is archived at UC Irvine. It thoroughly covers the years from 1896-1960 and was the inspiration for this current project to document and make accessible the history of the relationship between the two medical professions with full and unlimited scope of practice in California.

Forest J. Grunigen, M.D.
1905-1999

While not really a historical person yet—so many of his colleagues and friends seem to have seen him "just yesterday"—a summary of his career as one of the most influential physicians in both medical professions deserves a special place in California's medical history. Dr. Grunigen was recognized as an outstanding physician as well as an inspiring leader.

His earliest years were unique, as he grew up in Sequoia National Park. He entered the College of Osteopathic Physicians and Surgeons in 1928 and earned the D.O. degree in 1931. He completed his internship, followed by a 2-year residency in urology, at the Unit II of the Los Angeles County Hospital.

As post-graduate training and residencies in osteopathy were hard to find in California at that time, Dr. Grunigen trained in Linz and Vienna in Austria in 1938 and '39 at specialty hospitals, at Johns Hopkins in 1940, in St. Louis in 1942, at the University of Michigan in 1945, and at Mayo Clinic in 1956. Upon his return to California, he established his private practice in Hollywood and soon became a renowned urologist. He still managed, though, to hold a teaching appointment at the College of Osteopathic Physicians and Surgeons until 1961 and to devote much of his time to serve on committees and administrative groups within the American Osteopathic Association. The archives at the American Osteopathic Association compiled this information:

- AOA Committee on Professional Liability Insurance, Chairman, 1946, 1949, 1950/ Member, 1952/ Chairman, 1954, 1955, 1956/ Member 1957, 1958, 1959
- AOA Committee on House of Delegates Procedure, Member, 1947
- AOA Bureau of Public Education and Health, Vice Chairman, 1949, 1950, 1951, 1952
- AOA Osteopathic Progress Fund Committee, Member, 1949, 1950, 1953
- AOA Subcommittee on Fund Raising, Member, 1949, 1950
- AOA Advisory Board for Osteopathic Specialists—Executive Committee, (Member representing Board of Trustees—1952, Vice Chairman-1953)
- AOA Committee on Life Insurance, Chairman, Member, 1952
- AOA Committee on Distinguished Service Certificates, Chairman, 1953, 1954
- AOA Committee on Medical Economics, Member, 1953
- AOA Study Committee on Insurance Problems and Labor Contacts, Member, 1953
- AOA Bureau of Professional Development, Vice Chairman, 1954, 1955, 1956
- AOA Committee on Editorial Department Structure, Member, 1957
- AOA Bureau of Insurance, Member, 1960

Upon the conversion of his *alma mater* (COP&S) into an allopathic college, the California College of Medicine, he obtained the M.D. degree in 1962 and proceeded to teach at the California College of Medicine and, upon its move to the University of California, Irvine, College of Medicine, from 1968 until 1984.

For decades he pursued a merger between the osteopathic and allopathic medical professions in California, thus setting the stage for a nation-wide recognition of osteopathic medicine as equally competent as allopathy. His hope was that the University of California, Irvine (UCI) with its strong infrastructure for conducting scientific research would provide opportunities to demonstrate scientifically the effectiveness of musculoskeletal manipulation. Throughout his long life he continued to search the world over for researchers who were most respected for their work in basic science and investigations into the efficacy of osteopathic manipulation.

While attending to his patients in his specialty practice in urology in Los Angeles for 35 years, he still held many prestigious positions over the span of 50 years. Starting as president of the California Osteopathic Association in 1943, followed by his position as chair of the Fact Finding Committee of the California Osteopathic Association until 1961, he held four consecutive appointments by the Governor till 1970.

Dr. Grunigen advanced into important positions. In 1962, he became Councilor to the California Medical Association. In four consecutive appointments by the California Governor, he was appointed as a member of the Advisory Council on Hospital Facilities from 1946 to 1964, and as a member of the Governor's Survey on Efficiency and Cost Control in 1967. In 1969 he became president of the State Board of Medical Examiners (BME)—the first former D.O. to preside over the allopathic Medical Licensing Board. In 1974, he created the position of a State Medical Consultant to the BME and was the first to be appointed in that position from 1971 to 1974.

Starting in 1974 he was for 20 years the Special Assistant to the Dean and Executive Director of the Support Foundation of the Board of Trustees at the College of Medicine at the University of California, Irvine. No wonder so many still value his support as colleague and friend!

In 2001, the medical library at the University of California, Irvine, Medical Center in Orange, California was dedicated as the *Forest J. Grunigen, M.D. Library and Medical Education Center.*

Senator Stephen Teale, M.D.
1912-1997

In 1943, Stephen Teale graduated from the College of Osteopathic Physicians and Surgeons (COP&S) with the D.O. degree. Together with his wife Barbara who was also an osteopathic physician and graduate of COP&S, he practiced medicine in the Sierra Nevada mountains. He was a California State Senator from 1953 to 1972.

As a senator he wrote the legislation for closing the Osteopathic Licensing Board, called proposition 22, put on the state ballot in 1962. There were other facets to the Proposition 22 as well. He was the only physician in the legislature and chairman of the Senate Finance Committee—both titles carrying prestige and influence. In 1962, proposition 22 passed, curtailing the osteopathic profession in California by eliminating the licensing power of its independent Board of Osteopathic Examiners. Proposition 22 enabled D.O.s to practice alongside MDs as long as they accepted the MD degree and deleted their D.O. degree.

Senator Teale also chaired the Budget Committee of the California State Senate and was directly responsible for COP&S becoming the California College of Medicine (CCM) in 1962. Working closely with Dr. Bostick and Dr. Grunigen, he moved CCM into the UC system in 1964. Senator Teale had obtained the M.D. degree from the California College of Medicine in 1962.

In Sacramento's political circles, Senator Teale was mainly known for re-apportioning the state's senate districts and for his efforts to develop computerized data systems. The government's Data Center bore his name until recently. He worked in the legislature for nearly 20 years and retired in 1972. Upon his retirement he was appointed to the Post Secondary Education Committee.

Warren L. Bostick, M.D.
1914-2006

Dr. Bostick was a pathologist with a distinguished career at the University of California, San Francisco in the 1950s. He also had a prominent career at the California Medical Association as its president from 1961 to 1962 where he was active in gaining recognition from the state legislature for D.O.s in California to receive the M.D. degree.

In the 1950s he worked closely with Forest Grunigen, D.O. and Dorothy Marsh, D.O. at the California Osteopathic Association to develop a merger between the osteopathic and allopathic professions. In the early 1960s, Dr. Bostick worked with Senator Teale to turn the College of Osteopathic Physicians and Surgeons into a mainstream medical school, with the goal to have it located at the University of California, Irvine, which at that time was in the planning stage. When the College of Osteopathic Physicians and Surgeons became the allopathic California College of Medicine (CCM), he succeeded Dean Wells in 1963 as Dean of CCM.

In 1964, Dr. Bostick came to the University of California, Irvine (UCI) to become the founding Dean of the UCI College of Medicine, the former College of Osteopathic Physicians and Surgeons, turned California College of Medicine in 1962. He was Dean of the College of Medicine until he resigned in 1973. He continued his career as a Professor of Pathology, though, and made significant contributions to the Department of Pathology and to the College of Medicine until his death in 2006.

Grace Bell, M.D.
1897-1989

Dr. Bell was born in 1897 in San Jose into a family with several children. Her parents were prune farmers who raised their children with the expectation to obtain a good education and to become professionals. Thus, Grace Bell set out to study physics and biochemistry at UC Berkley from 1915 to 1919. She had intended to study (allopathic) medicine but an encounter with an inspiring osteopathic physician led her to enroll at the College of Osteopathic Physicians and Surgeons (COP&S). While still a student at COP&S she already taught biochemistry there. She graduated in 1925 and married Dr. John Bell, also a graduate of COP&S—a marriage that would last nearly 50 years until John Bell's death.

Initially, they had a practice together but Grace Bell soon started teaching at COP&S full-time and became a much admired professor of biochemistry. She felt more successful mentoring students than seeing patients, as she described herself as sympathizing and worrying too much about her patients. Her husband proceeded to become an anesthesiologist.

Dr. Bell soon became professor and executive of the department of Biochemistry, a position she held for 30 years. During all these years, she educated probably 3,000 students most of whom became osteopathic physicians.

In 1948, she obtained a master's degree in biochemistry from USC. She developed a nutrition clinic to counsel patients on the dietary management of diabetes and obesity, possibly anticipating the health problems that lay ahead for the nation's population.

In 1955 she became the first and only female dean at COP&S; in fact, she was the first Dean of a co-educational medical school in America. She took the M.D. degree in 1962 from the California College of Medicine. With her name at the top of the alphabet, she was the first to receive the M.D. degree.

In 1955 she was approached by President Henley to serve as dean for COP&S. While she did not feel up to the task immediately, she eventually agreed to become acting dean for two years and subsequently dean of COP&S. As in 1962 the College became the allopathic California College of Medicine (CCM), she was one of the few women in history to be distinguished as a dean of an American school of medicine. She was the only person in history to be a dean of both an osteopathic and an allopathic medical school, a feat that she accomplished in one year. (Nettie Bolles, D.O. was president of her college in Colorado from 1897-1904, not the dean, though).

In 1963 Dr. Bell became Associate Dean of CCM under Dean Wells who had been appointed in 1962. They both presided over the ceremony that granted the M.D. degree to nearly 2000 COP&S alumni, as well as other D.O.s already licensed in California, later that month.

In 1978 Grace Bell, M.D. was asked to participate in the organization of the new osteopathic college in California, the College of Osteopathic Medicine of the Pacific, but she declined. Not much is known about Dr. Bell's professional activities in the subsequent years. A Grace Bell Distinguished Chair in Biological Chemistry was developed at the College of Medicine, University of California, Irvine, as part of her endowment in biological chemistry.

Dr. Bell lived to be in her nineties. She had decided that her files, housed in the Archives at UC Irvine, were to be locked until 2015.

Dorothy Marsh, M.D.
1915-2005

While several women have been outstanding leaders and clinicians in osteopathy, Dr. Dorothy Marsh stood out among them as an obstetrician and leader. She passed away on April 10, 2005 after a long and productive life.

Dr. Marsh graduated from the College of Osteopathic Physicians & Surgeons, at Los Angeles in 1938 where she earned the degree Doctor of Osteopathy. In 1962 she obtained a Doctor of Medicine degree from the newly formed California College of Medicine. In her specialty practice of OB/GYN in Glendale, California, she delivered more than 8,000 babies in her 50 years of practice.

Dr. Marsh was actively involved in formulating policy within the practice of medicine. She served on the Insurance Review Committee of the Los Angeles County Medical Association, the Utilization Review Committee and Bylaw Committee of the Glendale Adventist Medical Center, Chairperson of the American Osteopathic Board of Certification, a member of the Intra Agency Council of California's Public Health Department. She was a Trustee and then President of the California Osteopathic Association during the merger of the osteopathic and allopathic professional organizations in 1960 and 1961. She also held various teaching positions at the College of Osteopathic Physicians & Surgeons and at the University of California, Irvine School of Medicine.

Among her many awards and achievements, Dr. Marsh is listed in "Who's Who of American Women" and has been a dedicated advocate of professional excellence. Additionally, the Dorothy J. Marsh Chair in Reproductive Biology was established in her name by the University of California, Irvine, School of Medicine.

Dr. Dorothy J. Marsh—A Remembrance, was the theme of a reception to honor Dr. Marsh. The event was held at the University of California, Irvine School of Medicine in Irvine Hall on June 24, 2005. Distinguished speakers included Thomas C. Cesario, M.D., Dean of the UCI School of Medicine; Dr. Philip Disaia, M.D., The Dorothy Marsh Chair in Reproductive Biology, and Dr. Richard Kammerman who had been one of her students.

Louisa Burns, D.O., M.S.
1869-1958

Dr. Burns was born in 1869 in Indiana. She received her D. O. degree from the Pacific College of Osteopathy in 1903. She was a Professor of Physiology at the Pacific College from 1904 until 1915. At that time she started her association with the A.T. Still

Research Institute and served as its director for many years until the institute could no longer provide adequate financial support. In 1917, she moved her laboratory to *Sunny Slope* in Pasadena, California, and continued her animal experimentations which she published in scientific papers. Her work is summarized in the book *Pathogenesis of Visceral Disease Following Vertebral Lesions,* Chicago, Illinois: AOA 1948. Selections from her published work are included in the 1970 AAO yearbook as well (see Chapter 2 for a more detailed description of Dr. Burns' research career).

Louis C. Chandler, M.A., D.O.
1886-1950

Dr. Chandler was born in 1886 in Pennsylvania. He received his D.O. degree from the Los Angeles College of Osteopathy in 1913. He served as Sanitary Engineer with the Pennsylvania National Guard and as Food and Drug Chemist and Bacteriologist for the California State Board of Health. He was a member of the California State Board of Medical Examiners from 1921-1922. He taught at the Los Angeles College of Osteopathy in 1913-14 and at the College of Osteopathic Physicians and Surgeons (COP&S) from 1914 to the1940s, lecturing and writing on heart, lung, and nutritional diseases. He was president of COP&S as well as a member of its Board of Directors. He also was the director and a staff internist at Monte Sano Hospital. He served as chief of staff at the Los Angeles County Hospital Unit II in the 1930s. In spite of his many clinical and administrative obligations he found the time to author a text book on "*Clinical Toxicology*". His professional files are archived at Western University of Health Sciences in Pomona, CA.

Documentation

Published documentation

Bartosh, L. H. *The history of osteopathy in California.* The Journal of the Osteopathic Physicians and Surgeons of California, 1978, April/May, 30-33.

Buerger, A.A. and Tobis, J.S. (Eds.) *Approaches to the validation of manipulation therapy.* Charles C. Thomas Publisher, Springfield IL, 1977.

Cole, W.V. Historical basis for osteopathic theory and practice. In George W. Northup (Ed.) *Osteopathic research: Growth and development.* American Osteopathic Association, 1987.

Gevitz, N. *The D.O.s: Osteopathic Medicine in America,* The Johns Hopkins University Press, Second Edition, Baltimore 2004.

Gevitz, N. *The History of osteopathic medicine.* In Sirica, C.M. (Ed.) *Osteopathic Medicine: Past, Present, and Future.* Josiah Macy Jr. Foundation, New York NY, 1996.

Grunigen, D. and O'Connell, J. *A strength born of giants: The life and times of Dr. Forest Grunigen,* Raven River Press, Van Nuys, California, 2002.

Hruby, R.J. *Contemporary practice and philosophy of osteopathy.* In Sirica, CM (Ed.) *Osteopathic Medicine: Past, Present, and Future.* Josiah Macy Jr. Foundation, New York NY, 1996.

Lay, E. M. *Recollections. AOA Journal,*1998, spring issue, 25-28.

Riedell, E. H. *Babies by the dozen: Free home delivery, 1941.* Fithian Press, Santa Barbara CA, 1998.

Seffinger, M. A. and Hruby, R.J. *Evidence-based manual medicine: A problem-oriented approach.* Saunders/Elsevier, Philadelphia, PA, 2007.

Tobis, J.S. and Hoehler, F. *Musculoskeletal manipulation: Evaluation of the scientific evidence.* Charles C. Thomas Publisher, Springfield, IL, 1986.

Ward, R. C. *Foundations for Osteopathic Medicine,* Lippincott Williams & Wilkins, 2003.

Documentation obtained in Archives

Special Collections and Archives, The University of California Irvine Libraries, Irvine, California.

Dain Tasker, D.O.: *"History of Osteopathy in California"*

> Chapters 1-15 cover the years **1896 to 1910**;
> Chapter 20 covers the year **1914**;
> Chapters 66-70 cover **1948 to 1949** and Dr. Tasker's autobiography entitled:
> **"Fifty Golden Years"**
> Chapters 77-79 were added in 1961 and address merger-related issues

Forest Grunigen files on the California Osteopathic Association. AS-083.

California College of Medicine Records. AS-027.

Clinical Osteopathy.
>This journal was the official organ of COA, in collaboration with COP&S. It was formerly called *The Western Osteopath.*

Clinical Osteopathy, 1934:
>October issue: article by **T.J. Ruddy, D.O.**
>November issue: description of a new patient plan for the **Osteopathic Unit of the L.A. County General Hospital**

Clinical Osteopathy, 1935:
>January issue: paper by **Grace Bell, D.O.**
>March and April issues: two papers by **Louisa Burns, D.O.**
>June issue cites the graduation by **Sam Reese, D.O.** and **H. Norcross, D.O.**
>September issue lists the new admission requirements for COP&S.

Clinical Osteopathy 1936:
>January, February, and May issues: articles by **Dain Tasker, D.O.**;
>May issue cites Los Angeles area to have the greatest concentration of D.O.s anywhere, with **1/6 of D.O.s worldwide** practicing in California;
>September issue cites **1,487 D.O.s in California**, with 52.4% being members of COA, compared to their 33% membership with AOA;
>Osteopathy code of ethics is reprinted throughout several issues.

Clinical Osteopathy 1937:

>January, February, March and April issues published "A study of osteopathic fundamentals" as stated by Dr. **A.T. Still;**
>May issue has several articles on manipulation and a plea by **W.W.W. Pritchard, D.O.** *"why not brush up a bit on your technique, keep faith with ourselves, our patients and our profession"* . . . *"There is no reason to be ashamed of being an Osteopathic Physician and Surgeon."*
>The August issue shows a group photo of "Doctors attending the 1937 postgraduate week at COP&S." There were about 8 women among the 48 doctors.

Clinical Osteopathy 1938:
>March issue cites the celebration of **the10th anniversary of the L.A. County Osteopathic Hospital** which had opened in February 1928. *"This was*

the climax of a hard fight by the profession in California for recognition and the opportunity to demonstrate to the public what osteopathy can do for human ills . . . . The almost too rapid growth of the Unit created problems" (it didn't say which problems were created).

The May issue advises to keep a case history on every patient to protect against malpractice claims. The topic of **malpractice** comes up frequently in this year and subsequently.

Clinical Osteopathy 1939

The January issue announces an osteopathic hospital in Oakland

The February issue talks about the **California Board of Osteopathic Examiners,** organized in 1922. In early 1923 there were 924 licentiates in the State of California. At the end of 1937 there were **1,718 licentiates.**

Clinical Osteopathy 1940

The March issue mentions the College clinic again: Patients who cannot afford the County Hospital get good care at the clinic. Every patient receives a social service check-up. The issue also mentions a **Riverside Osteopathic Hospital.** The hospital has been in operation for 11 years. There were 213 admissions in 1939 and 55 infants were born.

The May issue mentions 26 participants in a postgraduate course on **manipulation.**

The June issue mentions the L.A. College to have a new president, **Ballentine Henley**, MA, MS, LLD. He was formerly the acting Dean of the School of Government at USC. He taught administrative law, jurisprudence, and public relations.

The July issue has news from the AOA convention: All 14 representatives of the CA House of Delegates were present, including **Glen Cayler, D.O**. Alternates included **Frank MacCracken, D.O**.

The September issue mentions an article on osteopathy in Life magazine and comments that *"**Dr. Fishbein of the AMA** was most annoyed by the article* [in Life magazine], *especially by the quote 'In 33 states, qualified doctors of osteopathy are permitted to practice on equal footing with doctors of medicine.'* The article continues: *" Dr. Fishbein in his JAMA editorial flatly denies that there are more than 5 states that allow D.O.s to prescribe without restriction. Apparently he does not expect having to prove his statement in court."*

The October issue shows the membership roster of COA, including **Betty, Daisy and Frank E. MacCracken, R.E. Eby, Cora and Dain Tasker, and Glen Cayler.**

The December issue has a historical piece by **Mark Twain** defending osteopathy, stating that he has the right and liberty to choose who treats him.

Four of 27 **AOA approved hospitals** nationwide are in California: The Doctors Hospital in Los Angeles, the L.A. County Hospital, Magnolia Hospital in Long Beach, and Monte Sano Hospital in Los Angeles.

Clinical Osteopathy 1941

The January issue announces the opening of the **San Diego Hillside Osteopathic** hospital. There were over 50 D.O.s in the San Diego area.

Ten issues, starting in 1940, are presenting reports on **osteopathic techniques**, including numerous photos.

The April issue has a letter explaining the *"reason for dissatisfaction in the profession is the fundamental disparity between increased training and license compared to low political, social and postgraduate opportunity."* The letter also states "Many D.O.s are non-members [in COA] because **they want an M.D. degree and the enlarged horizon it implies. If we do not settle the latter problem, it will settle us.**"

The September issue announces a 10-week course on public speaking by **Dr. Henley.**

The December issue as well as other issues, have WWII as the topic, including a paper by Lowell Kearl, D.O. on **osteopathic management of trauma.** The issue lists the 1940 membership in COA, including **Dr. Forest Grunigen, Dr. Dorothy Marsh, Dr. Sam Reese, and Dr. Howard Norcross**.

Clinical Osteopathy 1942

The February issue lists 1,890 licentiates in California.

All issues feature articles on osteopathic care related to war injuries.

The May issue features a **photo of Forest Grunigen, D.O. as President Elect of the COA**

Clinical Osteopathy 1945

The January issue mentions the L.A. County Osteopathic Hospital Interns' Alumni Association and *"**Dr. Grunigen**, the first one of the gang to make the top spot in the COA . . ."*

The February issue lists over **10 osteopathic hospitals** in the greater Los Angeles area as members of the California Osteopathic Hospital Association;

The August issue mentions the marriage of **Stephen (Tiny) Teale** and Barbara Baker;

In the October issue the **Advisory Board for Osteopathic Specialists** advocates recognition through specialty certification. The Long Beach Osteopathic Hospital aims to build a bigger hospital.

"*A tribute to a fallen leader*". Obituary for Dain L. Tasker, M.D., prepared in 1964 by Munish Feinberg, M.D., historian of the Forty-First Medical Society of the California Medical Association.

"*History of CCM, 1896-1914*", a document prepared in 1964 by Drs. DeStefano, Lee, and Schwartz

"*Historical Outline UCI—College of Medicine*", a typed list of dates and their respective events from the 1932 to 1960s; no authors cited

"*An Appeal to Reason*", undated, 18-page document printed by the "Committee for the Standardization of Medical Education and Practice in California", authors listed as Emerson J. Hutchinson, D.O., Chairman; Charles S. Nicholas, D.O., Vice-Chairman; and Jack Stein, D.O., Secretary Treasurer

"*A History of the Pediatrics Department, California College of Medicine, University of California, Irvine, Draft # 1*", *2/2/78,* **Prepared** by Dr. Betsy R. MacCracken with the assistance of Drs. Fred Stone, Mary O'Meara Pepper, Wayne Peyton, Jane Hamilton and Grace Bell

"*Grace Beekhuis Bell, M.D.*" *by Linda* Burnham, March 1977, Dean's Office, College of Medicine, the University of California Irvine

"*College of Medicine, University of California: History—Academics—Politics: The Merging Professions*" by Warren L. Bostick, M.D., 1994. Centennial Edition, printed in-house.

Cayler Report to COA:

"*September 12—Meeting of the Bureau of Public Affairs, COA Delegation to the House of Delegates of the AOA, with the Board of Trustees of the COA.*"
"*Beginning of Dr. Cayler's Report to the Board of COA.*". No year of documentation is provided.

Archives at the Harriet K. & Philip Pumerantz Library, Western University of Health Sciences, Pomona, California:

Louis C. Chandler, D.O. (1895-1950), Papers, Collection Number: 002
In addition the archivist at the Harriet K. & Philip Pumerantz Library has catalogued massive amounts of the institution's holdings of documents on osteopathy, including books, private files, and photographs.

Archives at the American Osteopathy Association in Chicago:

OPSC Charter:
> OPSC became a charter to represent the Osteopathic Association of California, as the amalgamation of AOA with AMA was pursued by Counselor Hufstedler and Dorothy Marsh, D.O. At the AOA convention in 1960, Richard Eby, D.O. had objected to the amalgamation and the charter became important to represent the Osteopathic Association in California.

AOA policy on individual requests by former D.O.s to reverse their decision and to re-gain their D.O. degree:
> In 1963, AOA developed a policy about individual reversing requests. AOA required the return of the new M.D. diploma but this request was not adhered to. There are no data published on the number of applicants who wanted to reverse their switch to the M.D. degree. An additional document provides information about OPSC offering help to AOA to assist with these individual reversing requests.

AOA document on defining osteopathic medicine:
> As M.D.s apparently differentiated in the early 1960s between "scientific D.O.s" and "touching (manipulation) D.O.s", AOA provided a document to explain the full scope of osteopathic medicine.

Profile of a Merger. A Report to the American Osteopathic Association, prepared by Market Facts, Inc, Chicago IL, February 1966.

The AMA and the osteopaths: A study of the power of organized medicine, by Erwin A. Blackstone. *The Antitrust Bulletin*, Volume XXII, 405, 1977.

Documents developed in California in the late 1950s and early 1960s:

> **Doctors of Medicine and Doctors of Osteopathy in California: Two Medical Professions Face the Problem of Providing Medical Care.** By Arnold I. Kisch, M.D., Assistant Professor of Medical Care Organization and Arthur J. Viseltear, Ph.D., Assistant Research Historian, School of Public Health, University of California, Los Angeles. Published by the U.S. Department of Health, Education, and Welfare, the document is identified as "Medical Care Administration—Case Study No. 2. A preliminary edition— For evaluation purposes only and prepared for a limited audience . . . primarily for teaching purposes, student discussion and analysis in seminars."

> **Dain Tasker, D.O., historian** on osteopathic medicine, ended his manuscript, "*A History of Osteopathy in California*" in the late 1950s but provided additional

Statements in 1960 in chapters 77 through 79, housed at the UC Irvine Libraries, Special Collections & Archives.

Outline for a history of osteopathy in California, possibly prepared for Dr. Bostick's book (no authors and date cited for the document), housed at the Special Collections & Archives of the UC Irvine Libraries.

Photographs of OPSC presidents, displayed at the College of Osteopathic Medicine of the Pacific at Western University of Health Sciences, Pomona

"Bonesetting, Chiropractic and Cultism": This manuscript contains a misleading yet often quoted statement about osteopathy.

Anti-Trust Bulletin: This document was obtained from the Trade and Trust Journal.

Publication in *Social Science and Medicine*, 1981: The paper is entitled *"The organization and rejuvenation of Osteopathy: A reflection."* This publication provides an overview on facts from the early 1960s to the late 1980s.

Affidavit dated March 1967: This document provides a snapshot view of events occurring at that time.

Letter by Frank McCracken, D.O., entitled "Why can't we merge?" Grace Bell, D.O. responded to this challenging key letter and outlined the steps required to convert to the M.D. degree. These documents are housed in the archives at Western University, as part of files that were donated by Louis Chandler, D. O. Dr. Chandler graduated in 1913 and collected important documents regarding his profession.

Index of Documents collected by Dr. Forest Grunigen and Dolores Grunigen (informally indexed on 12-18-06)

1997: 41st Medical Society dissolved:

Letter to Dr. Grunigen by administrator

Certificate of Dissolution, signed by Paul Yates, M.D., President, and Jordan Phillips, M.D., stating that monies were transferred to the 41st Medical Trust Endowment

1961 Agreement between CMA and COA to merge

1998 folder about 41ˢᵗ TF efforts to establish research on manipulation:
- Proposal by neurologists and a physiatrist: Wolfgang Gilliard, D.O., Bill Anderson, M.D., Philip Greenman, D.O.
- Proposal by Dr. Hong, with outcome assessments proposed by Dr. Reinsch

Vincent Carroll, M.D. 1904-1986:
- A brochure about Dr. Carroll with color photo

Stephen Teale, M.D. 1916-1997:
Obituary published in the *Sacramento Bee*, February 3, 1997 (Dr. Teale died February 1ˢᵗ, 1997)

Forest Grunigen, M.D., curriculum vitae

Informal History of the University of California Irvine, manuscript by Stephen Man:
This partly fictional story was written from a medical student's perspective and might have been published as *The Healing Circle*, Dolores Grunigen recalled.

1986 documentation about the Osteopathic Licensing Board

1979 Senate Bill 1199

Merger-related materials:
- The publication by Kisch and Viseltear
- A proposal (undated) entitled Unification II

Establishment of the Dorothy Marsh Endowed Chair

Development of the 41ˢᵗ TF: written on December 31, 1964, this document was created 1 day prior to the UC Regents taking over CCM.

Second Amendment to Affiliation Agreement, created on 9-14-1967, this document includes valuable historical information

Further research proposals submitted to the 41ˢᵗ TF committee:
- Robert Blanks, Ph.D., examining chiropractic manipulation
- Yu Zhu, M.D.: the proposal by his group was funded by the 41ˢᵗ TF, together with matched funding by the AOA, as requested by Dr. Seffinger

Several folders contain documentation regarding a hospital for UCI College of Medicine

Grace Bell, M.D.:
In 1986, her private records were given to Dr. Grunigen. Dr. Bell lived to be in her 90s.

Documentation regarding the Grace Bell, M.D. Endowed Chair in Biological Chemistry at UCI is included as well as a Bio sketch and a photo, taken in 1986.

1978 Physical Medicine & Rehabilitation Manipulation Project: A conference was conducted by Dr. Tobis and Dr. Buerger. Murray Goldstein, D.O. provided consultation in 1976

Scott Haldeman, M.D., Ph.D. was accepted to residency: He conducted a workshop on manipulation at Michigan State University, as a follow-up to Dr. Tobis' conference.
Dr. Haldeman published his study on manipulation, an example for the nation-wide interest in manipulation generated by the 41st Trust Fund.

August 1981, CMA position on Osteopathy: *"Osteopathy—where we stand."*
The Saga of Osteopathy, a reprint of a publication in the Western Journal of Medicine, 1975

Legal Documentation about the M.D.–D.O. Relationship in California:

CA Statutes 1962:
First Extraordinary Session, Chapter 46: An act to amend Section 2310 of, and to repeal Section 2492 of, the Business and Professions Code, relating to physicians and surgeons.

CA Statutes 1962:
Chapters 48 to 50

CA Statutes 1963:
Chapter 1933: An act to add Article 3 (commencing with Section 23471) to Chapter 3 of Division 17 of the Education Code, relating to higher education.

CA Statutes 1963:
Chapter 942. Section 2396.5 is added to the Business and Professions Code, to read: In addition to those persons authorized by Section 2396 to use the term or suffix "M.D.," those persons who meet all of the requirements of subdivisions (a), (b), and (c) of this section may use such term or suffix

CA Statutes of 1981:
> Chapter 652: An act to amend Section 69670 of the Education Code, relating to postsecondary education

CA Statutes of 1982:
> Chapter 446: An act to add Section 5 to an initiative act entitled the "Osteopathic Act," approved by the electors November 7, 1922, relating to physicians and surgeons.

CA Statutes of 1984:
> Chapter 294: An act to add Section 2064.1 to the Business and Professions Code, relating to medicine to read: *Notwithstanding the provisions of Section 2064 or any other provisions of this chapter, a regularly matriculated student undertaking a course of professional instruction in a medical school approved by the American Osteopathic Association or the Board of Osteopathic Examiners is eligible for enrollment in elective clerkships or preceptorships in any medical school or clinical training program in this state.*

CA Statutes of 1987:
> Chapter 909: An act to amend Section 2453 of the Business and Professions Code, relating to healing arts.

CA Statutes of 1988:
> Chapter 663: An act to amend Section 2453 of the Business and Professions Code relating to healing arts.

CA Statutes of 1988:
> Chapter 325: An act to add Section 2457.5 to the Business and Professions Code, relating to osteopathic physicians and surgeons.

CA Statutes of 1989:
> Chapter 425: An act to add Section 2064.2 to the Business and Professions Code, relating to the practice of medicine to read:
>
> 2064.2. No medical school or clinical training program shall deny access to elective clerkships or preceptorships in any medical school or clinical training program in this state solely on the basis that a student is enrolled in an osteopathic medical school.

1992 Summary Digest:
> Chapter 619 (AB 2372) Frizzelle. Medical practice: osteopathic physicians and surgeons: discrimination.

List of Figures

Figure 1: "The 41st Medical Trust Committee, 2007: Standing from left to right: Richard Kammerman, M.D., Jen Yu, M.D., Ph.D., Robert Steedman, M.D. Seated from left to right: Victor Passy, M.D., Dolores Grunigen, B.A., Stanley van den Noort, M.D.", courtesy Foundations Relations, UC Irvine

Figure 2a: "Pacific Sanitarium and School of Osteopathy in Anaheim, 1896", Special Collections and Archives, the UC Irvine Libraries

Figure 2b: "Pacific School of Osteopathy in Los Angeles, 1898", Special Collections and Archives, the UC Irvine Libraries

Figure 3: "Louisa Burns, D.O.", Special Collections and Archives, the UC Irvine Libraries

Figure 4: "Dain Tasker, D.O., historian for the osteopathic medicine profession", Special Collections and Archives, the UC Irvine Libraries

Figure 5a: "Los Angeles County Hospital, Unit II, 1933", Special Collections and Archives, the UC Irvine Libraries

Figure 5b: "Glen Cayler, D.O., Children's Ward, Los Angeles County Hospital, Unit II, 1930s", Courtesy of the Darby Family Collection

Figure 6: "Merrill Sanitarium: Myrtle and Carle Phinney; Kappy and Edward Merrill, 1930", Special Collections and Archives, the UC Irvine Libraries

Figure 7: "Studying Osteopathy: Glen Cayler and students at COP&S, 1920s", Courtesy of the Darby Family Collection

Figure 8: "Dr. Miller, Orthopedics, 1951", Special Collections and Archives, the UC Irvine Libraries

Figure 9: "COA Convention, Coronado, 1930s", Special Collections and Archives, the UC Irvine Libraries

Figure 10: "Dean Grace Bell, D.O., early 1950s", Special Collections and Archives, the UC Irvine Libraries

Figure 11: "Carle Phinney, D.O., 1938", the Harriett and Phillip Pumerantz Archives, Western University of the Health Sciences, Pomona CA

Figure 12: "Senator Steven Teale, D.O.", Special Collections and Archives, the UC Irvine Libraries

Figure 13: "Dorothy Marsh, D.O. and Warren Bostick, M.D., May 17, 1961, signing the merger agreement", Special Collections and Archives, the UC Irvine Libraries

Figure 14: "Dorothy Marsh, D.O., COA Convention, Coronado, 1930s", Special Collections and Archives, the UC Irvine Libraries

Figure 15: "Dr. Wayne E. Pollock, Dr. Joseph P. Cosentino (COA President), Dr. Ballentine Henley, Dr. Omar Wheeler (CMA President), June 17, 1962, Commencement", Rothschild Photography, Los Angeles, Special Collections and Archives, the UC Irvine Libraries

Figure 16: "Dr. Michael Moulton and Dean Grace Bell being presented with the senior class gift at the Senior Breakfast, 1962", Rothschild Photography, Los Angeles, Special Collections and Archives, the UC Irvine Libraries

Figure 17: "Dedication of the University of California Irvine campus by U.S. President Lyndon B. Johnson, 1964", Special Collections and Archives, the UC Irvine Libraries

Figure 18: "Founders of the College of Osteopathic Medicine of the Pacific, 1977: From left to right: Saul Bernat, Ph.D., Donald Dilworth, D.O., Viola Frymann, D.O., Philip Pumerantz, Ph.D., Richard Eby, D.O., Ethan Allen, D.O.", the Harriett and Phillip Pumerantz Archives, Western University of the Health Sciences, Pomona CA

Figure 19: "Student learning the scapular myofascial release OMT procedure during osteopathic manipulative medicine class at the College of Osteopathic Medicine of the Pacific". Photo courtesy of Jess Lopatynski, photographer, Western University of Health Sciences, Pomona, CA.

Figure 20: "Dolores Grunigen at the Forest J. Grunigen M.D. Medical Center Library in Orange CA, 2007", courtesy Dolores Grunigen.

INDEX

Bold refers to image page number
Italics refer to biography page numbers

Interview participants:

Historical persons:

Acknowledgements

We want to express our deep appreciation to the 41st Medical Trust committee members for their support in enabling this endeavor to become a reality. Their imprimatur created the trust among the interviewed individuals to tell their story freely of the M.D.-D.O. relationship in California. We sincerely thank our interview participants for their time to meet with Dr. Seffinger, to review their transcripts, to search for documents if needed, and to provide their historical narratives for this project. Their contributions made this work meaningful.

The assistance provided by the Alumni Office of the University of California (UC) Irvine School of Medicine, the medical librarian Linda Murphy, MSL and the Special Collections and Archives of the UC Irvine Libraries, and the Archives of the Harriet K. & Philip Pumerantz Library at Western University of Health Sciences was invaluable in identifying important documents and photographs that validate the story described in this book. The College of Osteopathic Medicine of the Pacific has been generous in providing expertise and resources.

This manuscript would not have been possible without the untiring dedication of the transcriptionists who spent countless hours typing the oral interviews. For this we are deeply indebted to George C. Lin, D.O., Elizabeth (Becky) Allen and Sayuri Seffinger.

We wish to express our indebtedness to Dolores Grunigen for sharing her late husband's legacy with us as an essential component of this project. We deeply appreciate Dr. Victor Passy and Dr. Richard Kammerman for their patience and kindness in guiding our team. We are grateful to Dr. Jen Yu, Chair of the Department of Physical Medicine & Rehabilitation at UC Irvine, for providing his departmental support and his patient and repeated thorough reviews of the manuscript. His respectful and thoughtful attitude toward this project sustained our perseverance.

www.ingramcontent.com/pod-product-compliance
Lightning Source LLC
Chambersburg PA
CBHW031825170526
45157CB00001B/184